Reshaping Food Systems to Improve Nutrition and Health in the Eastern Mediterranean Region

Ayoub Al-Jawaldeh and Alexa L. Meyer

OpenBook Publishers

https://www.openbookpublishers.com

© 2023 Ayoub Al-Jawaldeh and Alexa L. Meyer

This work is licensed under an Attribution-NonCommercial 4.0 International (CC BY-NC 4.0). This license allows you to share, copy, distribute and transmit the text; to adapt the text for non-commercial purposes of the text providing attribution is made to the authors (but not in any way that suggests that they endorse you or your use of the work). Attribution should include the following information:

Ayoub Al-Jawaldeh and Alexa L. Meyer, *Reshaping Food Systems to Improve Nutrition and Health in the Eastern Mediterranean Region*. Cambridge, UK: Open Book Publishers, 2023, https://doi.org/10.11647/OBP.0322

The images in this publication have been created by the authors and they are released under the same licence as the rest of the book, except for Figure 1. Copyright and permissions for the reuse of this image is provided in the caption and in the list of illustrations. Every effort has been made to identify and contact copyright holders and any omission or error will be corrected if notification is made to the publisher.

Further details about the CC BY-NC license are available at http://creativecommons.org/licenses/by-nc/4.0/

All external links were active at the time of publication unless otherwise stated and have been archived via the Internet Archive Wayback Machine at https://archive.org/web

Digital material and resources associated with this volume are available at https://doi.org/10.11647/OBP.0322#resources

ISBN Paperback: 978-1-80064-863-0
ISBN Hardback: 978-1-80064-864-7
ISBN Digital (PDF): 978-1-80064-865-4
ISBN Digital ebook (EPUB): 978-1-80064-866-1
ISBN Digital ebook (AZW3): 978-1-80064-867-8
ISBN XML: 978-1-80064-868-5
ISBN HTML: 978-1-80064-869-2
DOI: 10.11647/OBP.0322

Cover image: Markus Spiske, Farmer's Market (2020), https://unsplash.com/photos/Lq--OvaORRQ). Cover design: Jeevanjot Kaur Nagpal

Contents

About the Authors	ix
Introduction	xix
Part 1: Food Systems: Concept, Definitions, and Approaches	**xxv**
1.1. The Food Systems Approach: Definitions and Concept	1
1.2 Challenges to Current Food Systems	7
1.3 Food Waste and Losses and Water Use	13
1.4 Sustainable Food Systems for Healthy Diets of the Future	23
Part 2: The Nutritional and Health Situation in the Countries of the WHO Eastern Mediterranean Region	**29**
2.1 Undernourishment in the WHO Eastern Mediterranean Region	31
2.2 The Increasing Problem of Overweight and Obesity	43
2.3 Micronutrient Deficiencies	53
2.4 Young Children and Infant Feeding Practices: Rate of Exclusive Breastfeeding, Early Breastfeeding Initiation and Complementary Feeding	63
2.5 Dietary Intake and Consumption Patterns of Adults and Adolescents	71
Part 3: Food System Actions as 'Game Changers' with a Special Focus on Regional Aspects and Effects	**79**
Goals and Objectives: Improving Food Environments and Empowering Consumers in their Food Demands to Make Diets Healthier and More Sustainable	81

3.1 Fiscal Policies for Healthy and Sustainable Diets	83
3.2 Regulation of Marketing of Foods and Non-Alcoholic Beverages as well as Breastmilk Substitutes through Traditional and Digital Media	95
3.3 Food Labelling with Focus on Front-of-Pack Labelling	125
3.4 Reformulating Food Products	143
3.5 Public Food Procurement and Service Policies to Support Healthy Sustainable Diets	179
3.6 Food Fortification, Including Biofortification	205
4. Conclusion and Outlook	243
References	247
Index	285

About the Authors

Ayoub Al-Jawaldeh is an international expert in nutrition and the author of more than 150 publications and books on nutrition, food systems and Non-communicable diseases (NCDs). He has worked with the World Health Organization as a Regional Adviser in Nutrition in the Eastern Mediterranean Region since 2009, and prior that he was a leading member of the United Nations World Food Programme for 20 years, focusing on countries including Egypt, Iran, Afghanistan, Sudan, Malawi, and Iraq. In his work he manages multiple international executive functions, including nutrition policies and strategies, research and capacity-building programmes that address the double burden of malnutrition, including maternal and child nutrition, diet-related risk factors for non-communicable diseases, and nutrition for emergencies in the Eastern Mediterranean Region.

Alexa L Meyer graduated with a PhD in nutritional sciences and worked as a scientific assistant at the University of Vienna, Austria, contributing to the European Nutrition and Health Report 2009, the Austrian Nutrition Report 2012, and the Palestinian Micronutrient Survey 2013 in cooperation with the Ministry of Health of the State of Palestine. She is also the author or co-author of several scientific papers, book chapters, and books on nutritional immunology, food composition as well as public health nutrition. Currently, she works at the Geriatric Care Hospital "Haus der Barmherzigkeit" in Vienna.

List of Tables

Table 1	Estimated amount of food waste in the countries of the WHO Eastern Mediterranean Region at the household, food service and retail level. Source of data: UNEP. Food Waste Index Report 2021.	16
Table 2	Prevalence of low birth weight (<2.5 kg) by country and year.	32
Table 3	Prevalence of wasting, stunting and underweight in children under 5 years by country. Source of data: UNICEF/WHO/World Bank (2021) Joint Child Malnutrition Estimates using data from national surveys, except for Lebanon, Somalia and Sudan (see below).	34
Table 4	Prevalence of underweight in school children and adolescents by country and sex (in %). Source of data: WHO Global Health Observatory.	14
Table 5	Prevalence of underweight (BMI<18.5 kg/m^2) in adults (≥18 years) in 2016 (in %, age-standardized estimate). Source of data: WHO Global Health Observatory.	38
Table 6	Prevalence of overweight and obesity in adults (≥18 years) by country and year. Source of data: WHO Global Health Observatory unless otherwise indicated.	44
Table 7	Prevalence of overweight in children under the age of 5 years by country. Source of data: UNICEF/WHO/World Bank Joint Child Malnutrition Estimates Expanded Database: Overweight (Survey Estimates), May 2022, New York, unless otherwise indicated.	46
Table 8	Prevalence of overweight and obesity in school-age children (5–9 years) sex and country (in %). Source of data: WHO Global Health Observatory, data from 2016.	48
Table 9	Prevalence of overweight and obesity in adolescents (10–19 years), sex and country (in %). Source of data: WHO Global Health Observatory, data from 2016.	49

Table 10	Haemoglobin concentrations in the blood at sea level to define and classify anaemia (g/dl). WHO VMNIS, 2011.	54
Table 11	Prevalence of anaemia in different population groups in the countries of the WHO Eastern Mediterranean Region. Al-Jawaldeh et al., 2021, based on the latest available estimates*.	55
Table 12	Median urinary iodine excretion and deduced iodine status by country of the WHO Eastern Mediterranean Region. Surveys were conducted in school-age children unless otherwise indicated (Source of data: Iodine Global Network, 2021).	58
Table 13	Percentage of children exclusively breastfed during their first 5 to 6 months of life by country and year in the WHO Eastern Mediterranean Region.	64
Table 14	Types of taxes on unhealthy foods. Based on WCRF, 2018.	89
Table 15	Taxation of foods and beverages containing added sugars in countries of the WHO Eastern Mediterranean Region. Source of data: Popkin & Ng, 2021; Zargaraan et al., 2017.	92
Table 16	Recommendations on the marketing of foods and non-alcoholic beverages to children. Adapted from WHO, 2010 and WHO-EMRO, 2018.	97
Table 17	Nutrient profile model for the WHO Eastern Mediterranean Region (modified from WHO EMRO, 2017a).	102
Table 18	Steps in setting up a national Code monitoring system. Based on WHO/UNICEF, 2017a.	115
Table 19	Status of implementation of the International Code on the marketing of breastmilk substitutes and products covered in countries of the WHO Eastern Mediterranean Region. Source of data: WHO, 2020.	118
Table 20	Implementation of selected provisions of the International Code on marketing of breastmilk substitutes and products covered in countries of the WHO Eastern Mediterranean Region. Source of data: WHO, 2020.	120
Table 21	Classification of front-of-pack labelling systems.	129
Table 22	Major strengths and weaknesses of common front-of-pack nutrition labelling systems.	132
Table 23	Salt intake in adults, children, and adolescents in the countries of the WHO Eastern Mediterranean Region based on urinary Na excretion. Source: Al-Jawaldeh et al., 2021b unless otherwise indicated.	149

List of Tables

Table 24	Policies on the reduction of salt in bread and other selected food sources in countries of the WHO Eastern Mediterranean Region.	156
Table 25	Mandatory limits, bans and labelling of trans-fats in foods in the countries of the WHO Eastern Mediterranean Region in 2021. Source of data: WHO, 2021b.	170
Table 26	Aspects of healthy public procurement to be considered in the situation analysis.	187
Table 27	Guiding principles for healthy public food procurement and service policies. Source: Adapted from WHO, 2021c. This is an adaptation of an original work, "Action framework for developing and implementing public food procurement and service policies for a healthy diet. Geneva: World Health Organization; 2021. Licence: CC BY-NC-SA 3.0 IGO." This adaptation was not created by the WHO. The WHO is not responsible for the content or accuracy of this adaptation. The original edition shall be the binding and authentic edition.	188
Table 28	Examples of process and outcome indicators for policy evaluation. Adapted from WHO, 2021c. This is an adaptation of an original work, "Action framework for developing and implementing public food procurement and service policies for a healthy diet. Geneva: World Health Organization; 2021. Licence: CC BY-NC-SA 3.0 IGO." This adaptation was not created by the WHO. The WHO is not responsible for the content or accuracy of this adaptation. The original edition shall be the binding and authentic edition.	190
Table 29	Challenges to the implementation of healthy school feeding programmes.	199
Table 30	Policies relating to public food procurement in different settings in countries of the WHO Eastern Mediterranean Region.	201
Table 31	Status of salt iodization in the WHO Eastern Mediterranean Region. Source of data: Doggui et al., 2020; UNICEF, 2021b.	221
Table 32	Average levels of nutrients recommended by the WHO to consider adding to fortified wheat flour depending on extraction, fortificant chemical form and per-capita flour availability. Modified from WHO et al., 2009.	223

Table 33 Status of industrial processing and fortification of wheat 226
flour (and rice) in the countries of the WHO EMR. Source
of data: Global Fortification Data Exchange; WHO EMRO,
2019b.

Table 34 Advantages and disadvantages of biofortification techniques. 240

List of Illustrations

Fig. 1	The UN Food Systems Summit's Action Tracks. Source: UN, 2021.	xx
Fig. 2	A schematic overview of activities, drivers, and outcomes of food systems and their interaction with each other.	3
Fig. 3	Characteristics of optimal food systems for the future. Based on IFPRI, 2021.	11
Fig. 4	Food losses by region as a percentage of total food production. Source of data: FAO Food Loss Index, 2020.	14
Fig. 5	Effect of fiscal policies on the food system. Based on FAO, UNEP & UNDP, 2021.	87
Fig. 6	Stakeholders in the development and dissemination of marketing and determinants of its impact.	99
Fig. 7	Legal status of the International Code of Marketing of Breast-Milk Substitutes by WHO region in 2020. Source of data: WHO, 2020; WHO-GINA, 2012.	117
Fig. 8	The WHO's Principles for the implementation of FOPL systems (WHO, 2019b).	137
Fig. 9	FOPL systems currently used or planned to be used in the countries of the WHO Eastern Mediterranean Region. Clockwise from top left: traffic-light system from Iran; traffic-light system from Saudi Arabia; Weqaya health logo from Abu Dhabi; Healthy tick symbol currently tested and envisaged in Tunisia; Nutri-Score tested and envisaged in Morocco.	139
Fig. 10	Principal actors involved in and factors driving food reformulation.	146
Fig. 11	Age-standardized death rates per 100,000 attributable to systolic blood pressure ≥140 mm Hg in 2015 by region. Source of data: Forounzafar et al., 2017.	147
Fig. 12	The SHAKE Technical Package for salt reduction. Based on WHO, 2016b.	153

Fig. 13	Structure of common trans-fatty acids compared to the cis-unsaturated oleic acid.	165
Fig. 14	The REPLACE Action Package of the WHO. Based on WHO, 2021a.	167
Fig. 15	Number of countries by WHO region with mandatory policies for the elimination of TFAs in food. Best practice: Legislative or regulatory measures limiting industrially produced TFAs to 2 g per 100 g of total fat in all foods and settings and imposing a ban on the production and use of PHO as an ingredient in all foods. Other complementary measures: legislative or other measures that facilitate healthier choices with regards to industrially produced TFAs for consumers (like mandatory declaration of TFA on nutrition labels, front-of-pack labelling systems including TFAs, or product reformulation) or impose mandatory limits on industrially produced TFAs in foods in specific settings like public schools only. National policy commitment: national policies, strategies or action plans expressing a commitment to reduce industrially produced TFAs in the food supply. Source of data: WHO, 2021b.	169
Fig. 16	Public food procurement as part of a sustainable healthy food system.	181
Fig. 17	Long-term benefits from school feeding. By the authors using free vectors from OpenClipart-Vectors, AnnaliseArt and Tumisu on Pixabay, https://pixabay.com/de/	194
Fig. 18	Monitoring and evaluation of food fortification and its public health effects. Based on Allen et al., 2006.	210
Fig. 19	Salt iodization in the WHO regions by legislation status (% of countries). Source of data: Global Fortification Data Exchange.	214
Fig. 20	Percentage of countries practising wheat flour fortification by WHO region and legislation status. Source of data: WHO EMRO, 2019b; Global Food Fortification Data Exchange.	224
Fig. 21	Wheat flour fortification in the WHO Eastern Mediterranean Region. Source of data: WHO EMRO, 2019b; Global Food Fortification Data Exchange.	224
Fig. 22	Frequency of micronutrients added to wheat flour in the countries of the WHO Eastern Mediterranean Region. Source of data: Global Fortification Data Exchange.	231
Fig. 23	Mechanisms of biofortification.	237

Fig. 24 Countries of the WHO Eastern Mediterranean Region with biofortified crops released or in testing. Abbreviations: Zn W: zinc-fortified wheat, Zn Fe L: zinc- and iron-fortified lentil, Fe PM: iron-fortified pearl millet, VA M: pro-vitamin A-fortified maize, VA SP: pro-vitamin A-fortified orange sweet potato, (R): released, (T): tested. Source of data: HarvestPlus. 241

Introduction

Healthy, wholesome nutrition in adequate quantities is a prerequisite for health and wellbeing and, thereby, human productivity. Eliminating malnutrition and food insecurity and increasing access to healthy food have become high priorities in the fight against poverty. In 2014, the Rome Declaration on Nutrition and the accompanying Framework for Action that were issued at the Second International Conference on Nutrition (ICN2) initiated a number of efforts towards a world without hunger (ICN, 2014a; ICN, 2014b), culminating in the proclamation of the United Nations Decade of Action on Nutrition 2016 to 2025 (UN General Assembly, 2016).

Despite many efforts, the prevalence of hunger and undernourishment has remained high and has even slightly increased as a result of increasing conflicts, climate change and the global COVID-19 pandemic (FAO, IFAD, UNICEF, WFP and WHO, 2021). The current war in Ukraine, a major exporter of wheat, corn, and sunflower oil, threatens to further delay the eradication of hunger in the world, as volumes of these commodities are expected to decline and prices to rise significantly (FAO, 2022).

At the same time, the problem of overnutrition has been increasing for many years. The number of overweight and obese people is now exceeding that of undernourished people and nutrition-related non-communicable diseases are currently the most common cause of death in all regions of the world (WHO, 2019a; WHO Global Health Estimates 2019).

Against this background, the fight against malnutrition is also a central element of the United Nations' Agenda for Sustainable Development 2030 to end poverty and promote global development. In addition to the Sustainable Development Goal (SDG) 2 that is directly aimed at ending hunger and all forms of malnutrition by 2030, other SDGs are related to

© 2023 Al-Jawaldeh and Meyer, CC BY-NC 4.0   https://doi.org/10.11647/OBP.0322.18

nutrition, such as SDG 3 to improve health and wellbeing and SDG 12 to make consumption and production systems more sustainable (https://www.un.org/sustainabledevelopment).

Making healthy, sustainable diets accessible for everyone requires profound changes in the current methods of producing and consuming food, also in the face of climate change. Therefore, the United Nations have convened a Food Systems Summit in September 2021 to offer a platform for exchange and cooperation between countries and actors in the food system (more detail can be obtained from https://www.un.org/en/food-systems-summit/).

In alignment with the SDGs, the actions stimulated by the UN Food Systems Summit are organized into five Action Tracks as shown in Figure 1.

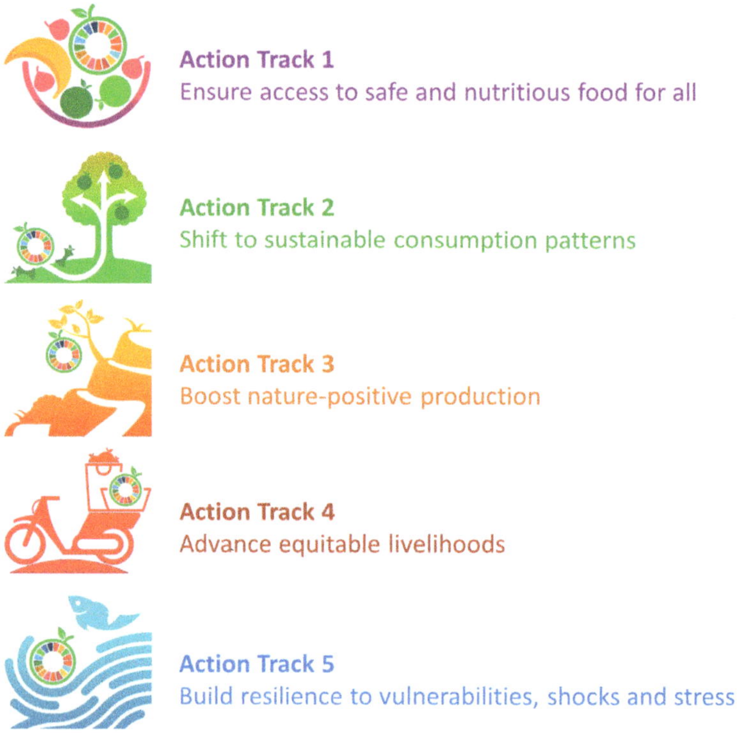

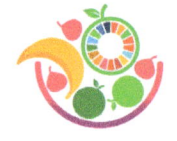

Action Track 1
Ensure access to safe and nutritious food for all

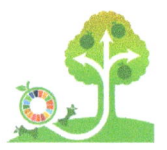

Action Track 2
Shift to sustainable consumption patterns

Action Track 3
Boost nature-positive production

Action Track 4
Advance equitable livelihoods

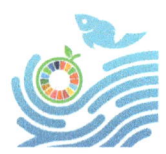

Action Track 5
Build resilience to vulnerabilities, shocks and stress

Fig. 1 The UN Food Systems Summit's Action Tracks. Source: UN, 2021.

True to its mission "to promote health, keep the world safe and serve the vulnerable — so everyone, everywhere can attain the highest level of health", the World Health Organization has taken on a role as the anchor agency of Action Track 2: Shifting to Sustainable and Healthy Consumption Patterns.

The focus of this Action Track is on three major objectives:

- Motivating and empowering consumers to make informed, healthy, safe and sustainable choices for their diets;
- Making sustainable and healthy food more available, accessible, and affordable; and
- Reducing, measuring and regulating food waste in the food retail, service, and at household level.

To support its member states in the realization of this goal, the WHO suggests a package of six 'game changing' food systems actions:

1. Fiscal policies for healthy and sustainable diets;
2. Public food procurement and service policies for a healthy diet sustainably produced;
3. Regulation of marketing of foods and non-alcoholic beverages, including breastmilk substitutes;
4. Food product reformulation;
5. Front-of-pack labelling; and
6. Food fortification.

These approaches were also promoted by the WHO Regional Office for the Eastern Mediterranean Region in its Strategy on nutrition for the Eastern Mediterranean Region, 2020–2030 (WHO EMRO, 2019a).

The World Health Organization's region of the Eastern Mediterranean encompasses twenty-two countries: the Islamic Republic of Afghanistan, the Kingdom of Bahrain, Djibouti, Egypt, the Islamic Republic of Iran, Iraq, Jordan, Kuwait, Lebanon, Libya, the Kingdom of Morocco, Oman, Pakistan, the Occupied Palestinian Territories, Qatar, the Kingdom of Saudi Arabia, Somalia, Sudan, the Syrian Arab Republic, Tunisia, the United Arab Emirates, and Yemen.

The region is characterized by a high diversity, especially with regards to economic development and income level, as it includes both, countries with low income like Afghanistan, Somalia, Sudan and Yemen, but also those with very high income like Oman, the Kingdom of Bahrain, Qatar, the Kingdom of Saudi Arabia, and the United Arab Emirates. This is also reflected in differences in the nutritional status and food security. Nevertheless, malnutrition in all its forms affects people in all countries of the region. Besides high prevalence of undernourishment in the countries with lower incomes, overweight and obesity are common in all countries and particularly in those with high incomes. The region is also characterized by a high dependency on food imports due to its environmental situation. This makes its countries vulnerable to global price volatility and supply insecurity for key agricultural commodities, as the war in Ukraine is currently demonstrating. Indeed, some countries in the region are among the main buyers of wheat from Ukraine, which will have unpredictable consequences for their food security while the war continues (FAO, 2022).

Like countries in many regions of the world, the nations of the Eastern Mediterranean Region have experienced or are still going through significant changes in their diets from traditional nutrition to more "Westernized" patterns, known as nutritional transition (WHO EMRO, 2019a). These changes are mainly driven by economic development and modernization, leading to increases in income, urbanization, digitalization, and altered lifestyles. While these are not generally negative and even improve food security and reduce undernourishment, the introduction of highly processed foods that replace traditional foods contributes to micronutrient malnutrition and increases the intake of sugar, salt, saturated and trans-fatty acids. Combined with reduced physical activity, this promotes the development of nutrition-related non-communicable diseases (Popkin, 2006 & 2015). Indeed, the burden of non-communicable diseases is high in the region, having caused an estimated 66.2% of all deaths in 2019. Although not all of these diseases are related to diet, cardiovascular diseases and strokes as well as some nutrition-related cancers contribute significantly to the death toll (WHO Global Health Estimates 2019). In the Diabetes Atlas 2021, the highest age-adjusted prevalence of diabetes mellitus (16.2% of the adult population) was reported for the Middle Eastern and Northern African

Regions that correspond broadly to the WHO's Eastern Mediterranean Region. In addition, this region is projected to have the second highest increase in diabetes prevalence from 2021 to 2045 at 87% (from 73 million to 136 million). Two of the region's countries, Pakistan and Egypt, are among the ten countries with the highest number of diabetics (International Diabetes Federation, 2021).

Improving the diets of people of all ages in the Eastern Mediterranean Region is a crucial step towards better health. After a short overview of the food systems and nutritional situation in the region, this book outlines the status and progress of the WHO's six game-changing actions within the frame of the UN Food Systems Summit, and looks at opportunities to make food systems in the Eastern Mediterranean Region healthier and more sustainable.

PART 1

FOOD SYSTEMS: CONCEPT, DEFINITIONS, AND APPROACHES

1.1. The Food Systems Approach Definitions and Concept

The concept of a food system involves the full food and nutrition chain from production to consumption, as well as their impact on the environment. A more comprehensive approach to efficiently combat food insecurity that would not just target primary food production but also social, political, economic and environmental aspects, among others, was suggested some years ago and has since gained increasing attention when it comes to making diets healthier and more sustainable. What people eat is indeed influenced by a multitude of factors, not just the availability of food. Efforts to improve not only food security but also diet quality with regards to healthiness must focus on the entire life cycle of food, from the field, farm or water in which it is produced to the disposal of the waste it creates, and including various influential factors and drivers and the sociocultural environment (UNEP, 2016; Global Panel, 2016 and 2020).

Already in 2013, the Food and Agriculture Organization of the United Nations (FAO) dedicated its annual report on 'The State of Food and Agriculture' to the subject of 'Food Systems for Better Nutrition'. Food systems were defined as:

> the entire range of activities involved in the production, processing, marketing, consumption and disposal of goods that originate from agriculture, forestry or fisheries, including the inputs needed and the outputs generated at each of these steps [and also involving] the people and institutions that initiate or inhibit change in the system as well as the sociopolitical, economic and technological environment in which these activities take place (FAO, 2013a).

Food systems are variable and specific to the environment in which they are set. They also change over time with the appearance of new actors and situations. However, at the centre of each food system is a set of activities that constitute the food supply chain, ranging from production, processing, transforming, storage and transport to retail and consumption.

The great variety of food system activities entails an equally large number of actors, beginning with food producers—including individual farmers and fishers—to large agribusiness enterprises, multinational food companies, large retailers that are also increasingly involved in food production, the transport and packaging sector, and finally the consumers. Besides these direct actors, others including governments, civil society, non-governmental organizations (NGOs), legislators, policy makers, counsellors and/or lobbyists shape the food environment by determining the regulatory and legislative background, as well as the infrastructure and the socioeconomic environment, and by raising awareness of specific issues. An important point to keep in mind is that, in the end, all actors are also food consumers (UNEP, 2016; van Berkum et al., 2018).

The interaction of consumers with the food supply chain occurs within the food environment that constitutes the physical, social and economic conditions that determine food choices of the consumers. This environment includes the physical places where food is bought and eaten like markets, stores, restaurants etc., but it also involves regulatory elements such as the laws that regulate food quality, labelling, food prices and infrastructure elements that create an enabling environment for food system activities.

A schematic representation of major activities, drivers and outcomes of food systems is given in Figure 2.

Food system activities have a number of outcomes. Firstly, they affect the supply of food to the population, thereby determining food security. However, they have other effects on socioeconomic and environmental aspects that also influence food security and the sustainability of a given food system. All along the value chain, food production is a source of income and employment not only for farmers and fishers but increasingly for those working in the processing, transportation, packaging and retail sectors. In modern food systems, these latter constitute the largest

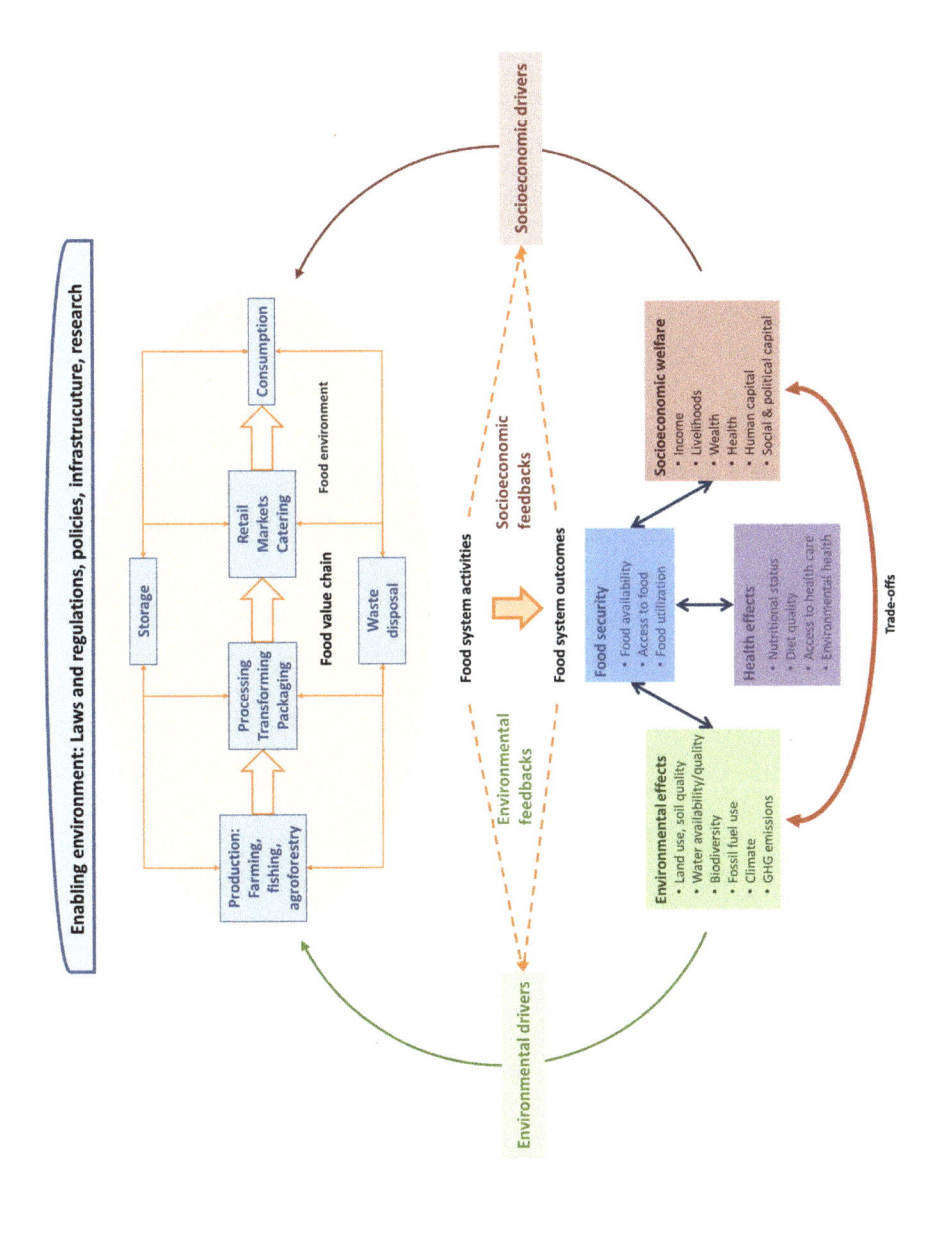

Fig. 2 A schematic overview of activities, drivers, and outcomes of food systems and their interaction with each other.

fraction of employers within the food supply chain. Additional revenues arise from sales of inputs like seeds, plants, fertilizers, pesticides and herbicides (UNEP, 2016, van Berkum et al., 2018).

In turn, climate and weather changes have effects on the food system, especially on crop production but also on storage and food loss. Socioeconomic factors and demographic trends such as population growth, changes in the age structure, increasing urbanization and rising income in many transition countries are other drivers of food activities, as are political and cultural aspects including food subsidies and other price policies, religious food laws and dietary trends. Scientific developments and new technologies have implications for different parts of the food chain, ranging from agricultural production (e.g., seed development, new varieties, harvest technologies etc.), processing, storage and transport to consumer choices and diets (UNEP, 2016, van Berkum et al., 2018).

The interaction of the different components of a given food system is important: as with any system, it should not just be considered as the sum of its parts. Interactions and dynamics between the different actors create new emergent properties that cannot be found in and explained by the single components or subsystems alone, but are characteristic of the whole system. The interactions produce feedback loops that can be positive (reinforcing) or negative (balancing) (Radzicki, 2007). Socioeconomic and environmental factors act as drivers of food system activities, creating feedback loops and multiplier effects. Incomes, for instance, have a strong influence on food choices, besides demographic developments and political and cultural settings. A favourable natural environment with fertile soils, sufficient access to clean water and other inputs are required for crop production, while environmental degradation and weather extremes due to climate change pose serious threats to food security (UNEP, 2016). Therefore, changes to the food system, even and especially if they are intended to improve the health and wellbeing of a population, have to be made in a sustainable way to limit negative effects on the environment and to reduce the production of greenhouse gases.

Food systems can be studied from different point of views, depending on the objectives and intended outcomes. However, some outcomes serve more than one purpose. For example, changes that would make a diet more sustainable and reduce its negative impact on the environment can also improve its healthiness, for instance by lowering the amount of animal products it contains. This will be discussed in more detail below.

Another important aspect of food systems is their variability and close relationship to the regional environment. Generally, a food system always has to be seen in its environment and context. Food systems from different parts of the world can of course be highly diverse, but so can systems within the same country. This makes it difficult to develop general models and solutions to improve food systems by making them more resilient and sustainable, and it is even more the case as food systems are changing rapidly, especially in countries experiencing nutritional transition.

Food systems are often categorized as "traditional" and "modern," with many stages in between. A food system can be described as traditional when the use of external inputs (like fertilizers or energy) and technologies, as well as crop yields, are low on the production side and the products are in most cases used by the producers themselves or sold locally. Agriculture in such a system is generally labour-intensive and most people employed in the food sector work in food production. Diets are predominantly plant-based with small amounts of animal products, and their composition varies with seasons.

On the other end of the spectrum are modern food systems that are dominated by industrial food production with high external input and degree of technologization. Farms are often large and tend to specialize in one or a few crops that are mostly grown in monoculture with high yields, and sold to processors or retailers. However, most incomes are generated through processing and retailing. Food reaches consumers in these systems mostly in a more or less processed or at least packaged state. The market is dominated by a few large retailers in the form of super- or hypermarkets that have their own brands of food. The distance between the site of food production and the place of its consumption is generally long, with the place of production often being located in other countries or on different continents. Modern food systems are therefore very sensitive to global price fluctuations and food crises, although these also affect more traditional food systems. Most food systems are intermediate forms between these two extremes with smaller food producers still playing a major role (Ericksen, 2008; UNEP, 2016).

1.2 Challenges to Current Food Systems

Until 2014, there was a steady decrease in the global number of undernourished people. Despite ongoing efforts to end world hunger, the numbers have stagnated since and have actually risen from 720 to 811 million undernourished people in 2020, corresponding to up to 161 million more people suffering from hunger (FAO, IFAD, UNICEF, WFP & WHO, 2021).

At the same time, the number of overweight and obese people is even larger, amounting to almost 2 billion people and to over 650 million adults (people aged ≥18 years) in 2016. This corresponds to 39% and 13% of the global population respectively. It is an issue that includes young people, affecting 39 million children under 5 years (2020) and 340 million school-age children and adolescents aged 5 to 19 years (2016) (WHO, 2021) and the associated non-communicable diseases place a heavy burden on those affected and on health systems. According to the Global Burden of Disease Study 2017 using data collected from 1990 to 2017 from 195 countries, unhealthy diets that are low in vegetables, fruits, wholegrain and dietary fibre caused about 11 million deaths and 255 million disability-adjusted life-years (DALYs) (GBD 2017 Diet Collaborators, 2019).

Adequately feeding a growing world population has become increasingly challenging. The latest report on the State of Food Security and Nutrition in the World by the FAO, IFAD, UNICEF, WFP and the WHO identifies three principal drivers of food insecurity: climate variability and weather extremes; conflicts; and economic slowdowns and downturns. The impact of the latter has become particularly apparent during the COVID-19 pandemic that has led a disruption of food supply chains and access to markets, as well as income losses during lockdowns (Al-Jawaldeh & McColl, 2020; FAO, IFAD, UNICEF, WFP & WHO, 2021; IFPRI, 2021). The Eastern Mediterranean Region has suffered repeatedly from political instability and conflicts that are also contributing to a decline in food security and increasing malnutrition.

Climatic conditions and the scarcity of cultivable land in the region make many countries highly dependent on food imports, as exemplified by cereal import dependency ratios of over 90% in the Gulf Cooperation Council countries, Djibouti, Jordan, Lebanon, and Yemen (FAO, 2017a). The region is therefore vulnerable to disruptions in global food trade and market price fluctuations, as revealed during the COVID-19 pandemic and more recently against the background of the war in Ukraine. These incidents show how closely interconnected modern food systems are under the influence of globalization.. Both Ukraine and its aggressor Russia are among the largest producers and exporters of wheat, with respective combined shares of 14% and 28% of global volumes (wheat and maslin) (FAO, 2022).

In 2020 and 2021, several of the top ten buyers of wheat from Ukraine were located in the Eastern Mediterranean Region (Egypt, Pakistan, Morocco, Tunisia, Yemen, Lebanon, and the Kingdom of Saudi Arabia), Egypt being the largest of all (UN Comtrade, https://comtrade.un.org/data/). Egypt, Sudan and Yemen, as well as many other countries from the Eastern Mediterranean and other regions, obtain more than 30% (and in some cases up to 100%) of their wheat imports from Russia and Ukraine (FAO, 2022). Some of these countries are already experiencing food insecurity, such as Yemen, Libya, Sudan, and Somalia.

In addition to wheat, Ukraine and the Russian Federation also produce and export significant amounts of maize and barley that are important feed commodities, as well as sunflower seeds, which are used for cooking oil but also as animal feed. Reduced supply and higher prices result in price increases for animal food products, further decreasing the affordability of these nutritious products. This poses a threat to adequate micronutrient supply, especially for vulnerable groups like young children, adolescents and the elderly. Losses are not only caused by direct damage to fields and crops from military activities but also from the destruction of infrastructure needed for crop processing, storage, and transportation (FAO, 2022).

The situation is further aggravated by the fact that the Russian Federation is also the largest exporter of nitrogen fertilizers and the second- and third-largest exporter of potassium and phosphorus fertilizers, respectively. The sanctions imposed on Russia will reduce the availability of fertilizers. In addition, the significant rise in prices for energy and gas will also increase the costs of fertilizer production in other countries. For 2022/2023, the global reference price for fertilizers is forecast to increase by 13% (FAO, 2022).

A simulation by the FAO projects a rise in the number of undernourished people in 2022/2023 by 7.6 million to 13.1 million, based on a moderate or severe scenario respectively. These two scenarios differ in terms of expected price increases for wheat and corn, as well as livestock products, and compensation by other producers for the shortfall in export volumes from Ukraine and Russia. For both models, the highest increase is expected in the Asia-Pacific Region, ranging from 4.2 to 6.4 million people, followed by Sub-Saharan Africa and the Near East & North African Region with projected 2.6 to 5.1 million and 0.4 to 0.96 million people, respectively. High prices for staple foods like wheat, maize, and sunflower oil will also increase the costs of food assistance to countries affected by crises and emergencies, further slowing the eradication of global hunger (FAO, 2022).

Current food systems have so far failed to address these challenges, both to ensure food security and the access to a healthy diet for everyone at affordable prices while at the same time providing sufficient incomes to food producers and limiting environmental damage (OECD, 2021). The situation is further complicated by the fact that it is not sufficient to supply the right amount of energy and nutrients, but to support a diet that is diverse, safe, healthy, sustainable, and also culturally acceptable (Global Panel, 2016).

Besides the three factors mentioned above, other aspects cause changes in diet composition and can interfere with efforts to improve the nutritional situation. Food systems and diets are evolving rapidly, and while changes to food habits and the introduction of new foods and preparation techniques as such are nothing new, they are occurring faster than ever before and some of them have negative effects on health (Global Panel, 2020).

Middle-income countries in particular are seeing increases in incomes that are also mirrored in food demand and consumption, including increased consumption of animal products, vegetable oils and processed foods and, albeit to a lesser degree, in fruits and vegetables (Gouel & Guimbard, 2017). While these changes at first lead to a decrease of undernutrition due to higher energy consumption and better supply of essential nutrients, they often result in increased overweight and obesity prevalence, and even in micronutrient malnutrition if more highly processed foods are consumed. The associated increase in the prevalence of nutrition-related non-communicable diseases puts a heavy burden on health systems (Popkin, 2006; WHO, 2013).

Increasing globalization and urbanization lead to greater distances between the producers of food and its consumers. Consumers thereby have less knowledge about the food they eat. This development also encourages the use of highly processed foods that have long shelf lives and are easier to transport than fresh commodities. It is also accompanied by the growing influence of some large-scale food producers, processors and retailers operating at regional or global level. Such actors are even harder to control by national policies and legislation. Globalization also exposes both producers and consumers to price variability and to global food crises. Urbanization has been associated with higher intake of processed foods and increased out-of-home consumption, especially among higher income groups, due to longer time spent working outside the home and less access to home cooking. However, urbanization and globalization also offer opportunities for improved nutrition, as residents of urban areas generally have access to a more diverse diet and also to refrigeration to allow for higher consumption of fresh products including fruits and vegetables. Globalization can contribute to a better and more stable supply of foods independent of national yields (UNEP, 2016; Global Panel, 2017).

Over the last few decades, agricultural policies and subsidies have not been aligned with nutrition and health objectives but have been largely dictated by economic factors, including a high demand for feed for large-scale livestock production in high-income countries. This has led to large increases in the production of staple grain, sugar and oil crops while that of many nutrient-dense vegetables and fruits has stagnated or declined. As a consequence, today's levels of food production would not support a healthy diet for the global population according to the recommendations of the WHO and nutritional entities. While there is greater awareness about this deficit, further efforts are needed to repurpose agriculture policies and reallocate subsidies to make diets more sustainable and nutrition-sensitive (UNSCN, 2014; FAO, 2017b; UNEP, 2020).

The challenges that food systems have to face can also be seen as an opportunity to induce changes towards better food security, more sustainability and improved health. A recent report by the International Food Policy Research Institute (IFPRI) on the impact of the COVID-19 pandemic on food systems identifies five properties that could make future food systems successful in enabling healthy food environments (Fig. 3).

With increasing threats from weather extremes and economic shocks, food systems have to be made more resilient. Solutions may for example be found in higher diversification, digitalization to improve information and communication, and investments in infrastructure for storage and transportation.

The efficiency of food systems can be improved in many aspects, from obtaining higher yields in food production by developing and applying new, climate-smart agricultural techniques and crop varieties with optimized properties; better use of natural resources like water, soils and minerals; improved infrastructure for food transport and storage; to food consumption that avoids food waste.

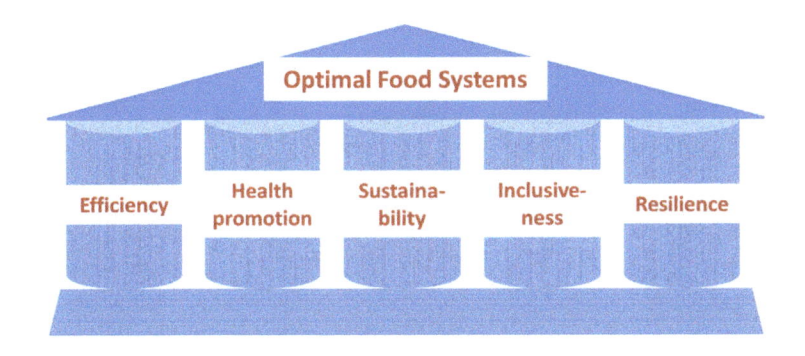

Fig. 3 Characteristics of optimal food systems for the future. Based on IFPRI, 2021.

Food systems should provide healthy diets for everyone, especially for marginalized groups that are at risk of malnutrition such as women of child-bearing age, children and adolescents, low-income groups and refugees. This is all the more relevant as women are to a large extent responsible for diet composition and food preparation as well as child nutrition (IFPRI, 2021).

These properties help to make food systems more sustainable and facilitate access to a healthy diet. This will be treated in more detail in the following subchapter.

1.3 Food Waste and Losses and Water Use

Another factor contributing to the unsustainability of food systems is the high proportion of food that is lost or wasted. An estimated 20 to 30% of produced food, or about 1300 million tonnes of edible food per year based on estimates for the year 2007, is lost or wasted across the food value chain. Food loss occurs upstream of the food value chain, on the field or during harvest or transportation due to spoilage or spilling, before products are produced or sold. In turn, food waste means that foods that would be edible are discarded by processors or consumers because their quality does not meet certain expectations or because they have expired. This therefore happens downstream of the food supply chain. Food loss and food waste are subsumed under the term food wastage (FAO, 2011). An analysis of data from 2007 found that food losses and waste account for about equal parts of total food wastage (approximately 54% and 46%, respectively) (FAO, 2013b).

However, more recent data suggests much higher food waste (931 million tonnes) that would also raise the total volume of food wastage (UNEP, 2016).

Food waste is particular high in high-income countries, while in low-income countries, food losses dominate due to poor harvesting techniques, pest management, insufficient storage capacities and transport infrastructure (UNEP, 2016). Nevertheless, large volumes of food are lost before food reaches retail level in all world regions (Fig. 4). In the North American and European Region, in 2020, the estimated share of food lost on the way from production to distribution to the market amounted to almost 10%. In the Northern African and Western Asian Region that approximately corresponds to the WHO Eastern

© 2023 Al-Jawaldeh and Meyer, CC BY-NC 4.0   https://doi.org/10.11647/OBP.0322.03

Mediterranean Region, food losses made up almost 15% (FAO, Food Loss Index, 2020).

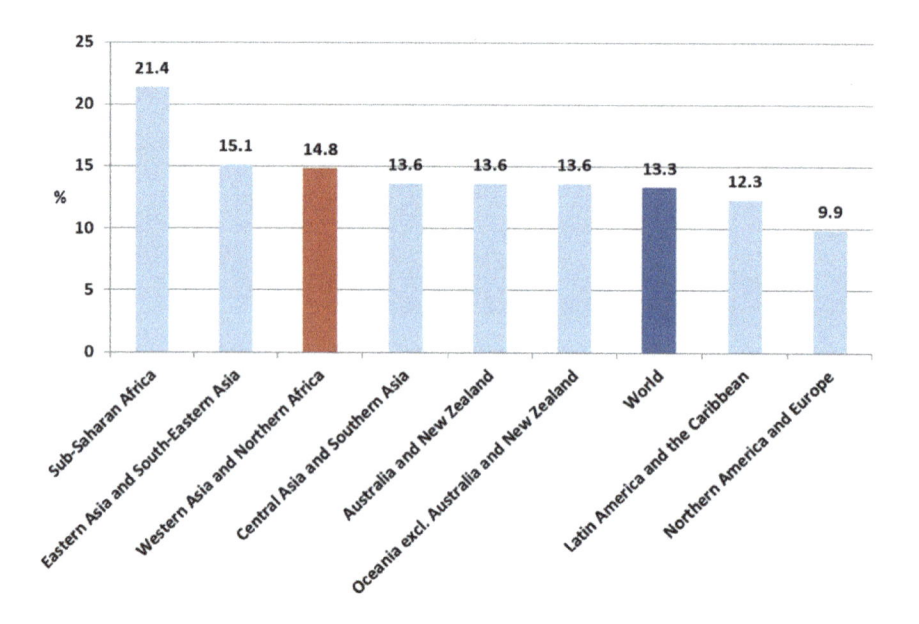

Fig. 4 Food losses by region as a percentage of total food production. Source of data: FAO Food Loss Index, 2020.

While losses at the level of agricultural production vary comparatively little, ranging from about 27 to 40% of total food wastage, large differences are seen at the post-harvest and storage phases that contribute significantly to food wastage in Sub-Saharan Africa and South and South-Eastern Asia. Together, agricultural and post-harvest losses make up the major part of total food wastage, accounting for 54% globally and higher contributions in less developed regions. In turn, in industrialized countries, a high proportion of food wastage occurs at consumption level (31–39% in middle- and high-income regions vs. 4–16% in low-income regions) (FAO, 2013b). The total amount of food wastage in industrialized regions is particularly high on a per-capita basis, amounting to about 300–340 kg/year compared to about 160 kg/year in South and South-Eastern Asia and 200 kg/year in Sub-Saharan Africa (FAO, 2013b).

A quantification of food waste at the global level as well as for individual countries was recently attempted by the United Nations

Environmental Programme (UNEP) to provide a basis for the monitoring of progress on Sustainable Development Goal 12.3 to "halve per capita global food waste at the retail and consumer levels and reduce food losses along production and supply chains, including post-harvest losses by 2030" (https://www.un.org/sustainabledevelopment). The results published in a Food Waste Index Report show that an estimated 931 million tonnes of food are wasted each year by households, retail establishments and the food service industry worldwide, with households accounting for the greatest part, corresponding to nearly two thirds (almost 570 million tonnes or 61%). On a per capita basis, on average 74 kg of food are wasted every year, and it is notable that this number varies little between countries with high and middle income levels (UNEP, 2021). An overview of estimated annual food waste levels in the countries of the WHO Eastern Mediterranean Region is shown in Table 1. However, measured data was only available for a small number of countries, so that most of these values are based on extrapolations and have only a low confidence level. Nevertheless, it is apparent that the greatest share of food waste occurs at the household level. This shows the importance of consumer education measures on the one hand to raise awareness about the issue of food waste and impart knowledge on how to avoid it, and on the other hand, of improving food storage at household level. The latter applies particularly to low- and lower-middle-income countries, where access to refrigerators and other technologies as well as regular power supply is low.

Different food commodities contribute differently to food wastage. Cereals have a high share due to the large production volumes of these crops. In turn, in the case of fruits, vegetables and starchy roots, their high perishability especially in warmer climate zones as well as high quality standards of importers, retailers and consumers in high-income countries are the main reasons for high wastage in this category (FAO, 2013b).

Food waste and losses also contribute to the carbon footprint of food production and consumption. Based on data for the year 2007, it has been estimated that global food waste and loss produce about 3.3 Gtonnes of CO_2 equivalents, which would rank third in the list of countries that contribute most to greenhouse gas (GHG) emissions (FAO, 2013b).

The high-income regions account for two thirds of the emissions, with the highest contribution coming from industrialized Asia. In turn,

Table 1 Estimated amount of food waste in the countries of the WHO Eastern Mediterranean Region at the household, food service and retail level. Source of data: UNEP. Food Waste Index Report 2021.

Country	Food waste (kg/capita/y)		
	Household	Food service	Retail
Afghanistan	82	28	16
Bahrain	132	26	13
Djibouti	100	28	16
Egypt	91	28	16
Iran	71	28	16
Iraq	120	28	16
Jordan	93	28	16
Kuwait	95	26	13
Lebanon	105	28	16
Libya	76	28	16
Morocco	91	28	16
Oman	95	26	13
Pakistan	74	28	16
Palestine	101	28	16
Qatar	95	26	13
Saudi Arabia	105	26	20
Somalia	103	28	16
Sudan	97	28	16
Syria	104	28	16
Tunisia	91	28	16
United Arab Emirates	95	26	13
Yemen	104	28	16

Colours of cells mark the level of confidence that the authors had in the respective data: green = high, yellow = medium, orange = low, red = very low.

the carbon footprint for food waste in the North African, Western and Central Asian Region, which includes the countries of the WHO Eastern Mediterranean Region, is comparatively small, amounting to slightly above 200 Mtonnes CO_2 equivalents per year. Emissions per capita are close to the global average of 500 kg CO_2 equivalents per year.

Greenhouse gases related to food wastage originate from different sources. At the level of agricultural production, emissions from the utilization of nitrogen fertilizers come from the direct release of nitrous oxide as well as the use of fossil energy for their production. Fossil fuels are also used in farming activities like ploughing and harvesting and for cultivation in heated greenhouses in colder climate zones. A major contributor to the carbon footprint of agriculture is the production of animal foods, which require fossil fuels and fertilizers in feed production and for animals' housing in some regions. Methane and nitrous oxide emissions from ruminants during enteric fermentation and animal manure are another direct source of GHG.

As the carbon footprint increases along the food value chain, it is highest when food is wasted during consumption, accounting for about 50% of the total food-waste-related carbon footprint in medium and high-income regions. However, agricultural food production is still the largest contributor in this phase too (FAO, 2013b).

By commodity, emissions are highest for wasted cereals, followed by vegetables and meat. However, cereals and vegetables also contribute the largest volume of food waste whereas it is much smaller for meat. Overall, animal products account for 33% of food-waste-associated GHG emissions, but only for 15% of food-waste volume, and while their relative contribution to the carbon footprint of food waste is highest in Latin America and North America and Oceania, it is notable across all regions (FAO, 2013b).

The environmental impact of food wastage is not limited to its carbon footprint but also affects land use, water and biodiversity. For 2007, the area of land used for the food wasted and lost globally was estimated at 1.4 billion ha, corresponding to about 28% of the total area of arable land or the second largest country of the world. It even exceeds the farmland of all countries. The highest land use by commodity results from wasted meat and dairy products. Most of this land is non-arable pasture. The region of North Africa, Western and Central Asia stands out as the region with the highest use of non-arable land for food wastage and most of this is related to meat and milk. The reason is that, due to the natural environment in this region, only a small part of the area is agricultural land (about 5% in the MENA region) and non-arable grasslands have a low productivity (Zdruli, 2014; FAO, 2013b). However, food wastage from meat and milk also uses much arable land for feed production, especially in industrialized regions. Notably, land use related to the wastage of vegetable food alone is highest in Sub-Saharan and North

Africa as well as Western and Central Asia due to the low productivity of agriculture in these parts of the world (FAO, 2013b).

Deforestation and the conversion of natural landscape into farmland also pose a threat to biodiversity. This is much more apparent in developing countries and in tropical and subtropical regions. Crop farming also has a higher impact than animal husbandry, with the former threatening 70% of all endangered species compared to 33% for keeping livestock. Intensive crop monocultures are especially harmful.

Moreover, food wastage results in a high water footprint. Indeed, food production and processing are major contributors to water use, and the sustainability of food systems is thus also determined by their impact on water resources. Agriculture alone accounts for about 70% of global freshwater extractions with much higher proportions in certain regions (FAO, 2011 and 2017b). The water footprint is defined as the volume of fresh water used directly and indirectly over the entire production and supply cycle of a product. It also includes water pollution, as grey water, and differentiates between use of ground and surface water and the consumption of rainwater (blue and green water, respectively) (Hoekstra et al., 2011).

In 2007, the blue water footprint of global food wastage amounted to about 250 km^3, more than twice the volume of the Dead Sea, and exceeding the blue water footprint for the consumed agricultural products of every single country (FAO, 2013b). Cereals and fruits were found to be the greatest contributors with 52% and 18% respectively, being both water-intensive crops. Regionally, North Africa and Western Asia have one of the highest blue water footprints, particularly considering this region's relatively small contribution to food wastage volume. Wastage of cereals accounts for the major part of the water footprint. Per capita, the region of North Africa, Western and Central Asia even has the highest food-waste-related blue water footprint with over 90 m^3 compared to the global average of about 38 m^3. This is all the more relevant considering the high water scarcity in this region (FAO, 2013b).

In addition to its environmental impact, food wastage leads to important economic losses and negative effects on public health. Based on food market prices for the year 2012, the cost of global food wastage was estimated at US$ 936 billion, corresponding to the GDP of the Netherlands or Indonesia. Food-wastage-related GHG emissions cause additional costs of about US$ 411 billion (FAO, 2015). The large amounts of food lost and wasted would be more than sufficient to eliminate hunger and malnutrition worldwide. A high proportion of wasted food consists of vegetables, fruits and meat. The loss of these nutrient-rich foods exacerbates the high prevalence of micronutrient deficiencies in many regions of the world (Miller &Welch, 2013).

In low-income countries, major causes of food wastage vary and include poor cultivation and harvesting technologies as well as inadequate storage facilities leading to spoilage of foods in the field or during post-harvest processing and storage. Lack of or poor access to transportation, processing and market infrastructure also results in food loss, especially at times of seasonal crop gluts. In high-income countries, on the other hand, food produced in excess to anticipate damage from adverse weather or pests is sometimes not harvested, or sold as feed to prevent price slumps. At the consumption level, exaggerated quality and aesthetic standards lead to the outgrading i.e., discarding of edible food. The ambition to always offer a wide range of products, even just before closing time, results in significant food wastage in retail (FAO, 2011).

Besides investments in better technologies and storage infrastructure, food loss can be reduced by facilitating market access for farmers, especially smallholders, through contract farming for retailers but also public food procurement (FAO, 2011). Recently, a number of retail chains have started campaigns to make suboptimal foods that are edible but do not meet aesthetic standards more acceptable to consumers and to sell them at lower prices (https://www.thelocal.de/20131013/52371/; https://www.ecowatch.com/french-supermarket-limits-food-waste-by-selling-ugly-produce-1881928868.html#toggle-gdpr). Consumer education plays an important role in preventing food waste to eliminate misconceptions about food expiry dates and product quality, and to raise awareness about food waste.

In 2014, on the occasion of the 32nd FAO Regional Conference for the Near East (NERC-32) a Regional Strategic Framework for Reducing Food Losses and Waste in the Near East & North Africa Region was issued to "assist member countries in addressing the key challenges of reducing food waste and losses by conducting comprehensive studies on [the] impact of food losses and waste on food security in the region and in establishing a plan to reduce food losses and waste in the region by 50% within 10 years". While linked to the FAO's *Global Initiative on Food Loss and Waste Reduction*, the framework takes into account the unique characteristics of the region in its recommended actions, including the socio-economic context, specific barriers to combating food losses and waste as well as the available resources, and efforts and achievements accomplished so far. National initiatives were already adopted in Egypt and the Kingdom of Saudi Arabia, and some very important measures were taken in Iraq, Iran, the United Arab Emirates, and Tunisia. Reducing food waste was also recognized in Oman as a central approach to improve the availability of healthy nutritious foods, namely fruits and vegetables and fish, and to enhance the country's self-sufficiency level in these commodities (Al-Jawaldeh et al., 2020a).

The Regional Strategic Framework includes four different components:

- Data gathering, analytical research and knowledge generation;
- Awareness-raising and promotion of good practices at all levels of the supply chain;
- Developing policies/regulations, and strengthening collaboration and networking; and
- Promoting investment and specific projects.

The aim is the development of well-coordinated multisectoral national action plans that adapt the regional strategy to the local circumstances. To support member states in this undertaking, the Regional Food Loss and Waste Network will provide a platform for information sharing and networking between national authorities and at the regional level, and it will assist with the monitoring of progress in the reduction of food loss and waste (FAO, 2015). Lebanon has established a food bank to collect wasted food of good quality and distribute it to charities and needy people (https://lebanesefoodbank.org/).

The water footprint of food systems is not only determined by food wastage. With the need to produce more food for a growing population under the pressure of climate change, water use is expected to increase globally. While it is generally assumed that water availability will suffice to produce food for a population of nine to ten billion people, water scarcity will occur and worsen in certain regions (FAO, 2015). Sustainable use of water is of particular importance for the Eastern Mediterranean Region, where arid climate zones predominate, especially in view of climate change. Key to sustainable water use is its efficiency. In agriculture, water use efficiency can be defined as the amount or value of crop being produced per volume of water applied. The use of inefficient irrigation techniques leads to large losses of water that often reach 50%. Unsustainable and inefficient water use results in the depletion of aquifers and non-renewable water resources, making them unavailable for current users like farmers and for future generations, and it forestalls the full exploitation of crop yield potential (UNEP, 2016).

Agriculture is also one of the largest contributors to water pollution, mainly due to the leakage of nutrients like nitrogen and phosphates that are applied as fertilizers or excreted by livestock into ground and surface water, causing eutrophication. Contamination of water with pesticides and herbicides, as well as hormones and drugs applied in livestock farming, poses a serious threat to human and animal health as well as to biodiversity (Mateo-Sagasta et al., 2017).

Making water use in food production more sustainable is a prerequisite for ensuring food security in the context of climate change. This involves the use of efficient irrigation using drip and trickle techniques that apply water more precisely to where it is needed. However, this requires investments to be made available to farmers and must be adapted to the local environment to prevent unwanted negative effects. For instance, higher yields from improved irrigation may instigate farmers to increase production, resulting in higher water withdrawals and overexploitation of aquifers (FAO, 2015; FAO, 2017c). Another approach is the devolvement of authority and responsibility for irrigation management from public entities to non-governmental institutions such as farmer associations. This approach, termed as irrigation management transfer, has been implemented in a number of countries with more or less success. While it can result in reduced bureaucracy, greater self-reliance of farmers, increased productivity and better efficiency of water use, property rights to land and water must be well-defined and legally ensured by governmental institutions (Garces-Restrepo et al., 2007; FAO, 2017c). Increasing competition for limited water resources requires innovative water governance to regulate water allocation and ensure its equitable distribution, while at the same time limiting contamination. This involves reducing the use of pesticides and herbicides as well as of animal density in livestock keeping, the promotion of organic farming, and improved manure management and fertilizer application (FAO, 2015). Importantly, free access to clean, safe water and adequate sanitation infrastructure is key to the prevention of infections and better health, which also improves nutritional status as poor access to safe drinking water and insufficient sanitation are contributors to high anaemia prevalence (Al-Jawaldeh et al., 2021a).

1.4 Sustainable Food Systems for Healthy Diets of the Future

The challenges outlined in the previous section make it clear that food systems of the future must be capable not only of supplying enough food in terms of energy and single nutrients, but rather supporting a diet that is healthy and environmentally and socioeconomically sustainable, while taking into account cultural aspects. The level of impact of these factors varies between different food systems and their interactions can be very complex. A food systems approach therefore must take into account the local circumstances and distinctions that apply, as well as the different objectives and interests of the various actors and the conflicts these can cause. Achieving this goal requires a multi-sectoral approach that includes all the parties involved in the food system.

A healthy diet can be defined in different ways. It should be diverse and based on foods that are only minimally processed and predominantly of plant origin like fresh vegetables and fruits, starchy tubers, pulses and wholegrain, complemented by moderate amounts of animal products, nuts and seeds, and vegetable oils of high quality. The energy content of the diet should be balanced with the person's energy expenditure, and nutrient requirements should be met. A low intake of saturated fatty acids, salt and added sugars is recommended while trans-fatty acids that are particularly detrimental for health, most of which are contained in highly processed foods, should be completely avoided. Healthy nutrition best begins early in life: infants should be exclusively breastfed until 6 months of age, and breastfeeding should begin within one hour of giving birth. After 6 months, infants need adequate, nutrient-dense and safe complementary food, while breastfeeding should ideally be continued until 2 years of age. (WHO, 2020 https://www.who.int/news-room/fact-sheets/detail/healthy-diet).

Sustainable food systems function so as not to impair the fundamental economic, social and environmental aspects of current and future food security, but rather to strengthen them (HLPE, 2017). The environmental sustainability of a food system is determined by its effects on land and water use and quality, on biodiversity and its contribution to greenhouse gas emissions. In many regards, current food systems are not sustainable as they result in soil degradation, contamination of water and soil due to leakage of agrochemicals and minerals used as fertilizers, use of fossil fuels, and the loss of biodiversity, genetic resources and minerals that are not recycled (UNEP, 2016). The fact that the food supply chain contributes about a quarter to global anthropogenic greenhouse gas emissions highlights the urgency with which we must act to limit the environmental consequences of our systems of agriculture and food production (Poore & Nemecek, 2018). A great opportunity to increase the amount of available food and reduce the environmental footprint of food production lies in minimizing food loss and waste. Approaches at the agricultural production level include investing in harvesting technology, as well as transport and storage infrastructure to help prevent spoilage. However, at least in higher income countries, there is also a need to reduce food waste at retail and household level by changing consumers' attitudes about food and their shopping habits and increasing their knowledge about proper food storage and handling (FAO, 2018).

Moreover, sustainability is not only defined by its environmental impact but also has a socioeconomic component, since it can help to ensure equal access to food and the maintenance of sufficient incomes and livelihoods for food producers and others working in the food value chain (HLPE, 2017).

All these objectives are often in conflict with each other. Changes to the food system, even if they are intended to improve the health and wellbeing of a population, can in turn have negative impacts on other system outcomes. Trade-offs arise particularly between economic and environmental aspects. For example, growing more fruits and vegetables to increase their availability would result in more land being used for cultivation and a higher use of water for irrigation, with negative effects on the natural environment and biodiversity. Less intensive cultivation techniques like organic agriculture are associated with higher costs and labour expenses for farmers, while yields are generally lower. Nevertheless, more sustainable farming that aims for healthier nutrition also benefits farmers. A higher diversity in food production not only provides consumers with more diverse and healthier diets, but also raises the incomes of farmers when they grow crops like fruits and vegetables that are sold at higher prices than staple crops. Growing food locally improves food security and can help to reduce the carbon footprint of food, while supporting the livelihoods of local farmers. Indeed, studies have shown that consumers generally favour locally produced food and are willing to pay more for it (Fan et al., 2019). Although these studies were done in high-income countries, they may be applicable to other settings as well.

Estimates based on current consumption patterns in the EU and OECD countries suggest that if consumers followed dietary recommendations such as those by the WHO, their diets would result in a smaller water footprint and lower levels of greenhouse gas emissions than the current average diet in these areas, while further reductions could be achieved with meat-reduced or vegetarian diets. Different food groups vary widely in their effects on the environment with regards to energy use, greenhouse gas emissions and water footprint. This underlines the importance of a balanced diet that includes a wide variety of foods (Global Panel, 2016 and 2020; Kim et al., 2020).

For diets to become healthier and more sustainable, and at the same time accessible to everyone, all the actors in a given food system have to collaborate and policies and actions must be coordinated in order to account for the complexity of the interactions that drive food chain activities.

Besides actions aimed at increasing the production and availability of healthy foods like vegetables and fruits, interventions at the level of food processing, retail and consumption are most relevant.

With the proceeding transformation and modernization of food systems, the contribution of food processing and retail to value addition along the chain and to employment in the food sector is increasing. At the same time, they also contribute significantly to the environmental impact of food production. Energy consumption in the food chain is highest for processing, packaging, transport and retail, and these sectors also contribute markedly to greenhouse gas emissions (Global Panel, 2016).

Moreover, food processors and retailers, who determine the kinds of food offered and its marketing, are key players in making healthier food accessible, affordable and desirable to consumers. In low- and middle-income countries, rising incomes as well as urbanization have been associated with higher consumption and with the increasing desirability of highly or ultra-processed foods. Increasing consumer knowledge about health and sustainability can be effective in promoting healthier diets, helping to control this influence and empowering consumers to make informed food choices. Additionally, the food industry should be actively engaged and made aware of its responsibility to provide healthy food to consumers.

Measures that are particularly suited to achieve these objectives include:

- Imposing taxes on foods that should be consumed less, such as those rich in sugar, salt and/or trans-fatty acids, and subsidising healthy foods like fruits and vegetables. The implementation of these measures has been shown to encourage food producers to reformulate their products so that they comply with the guidelines on which the taxes are based;

- Regulating the marketing of highly processed food products, especially to children;

- Providing guidelines on healthy and sustainable consumption patterns;

- Setting limits for food components whose intake should be limited such as free sugars, salt, saturated fatty acids, and trans-fatty acids;

- Providing consumers with easily understandable information on the nutritional value and composition of food through labelling, preferably in the form of front-of-pack labelling.

Rising awareness about the need to change food systems so that healthy and sustainable nutrition is available for all people worldwide has led to a number of events intended to stimulate actions in this direction and provide help to governments and other stakeholders involved. One of them is the United Nations Food Systems Summit, convened in autumn 2021 to offer a platform of exchange between the players in the food system, foster public discourse about the role of food systems in achieving the SDGs, provide solutions and encourage actions to end hunger and malnutrition worldwide (https://www.un.org/en/food-systems-summit/).

True to its mission "to promote health, keep the world safe and serve the vulnerable — so everyone, everywhere can attain the highest level of health", the World Health Organization has taken the role as the anchor agency of Action Track 2: Shifting to Sustainable and Healthy Consumption Patterns. Work in this Action Track is focusing on generating game-changing solutions in three areas:

- Motivating and empowering consumers to make informed, healthy, safe and sustainable choices;
- Improving the availability and affordability of healthy, safe and sustainable diets; and
- Minimizing food waste in the food service, retail and home environments; measure and regulate consumer and retail food waste.

To make diets more sustainable and at the same time healthier, the WHO has decided to focus on a package of six 'game changing' food systems actions:

- Fiscal policies for healthy and sustainable diets;
- Public food procurement and service policies for a healthy diet sustainably produced;
- Regulation of the marketing of foods and non-alcoholic beverages, including breastmilk substitutes;
- Food product reformulation;
- Front-of-pack labelling; and
- Food fortification.

These measures are also among the priorities suggested by the WHO Regional Office for the Eastern Mediterranean in its Strategy on Nutrition for the Eastern Mediterranean Region, 2020–2030, to support the countries of the region on their way towards healthier and sustainable diets. They will be presented in more detail in Part 3 of this book, and the progress of their implementation in the countries of the WHO Eastern Mediterranean Region will be reviewed.

Before this, however, we will look at the current nutritional situation in the region in the following chapters.

PART 2

THE NUTRITIONAL AND HEALTH SITUATION IN THE COUNTRIES OF THE WHO EASTERN MEDITERRANEAN REGION

2.1 Undernourishment in the WHO Eastern Mediterranean Region

Malnutrition is still widely occurring in the region in all its forms. Like other parts of the world, the region is suffering from a triple burden of malnutrition, with undernourishment and micronutrient deficiencies that coexist with overweight and obesity.

Deficiencies in energy and macronutrient intake that result in underweight and, in children, in growth deficits, are particularly common in Eastern Mediterranean countries with lower income levels, and those experiencing political unrest and conflicts. High-quality protein is a particularly critical macronutrient, especially for children and adolescents as well as pregnant and lactating women, that is often deficient among people in these countries.

2.1.1 Low Birth Weight

Low birth weight, defined by the WHO as a bodyweight of less than 2,500 g in newborns regardless of gestational age (WHO ICD-10, 2016a), is one of the first manifestations of undernourishment. Besides its immediately detrimental effects on infant health by increasing morbidity and mortality, it is a risk factor for non-communicable diseases in adult life through foetal programming (Fall, 2013).

A 2018 review of the nutritional status in the EMR found an estimated weighted average prevalence of 19.31 % for the whole region, based on various studies and national data from 1999 to 2014 (Nasreddine et al., 2018).

The latest estimates from UNICEF and the WHO for 2015 give a prevalence of 17.1 % for the WHO Eastern Mediterranean Region with an uncertainty bound ranging from 9.2 to 32.4%. These estimates show a slowly decreasing trend since 2000 when the prevalence was 19.4% (UNICEF/WHO, 2019). The most recently available data for the countries of the WHO EMR are shown in Table 2. However, no recent data were available for Afghanistan, Libya, Sudan and Yemen.

Looking at the development over time, there has been a decrease of this prevalence in some countries like the UAE, Djibouti, Morocco and Oman with some differences between the databases. In turn, the percentage of low-weight newborns increased in other countries like Bahrain, Jordan, Saudi Arabia, Somalia, Syria, and Yemen, or remained stable in others (Nasreddine et al., 2018; UNICEF/WHO, 2019; Department of Statistics/DOS and ICF, Jordan, 2019; Saudi Arabia General Authority for Statistics, 2017). Overall, many countries of the region are not on track to reach the third target of the Comprehensive Implementation Plan on Maternal, Infant and Young Child Nutrition, i.e., a 30% reduction in low birth weight by 2025 (WHO, 2014; Global Nutrition Report 2020).

Table 2 Prevalence of low birth weight (<2.5 kg) by country and year.

Country	Prevalence (%)	Year of survey
Bahrain	11.9	2015 [1]
Djibouti	10.0	2014 [2]
Egypt	14.1	2014 [2]
Iran	7.0	2014 [2]
Iraq	14.8	2014 [2]
Jordan	16.7	2017/2018 [3]
Kuwait	9.9	2015 [1]
Lebanon	9.2	2015 [1]
Morocco	17.3	2015 [1]
Oman	10.5	2015 [1]
Pakistan	32.0	2014 [2]
Palestine	8.4	2015 [1]
Qatar	7.3	2015 [1]
Saudi Arabia	16.5	2017 [4*]
Somalia	24.3	2019 [5]
Syria	9.4	2014 [2]
Tunisia	7.5	2015 [1]
United Arab Emirates	16.6	2018 [6]

Source of data: [1]UNICEF/WHO, 2019. Low birthweight (LBW) estimates, 2019 Edition https://www.unicef.org/media/53711/file/UNICEF-WHO%20Low%20birthweight%20estimates%202019%20.pdf; [2]FAO: Food and nutrition in numbers 2014. Rome; 2014 http://www.fao.org/3/a-i4175e.pdf; [3]Department of Statistics/DOS and ICF (2019). Jordan Population and Family and Health Survey 2017–18. Amman, Jordan, and Rockville, Maryland, USA: DOS and ICF; [4]Saudi Arabia General Authority for Statistics. Household Health Survey 2017; [5]Ministry of Health FGS, FMS, Somaliland, UNICEF, Brandpro, GroundWork. Somalia Micronutrient Survey 2019. Mogadishu, Somalia; 2020; [6]United Arab Emirates Ministry of Health and Prevention. UAE National Health Survey Report 2017–2018. Dubai, 2018.

*Prevalence was assessed for the five years preceding the survey, i.e., 2013–2017.

2.1.2 Wasting, Stunting and Underweight in Children Under Five Years

Undernourishment in preschool children under the age of 5 years is generally assessed through three indicators: wasting defined as weight-for-height below 2 standard deviations (SDs) of the WHO reference growth standards' median, stunting defined as height-for-age below 2 SDs of the WHO reference growth standards' median, and underweight defined as weight-for-age below 2 SDs of the WHO reference growth standards' median (WHO, 2006).

The prevalence for each indicator by country is shown in Table 3. For the whole region, it was estimated that in 2020, wasting affected 3.0% of children under 5 years and stunting 26.2%. Marked differences exist between countries with different income levels. Thus, wasting and stunting prevalence was 3.5% and 5.0% respectively in high-income countries (excluding United Arab Emirates) compared to 6.2% and 23.5% respectively in middle-income countries and 12.5% and 33.5% respectively in low-income countries (UNICEF/WHO/World Bank, 2021; WHO Global Health Observatory).

Generally, the respective prevalence of wasting, stunting and underweight varies widely across the EMR. In the case of wasting, the rates reported in the most recent surveys range from 1.3% in the State of Palestine to 21.5% in Djibouti. For the whole region, the prevalence of stunting in 2020 was estimated at 7.4%. The most recent data from the countries of the region shows a range from 6.4% in Kuwait up to 46.4% in Yemen. Yemen also had the highest prevalence of underweight with 39.9%, while the lowest (1.6%) was reported from Tunisia. In Lebanon, before the recent crises, 9.3% of children under 5 years living in Beirut,

Table 3 Prevalence of wasting, stunting and underweight in children under 5 years by country. Source of data: UNICEF/WHO/World Bank (2021) Joint Child Malnutrition Estimates using data from national surveys, except for Lebanon, Somalia and Sudan (see below).

Country	Wasting	Stunting	Underweight	Year of survey
Afghanistan	5.1	35.1 (2020)	19.1	2018
Djibouti	10.1	20.9	29.9 (2012)	2019
Egypt	9.5	22.3	7.0	2014
Iran	4.3	4.8	4.1 (2010)	2017
Iraq	3.0	12.6	3.9	2018
Jordan	0.6	7.4	2.7	2019
Kuwait	2.5	6.4	3.0 (2014)	2017
Lebanon[a]	6.7	8.4	0.5	2022
Libya	10.2	38.1	11.7	2014
Morocco	2.6	15.1	2.6	2017–2018
Oman	9.3	11.4	11.2	2017
Pakistan	7.1	37.6	23.1	2018
Palestine	1.3	8.7	2.1	2019–2020
Saudi Arabia	n.d.	3.9	5.3 (2004)	2020
Somalia[b]	10.5	17.8	12.7	2019
Sudan[c]	13.6	36.4	29.2	2018–2019
Syria	11.5	27.9	10.4	2009–2010
Tunisia	2.1	8.4	1.6	2018
Yemen	16.4	46.4	39.9	2013

Source of data: [a]Hoteit et al., 2022a; [b]Ministry of Health FGS, FMS, Somaliland, UNICEF, Brandpro, GroundWork. Somalia Micronutrient Survey 2019. Mogadishu, Somalia, 2020; Al-Jawaldeh & Dureab, 2021.

the capital city, and the governorate of Mount Lebanon, which together include about half of the country's population (UN OCHA, 2018), were underweight (WAZ < -2SD to -3SD), 9.3% were stunted (HAZ < -2SD to -3SD), and 6.25% were wasted (WHZ < -2SD to -3SD). In children under 2 years, the prevalence of underweight was 7%, of stunting 12.5% and of wasting 12% (Abi Khalil et al., 2022). Amid escalating crises—the COVID-19 pandemic, economic depression and political unrest—a national representative survey from 2021 showed that the prevalence of underweight, stunting, severe stunting, wasting and severe wasting in children aged under 5 years was 0.5%, 8.4%, 3.4%, 6.7% and 1.7%, respectively (Hoteit et al., 2022a).

Besides the prevalence, data availability is variable as well. For instance, there are no recent nationally representative data on wasting, stunting and/or underweight in children under 5 years for Bahrain, Qatar, Saudi Arabia and the United Arab Emirates. Some of the data from other countries are also rather old, like those from Syria (2009–2010), Iran (2011), Djibouti (2012) and Jordan (2012). In the case of the Gulf Cooperation Council countries that find themselves in an advanced stage of nutrition transition, this lack of data may be due to a higher focus on overweight as the rapidly growing health problem. The Syrian data were obtained before the outbreak of the war. Recent surveys among refugee children indicate low rates of acute malnutrition (1.7%) but a high prevalence of stunting (12.6%) (UNICEF, 2021a). This is in accordance with surveys conducted from 2013 to 2014 among refugees living at different sites (camps and outside camps) in Jordan, Lebanon and Iraq (Moazzem-Hossain et al., 2016). In Jordan, the prevalence of underweight in children under 5 years ranged from 2.9 to 4% for overall underweight and from 0.3 to 0.4% for severe underweight; in Lebanon, the range was 2.5 to 3.9% for overall underweight and 0.5 to 1.1% for severe underweight, while the numbers were slightly higher in Iraq (6.3%, of which the measurement of 1.4% severe underweight was obtained on one site) (Moazzem-Hossain et al., 2016). Global acute malnutrition (GAM, i.e., weight for height z-score <2 and/or the presence of oedema) was found in about 1% of preschool children in Jordan, in 0.3 to 4.4% in Lebanon and in 4.1% in Iraq (Moazzem-Hossain et al., 2016). Severe acute malnutrition (SAM, i.e., WHZ<3) was rare (<0.5%) with somewhat higher prevalence at the Bekaa camp in Lebanon (1.7%) and at the Domiz camp in Iraq (1.1%). Again, stunting was encountered more frequently, ranging from 10.5 to 16.7% in Jordan, 14.1 to 21.0% in Lebanon, and 19% in Iraq. In this latter group, 5.2% of cases were severe (Moazzem-Hossain et al., 2016). More recent surveys conducted in 2017 in two refugee camps and in host communities in Jordan reported a prevalence of GAM of 1.8–2.7% and of SAM of 0–0.3%, while stunting was found in 6.4 to 19.2% of the included children under 5 years (UNHCR/UNICEF/WFP/Save the Children, 2017). In 6- to 59-month-old Syrian refugee children living in Jordan, Lebanon, Turkey, Greece,

Egypt and Iraq in 2015 to 2016, the mean prevalence of wasting was 3.7% (2.5–10.2%) and that of stunting was 9.1% (7.4–16.6%) (Pernitez-Agan et al., 2019).

A much higher prevalence of GAM was reported from Yemen in 2021, where food security has deteriorated due to the civil war that began in autumn 2014. In an Integrated Food Security Phase Classification Acute Malnutrition (IPC AMN) analysis in 2020, the estimated prevalence of combined GAM (cGAM, based on WHZ and/or MUAC and/or oedema) in children under 5 years ranged from 7 to 31% across the 35 zones included, while combined moderate acute malnutrition (cMAM) ranged from 6 to 23% and combined SAM from 1 to 9% (IPC, 2021).

When looking at trends over the last few years, while some countries made progress in addressing undernutrition in children under 5 years and are on track to reduce the prevalence of stunting by 50% by 2030, and to reduce and/or maintain the prevalence of wasting to less than 3%, the majority of these countries are currently failing to reach these goals. Most progress was achieved with regard to wasting, while the prevalence of stunting, despite a decreasing overall trend, remains high in many countries. Nevertheless, the average prevalence of wasting showed a slight increase between 2000 and 2018 (from 11.8% to 12.5%) in low-income level countries (UNICEF/ WHO/World Bank, 2021).

2.1.3 Underweight in School-Age Children and Adolescents

Besides children under 5 years, other groups vulnerable to malnutrition are school-age children and adolescents. Among the latter, girls in particular are often not optimally supplied with micronutrients like iron, zinc, folate and vitamin A (see below). In both age groups, underweight or thinness is generally defined as BMI-for-age Z-scores <2 compared to the standard, and severe underweight as BMI-Z <3 (de Onis et al., 2007).

Information on the anthropometric status of 5- to 19-year-old children and adolescents is provided by the WHO's Global Health Observatory, the most recent numbers dating from 2016.

For children aged 5 to 9 years, the overall prevalence for the whole Eastern Mediterranean Region is estimated at 11%: 12.6% in boys and

9.3% in girls. In 10- to 19-year-old adolescents, the respective rates are 10.8%, 13.7% and 7.6%.

Table 4 shows the prevalence by country. In most countries, the values are so low that underweight in school-age children and adolescents does present a major public health problem. Exceptions are seen in Afghanistan, Pakistan and Yemen. Slightly higher rates are also observed in Iran, Saudi Arabia and Somalia. In all these countries and many others, there is a difference between the sexes, with more boys being underweight than girls.

A high prevalence was also reported in the more recent Pakistan National Nutrition Survey 2018, which included adolescents aged 10 to 19 years, with 21.1% of boys and 11.8% of girls being classified as too thin—although the numbers are somewhat lower than those given by the Global Health Observatory (Ministry of National Health Services, Regulations and Coordinations, Government of Pakistan, 2018).

No data are available for the State of Palestine and Sudan after its separation in two countries in 2011. However, adolescents aged 15 to 18 years were included in the Palestinian Micronutrient Survey 2013. In the whole sample, 4.3% of boys had a BMI-Z-score <-2, whereas this was the case in only 1.6% of the girls. Severe underweight (BMI-Z-score <-3) was seen in 1.0% of the boys and 0.2% of the girls. The prevalence of underweight was higher in the Gaza Strip than in the West Bank (6.6% vs. 1.9% in boys and 2.5% vs. 0.5% in girls) (Ministry of Health-Palestine & UNICEF, 2014).

For Sudan, information on the anthropometric status of adolescents, albeit dating from 2012, is provided by the Global School-Based Student Health Survey (GSHS), a collaborative surveillance project developed by the WHO together with UNICEF, UNESCO and UNAIDS, and with technical assistance from the U.S. Centers for Disease Control and Prevention (CDC). In the 13- to 15-year-old participants, the prevalence of underweight was also relatively high at 16.5% in boys and in girls 13.7% (https://www.who.int/teams/noncommunicable-diseases/surveillance/systems-tools/global-school-based-student-health-survey).

For Afghanistan, the Afghan National Nutrition Survey 2013 reported a somewhat lower prevalence in adolescent girls aged 10 to 19 years, of whom 8.0% were underweight and 1.5% severely underweight, compared to 10.5% according to the Global Health Observatory. Underweight was more common in the younger girls aged 10 to 14 years than in the older ones (15 to 19 years) (10.2% vs. 4.1%) (Ministry of Public Health of Afghanistan, UNICEF, 2013).

Table 4 Prevalence of underweight in school children and adolescents by country and sex (in %). Source of data: WHO Global Health Observatory.

Country	Children 5–9 y		Adolescents 10–19 y	
	Boys	Girls	Boys	Girls
Afghanistan	22.1	12.2	23.6	10.5
Bahrain	5.8	6.3	6.9	5.4
Djibouti	6.8	4.0	7.7	3.4
Egypt	3.2	2.3	3.7	1.9
Iran	8.9	8.2	10.1	6.8
Iraq	5.7	4.4	6.7	3.8
Jordan	4.2	3.8	4.7	3.2
Kuwait	3.4	3.5	4.0	2.9
Lebanon	4.8	5.0	5.8	4.0
Libya	5.8	5.2	7.0	4.5
Morocco	6.9	5.5	8.0	4.6
Oman	6.5	7.3	7.8	6.4
Pakistan	22.0	17.0	23.7	14.4
Qatar	4.6	5.2	5.6	4.6
Saudi Arabia	8.1	7.0	9.0	6.2
Somalia	8.0	4.8	9.1	4.1
Syria	6.3	5.8	7.5	5.0
Tunisia	7.1	5.7	8.2	4.8
UAE	5.0	5.1	6.1	4.5
Yemen	15.5	11.3	17.3	9.8

Data on underweight in younger school-age children is rarely found in national nutrition or health surveys; however, there are some regional studies on this population group. A survey of 390 5- to 12-year-old children from Khartoum City, Sudan, found a prevalence of 10.3% of underweight, including 3.3% of severe underweight. In boys, the prevalence was 15.3% and 4.5% respectively, and in girls it was 4.8% and 2.1% respectively (Elrayah et al., 2018). In another study from Argo City in Northern Sudan, conducted in 2016, 8.3% of 1223 school children aged 6 to 14 years were underweight, of whom 3.7% were severely underweight. In those aged 6 to 10 years, the prevalence of total underweight was 9.2%, including 4.2% severe underweight. Again, underweight was more common in male children aged 6 to 14 years, of whom 11.5% had a BMI <-2 SDs and 5.4% <-3 SDs below the WHO median (Hussein et al., 2018).

In a study of in 1320 Palestinian school children aged 6 to 12 years from the governorate of Nablus, a comparatively high prevalence of underweight based on the reference values of the CDC (BMI under the 5th percentile) was found, with 7.3% of the participants affected, 10.1% of the girls and 4.6% of the boys. The prevalence varied between the different age groups (6, 7, 8, 9, 10, 11, and 12 years), but no consistent trend was visible. Moreover, in a review of the literature, the authors observed an increase compared to earlier studies in Palestine (Al-Lahham et al., 2019).

2.1.4 Underweight in Adults and Pregnant and Lactating Women

Underweight in adults is generally defined by a BMI<18.5 kg/m^2, with further classification as moderate and severe by BMI between 16.0 and 16.99 kg/m^2 and <16 kg/m^2, respectively.

Prevalence of overall overweight (BMI<18.5 kg/m^2) can be found in the WHO's Global Health Observatory database, with the most recent values dating again from 2016.

For the whole Eastern Mediterranean Region, an average prevalence of 7.3% is given, 7.4% in men and 7.2% in women. However, the prevalence differs widely between countries, as shown in Table 5. As for school-age children and adolescents, no data are available for the State of Palestine and for Sudan after 2011.

In a study of 7239 adults (≥18 years) from Sudan, underweight defined by a BMI<18 kg/m^2 was found in 4.2% of the participants. The prevalence was comparable between sexes, but slightly higher in men (4.6% vs. 4.0% in women). The highest prevalence was found in the youngest participants (18 to 25 years, 9.2%) as well as the oldest (>75 years, 6.3%) while underweight was least common in middle-aged Sudanese (46 to 55 years, 1.8%) (Ahmed et al., 2017).

More recent data is also provided by some national nutrition and health surveys. However, weight assessment in adults is often limited to certain age groups or at-risk populations such as women of reproductive age.

The National Nutrition Survey in Afghanistan 2013 included measurements in women of reproductive age and in older adults (≥50 years). Of women aged 15 to 49 years, 9.2% had a BMI<18.5 kg/m^2 with 2.7% having a BMI<17 kg/m^2. In persons aged ≥50 years, the overall prevalence of underweight was 8.7% with 1.3% being severely thin. In the oldest group (>60 years), the respective prevalence was 12.9% and 2.2%, mirroring the higher risk of malnutrition with increasing age (Ministry of Public Health of Afghanistan, UNICEF, 2013).

The Jordan Population and Family Health Survey 2017–2018 assessed the weight status of women of reproductive age (15–49 years). The prevalence of underweight was 3.2% in the whole group, with the highest value (8.1%) found in the youngest group (15 to 18 years) and a successive decline with age (Department of Statistics/DOS and ICF, 2019).

Table 5 Prevalence of underweight (BMI<18.5 kg/m^2) in adults (≥18 years) in 2016 (in %, age-standardized estimate). Source of data: WHO Global Health Observatory.

Country	Men	Women
Afghanistan	17.1	15.8
Bahrain	2.7	3.6
Djibouti	8.9	7.4
Egypt	1.8	1.1
Iran	3.5	4.0
Iraq	2.3	2.3
Jordan	1.0	1.4
Kuwait	0.8	1.3
Lebanon	1.3	2.5
Libya	2.0	1.9
Morocco	2.9	3.4
Oman	3.3	4.7
Pakistan	15.2	14.7
Qatar	1.2	2.0
Saudi Arabia	1.8	2.4
Somalia	12.1	9.4

Country	Men	Women
Syria	2.5	2.8
Tunisia	3.1	3.3
UAE	1.6	2.3
Yemen	5.4	8.0

In Oman's National Nutrition Survey 2017, 9.1% of the participating women of reproductive age (15 to 49 years) were underweight, with 1.6% severely underweight (Ministry of Health, Sultanate of Oman, UNICEF, 2017).

More comprehensive anthropometric assessments in adults were undertaken in countries with a high burden of overweight and obesity. In the Bahraini National Health Survey 2018, 1.9% of the total participants aged ≥18 years were underweight, with a higher prevalence among women (3%) than men (1%) and also among the younger participants (18–29 years, 4.6%) as well as in the oldest group aged ≥80 years (6.9%) (Ministry of Health, Kingdom of Bahrain et al., 2018).

The anthropometric status of Kuwaiti adults aged 18 to 69 years was evaluated in a nationally representative sample as part of the WHO STEPwise Approach to NCD Risk Factor Surveillance (STEPS) in 2014. The prevalence of underweight was very low in this group: 1.4% in women and 1.0% in men in accordance with the high prevalence of overweight and obesity (see below) (Weiderpass et al., 2014).

A STEPS Analysis was also undertaken in Lebanon in 2016. Underweight prevalence in adults aged 18 to 69 years was 2.1% in women and 0.8% in men. The survey also included a subsample of Syrian refugees living in Lebanon that was evaluated separately. In this group, 1.7% of the women and 1.6% of the men were underweight (Ministry of Public Health, Republic of Lebanon & WHO, 2017).

The Saudi Health Interview Survey 2013 reported a prevalence of underweight of 6.3% in women and of 7.1% in men aged 15 years and older. For both sexes, the highest prevalence was seen in the youngest age group (15 to 24 years) at 12.3% and 14.4%, respectively. Prevalence declined with age to rise up again in the oldest group (≥65 years) where it was 2.0% for both sexes (Ministry of Health, Kingdom of Saudi Arabia et al., 2013).

In the Tunisian Health Examination Survey 2016, underweight was observed in 2.3% of the enrolled women and in 2.9% of the men aged 15 years and older (République Tunisienne Ministère de la Santé & Institut National de la Santé, 2019).

The prevalence of underweight in pregnant and lactating women is much less frequently assessed. However, this population group was included in Oman's National Nutrition Survey. Underweight, defined by a mid-upper arm circumference (MUAC) <23 cm, was found in 5.0% of the whole sample but reached 28.3% in the pregnant adolescents aged 15–19 years (Ministry of Health, Sultanate of Oman, UNICEF, 2017).

In pregnant and lactating women from Yemen, the prevalence of acute malnutrition ranged from 11 to 44% in 2020 (IPC, 2021).

In the Palestinian Micronutrient Survey 2013, the prevalence of underweight was 3.1% in pregnant women before their 17th gestational week (aged 18 to 43 years) and 1.8% in lactating women (aged 18 to 48 years) based on measured anthropometric data (Ministry of Health-Palestine & UNICEF, 2014).

2.2 The Increasing Problem of Overweight and Obesity

Despite the high prevalence of underweight and micronutrient deficiencies, overweight and obesity are on the rise in the Eastern Mediterranean Region, especially, but not exclusively, in the wealthier countries and those where nutrition transition is more advanced. For the whole region, the WHO Global Health Observatory gives an estimated average prevalence of overweight (BMI≥25 kg/m²) of 45.4% in men and of 52.6% in women aged 18 years and older for the year 2016. Of these, an estimated 15.7% and 26.0% of men and women, respectively, are obese (BMI≥30 kg/m²).

As shown in Table 6, there is some variation between the different countries. The lowest prevalence is seen in Afghanistan, followed by Somalia and Sudan, with the latest data for the latter only available from 2011. The highest prevalence is found in the Gulf Council States as well as Egypt and Jordan. These countries also have a high percentage of obesity in their population. In the case of Bahrain and the United Arab Emirates, recent national surveys confirm the WHO estimates, even though a lower prevalence of obesity was reported for the United Arab Emirates.

No data were available for the State of Palestine. However, a survey of 357 18- to 50-year-old mothers from the Gaza Strip who were not pregnant at the time of the study showed a prevalence of overweight (BMI = 25.0–29.9 kg/m²) of 34.5% and of obesity of 29.6%. Of these 3.9% were morbidly obese (BMI≥40 kg/m²). The data were obtained in 2012 through measuring (El Kishawi et al., 2020). Other studies included other population groups that are treated below.

Table 6 Prevalence of overweight and obesity in adults (≥18 years) by country and year. Source of data: WHO Global Health Observatory unless otherwise indicated.

Country	Men Overweight	Men Obesity	Women Overweight	Women Obesity	Both sexes Overweight	Both sexes Obesity	Year
Afghanistan	16.5	3.2	18.5	7.6	17.5	5.5	2016
Bahrain	38.5	25.5	31.7	36.8	36.0	29.8	2016
Bahrain[1]	36.1	39.2	29.7	47.2	33.2	42.8	2018
Djibouti	23.7	8.6	26.3	18.3	25.1	13.5	2016
Egypt	45.6	22.7	28.4	41.1	31.5	32.0	2016
Iran	38.4	19.3	33.2	32.2	35.8	25.8	2016
Iraq	37.6	23.4	31.0	37.0	34.2	30.4	2016
Jordan	38.8	28.2	29.1	43.1	34.1	35.5	2016
Kuwait	39.1	33.3	29.5	45.6	35.5	37.9	2016
Lebanon	39.5	27.4	32.1	37.0	35.9	32.0	2016
Libya	38.4	25.0	30.4	39.6	34.3	32.5	2016
Morocco	37.0	19.4	31.8	32.2	34.3	26.1	2016
Oman	37.7	22.9	32.0	33.7	35.6	27.0	2016
Pakistan	19.7	6.0	20.0	11.3	19.8	8.6	2016
Qatar	38.5	32.5	30.2	43.1	36.6	35.1	2016
Saudi Arabia	37.5	30.8	29.5	42.3	34.3	35.4	2016
Somalia	16.4	3.9	23.6	12.3	20.1	8.3	2016
Syria	36.4	20.9	30.6	34.8	33.6	27.8	2016
Tunisia	38.0	19.1	31.5	34.3	34.7	26.9	2016
UAE	38.8	27.5	30.1	41.0	36.1	31.7	2016
UAE[2]	45.7	25.1	34.3	30.6	40.1	27.8	2017/18
Yemen	32.1	12.0	31.3	22.0	31.7	17.1	2016

Source of data: [1]Kingdom of Bahrain Ministry of Health, Information and eGovernment Authority, WHO: Bahrain National Health Survey 2018; [2]United Arab Emirates Ministry of Health and Prevention: UAE National Health Survey Report 2017–2018.

Few data are available on overweight and obesity in elderly adults in low-income countries. A study of 7239 Sudanese adults ≥18 years reported the prevalence for different age groups including those aged over 65 years. Of the 66- to 75-year-old participants 31.5% were overweight and 22.2% were obese (7.1% morbidly). In participants aged over 75 years, overweight prevalence was 32.1%, that of obesity 16.3% (2.6% morbid obesity) (Ahmed et al., 2017).

Nasreddine et al. (2018) observed an increasing trend in the prevalence of overweight and obesity in adults in the EMR. As can be seen in Table 6, throughout the whole region, women are more affected by obesity than men.

Even more concerning is the occurrence of overweight in children under the age of 5 years, defined as weight for height above two standard deviations from the median of the WHO Child Growth Standards (WHZ>2), which—as in other regions of the world—is also observed in the EMR. UNICEF, the WHO and the World Bank, in their Joint Child Malnutrition Estimates, give a prevalence of 7.7% for overweight in children under 5 years for the year 2020, with an increasing trend since 2000 when the estimated prevalence was 7.2%, and corresponding to a medium prevalence level (UNICEF/WHO/WB, 2021). Again, there is a large variation between the different countries, with the highest prevalence encountered in Libya where 29.6 % of preschool children are affected, compared to only 2.5% in Yemen and 3.2% in Sudan and Somalia (Table 7). Generally, overweight in preschool children is more common in North African countries. However, recent data are not available for all countries, with a lack particularly for the Gulf Council countries. Nevertheless, some information can be gained from studies conducted on smaller samples. In 2015 to 2016, anthropometric data were obtained from 147 18-month to 4-year-old nursery children from the capital district of Abu Dhabi in the United Arab Emirates within the frame of the NOPLAS (Nutrition, Oral health, Physical development, Lifestyle, Anthropometry, and Socioeconomic status) Project. The prevalence of overweight (WHZ>2) was 6.4%, 8.5% in children of Emirati nationality and 5.6% in children of other nationality (Garemo et al., 2018).

In Lebanon, a study conducted in 2019 in the capital city, Beirut, and the governorate of Mount Lebanon, which together harbour about half of the country's population (UN OCHA, 2018), found that 6.5% of

Table 7 Prevalence of overweight in children under the age of 5 years by country. Source of data: UNICEF/WHO/World Bank Joint Child Malnutrition Estimates Expanded Database: Overweight (Survey Estimates), May 2022, New York, unless otherwise indicated.

Country	% overweight (of whom obese)	Year of survey
Afghanistan[1]	4.0 (1.2)	2018
Djibouti	1.6	2019
Egypt	15.7	2014
Iran	2.9	2017
Iraq	6.1	2018
Jordan	9.2	2019
Kuwait	5.5	2017
Lebanon[2]	16.8 (8.9)	2021
Libya	29.6	2014
Morocco[3]‡	10.9 (2.9)	2017–2018
Oman	4.2	2016–2017
Pakistan[4]	9.5	2018
Palestine	8.5	2019–2020
Qatar[5]	16.1	2006
Saudi Arabia	6.1	2004–2005
Somalia[6]	3.2	2019
Sudan[7]	3.2 (0.9)	2018–2019
Syria	17.9	2009–2010
Tunisia	17.2	2018
Yemen	2.5	2013

[1]Afghanistan Health Survey 2018; [2]Hoteit et al., 2021; [3]Ministère de la Santé, DPRF/DPE/SEIS, Royaume du Maroc. Enquête Nationale sur la Population et la Santé Familiale (ENPSF) 2017–2018. Rabat, Maroc; [4]Ministry of National Health Services, Regulations and Coordinations, Government of Pakistan, Nutrition Wing. National Nutrition Survey 2018; [5]World Health Survey, Qatar 2006. Doha, Qatar: Supreme Council of Health, 2006; [6]Ministry of Health FGS, FMS, Somaliland, UNICEF, Brandpro, GroundWork. Somalia Micronutrient Survey 2019. Mogadishu, Somalia, 2020; [7]Federal Ministry of Health, Sudan. Simple Spatial Survey Method (S3M II) Report; Federal Ministry of Health, General Directorate of Primary Health Care, National Nutrition Program: Khartoum, Sudan, 2020.

‡ included children <6 y.

children under 5 years were at risk of being overweight (WHZ > 1 SD and ≤2 SD) and 24.45% were overweight (WHZ > 2 SD). In children under 2 years, the prevalence of overweight was 20% (Abi Khalil et al., 2022). In a more recent, nationally representative survey from Lebanon dating from 2021 and therefore reflecting the impact of the COVID-19 pandemic, economic depression and political unrest, the prevalence of overweight and obesity in children aged under 5 years was 16.8% and 8.9%, respectively (Hoteit et al., 2022a).

In another study conducted in 2 healthcare centres in Abu Dhabi in 2014 to 2015 the prevalence of obesity in children (defined as BMI≥95th percentile of the WHO growth curve) aged 2 to 4 years was 6.3% but no values for overweight were given (Al-Shehhi et al., 2020). More information on overweight and obesity prevalence in the Gulf States is available for school-age children and adolescents, and this will be treated at the end of this chapter.

The data for Syria precede the outbreak of the civil war. However, a survey conducted on the nutritional status of Syrian refugees in Jordan in 2017 reported a low prevalence of overweight, ranging from 1.0 to 1.6% and the absence of obesity in the included sample (UNHCR/UNICEF/WFP/Save the Children, 2017). A different picture was revealed by a study of Syrian refugee children aged 6 to 59 months from Jordan, Lebanon, Turkey, Greece, Egypt and Iraq in 2015 to 2016, of whom the vast majority (>99%) were not living in camps. In this population, the prevalence of overweight and obesity was much higher, with an average of 10.6%, ranging from 5.4% to 11.5% (Pernitez-Agan et al., 2019).

The WHO's Global Health Observatory also contains data on overweight and obesity in school-age children and adolescents, shown in Table 8 and Table 9. Based on the WHO growth curve for children and adolescents aged 5 to 19 years, overweight in this group is defined by a BMI-for-age that exceeds the median by more than 1 but less than 2 standard deviations and obesity by a BMI-for-age exceeding the median by more than 2 standard deviations (de Onis et al., 2007).

Table 8 Prevalence of overweight and obesity in school-age children (5–9 years) sex and country (in %). Source of data: WHO Global Health Observatory, data from 2016.

Country	Overweight		Obesity	
	Boys	Girls	Boys	Girls
Afghanistan	6.3	6.5	4.2	4.2
Bahrain	18.1	17.0	22.0	18.3
Djibouti	8.7	15.2	6.2	7.7
Egypt	19.6	17.0	20.5	23.2
Iran	15.1	14.8	13.1	9.8
Iraq	17.6	16.9	18.1	17.1
Jordan	18.4	17.6	15.4	14.4
Kuwait	19.6	18.2	24.8	21.2
Lebanon	19.6	17.8	20.9	15.4
Libya	18.1	17.4	19.3	16.4
Morocco	16.8	16.7	13.5	12.7
Oman	18.0	16.4	20.2	16.1
Pakistan	6.8	5.9	4.9	3.4
Qatar	19.1	18.4	26.2	19.2
Saudi Arabia	18.6	17.4	21.3	15.4
Somalia	6.6	13.2	3.0	5.1
Syria	16.9	16.5	15.5	13.5
Tunisia	16.0	16.0	10.7	10.1
UAE	18.5	17.7	22.7	18.1
Yemen	13.2	12.4	9.5	10.9

For the whole region, the average prevalence of overweight in primary-school-age children (5 to 9 years) in 2016 was reported as 22.6% in boys and 22.1% in girls, and that of obesity as 10.6% and 10.0% respectively. Of the region's adolescents (10 to 19 years), 18.5% of boys and 19.7% of girls were overweight and 6.8% and 7.0%, respectively, were obese. No clear pattern was seen concerning the frequency in boys vs. girls. Particularly high levels of overweight and obesity were observed in the Gulf countries, Egypt and Lebanon, and to a slightly lesser degree in Libya and Iraq. Obesity rates in these countries are among the highest in the world, underlining the severity of the problem.

Recent regional studies confirm these findings (reviewed by Al-Thani et al., 2017; Aljaadi & Alharbi, 2021). In a study conducted in Bahraini adolescents aged 12 to 15 years in 2017 to 2018, obesity prevalence ranged from 16.5% to 19.3% in boys and from 13.1% to 19.6% in girls (15 vs. 12 years each) showing a decreasing trend with age (Taher et al., 2019). In the city of Sharjah, in the UAE, a survey in 2017 found that 14.2% of the enrolled 6- to 11-year-old children were overweight and 14% were obese (Abduelkarem et al., 2020).

Table 9 Prevalence of overweight and obesity in adolescents (10–19 years), sex and country (in %). Source of data: WHO Global Health Observatory, data from 2016.

Country	Overweight		Obesity	
	Boys	Girls	Boys	Girls
Afghanistan	5.9	6.9	2.3	2.5
Bahrain	18.3	18.4	16.4	14.5
Djibouti	8.4	15.5	3.6	5.0
Egypt	20.5	18.7	13.2	17.1
Iran	15.7	17.1	9.3	8.1
Iraq	17.8	17.7	12.4	12.8
Jordan	18.2	18.2	11.7	11.6
Kuwait	19.3	20.4	25.7	19.7
Lebanon	19.6	18.7	14.5	10.0
Libya	18.2	18.4	13.6	11.8
Morocco	16.4	17.4	8.7	8.5
Oman	17.9	17.1	13.6	11.9
Pakistan	6.4	7.0	2.9	2.0
Qatar	19.4	19.6	19.9	14.5
Saudi Arabia	18.4	18.3	19.0	13.6
Somalia	6.3	13.5	1.6	3.2
Syria	16.8	17.2	10.3	9.4
Tunisia	15.7	17.6	6.9	8.1
UAE	18.6	18.9	16.3	13.1
Yemen	12.5	13.6	5.0	5.7

The prevalence of overweight is somewhat lower than in the WHO Global Health Observatory database, but this may be due to the fact that weight was categorized using the CDC standard that defines overweight as BMI exceeding the 85th percentile but below the 95th percentile and obesity as BMI equal to or over the 95th percentile. Comparisons of the WHO growth charts with the CDC and IOTF standards have shown some, albeit small, differences between these references (Kaigang et al., 2016; Aljaadi & Alharbi, 2021).

A high rate of overweight and obesity was also observed in studies in school-age children from Egypt, with obesity even more common than overweight in some age groups and at some locations. In 5 studies in primary school children (6–12 years) from 2010 to 2017, prevalence of overweight and obesity ranged from 11.1 to 23.7% and 8.2 to 19.5%, respectively. Overall, prevalence of overweight and obesity was comparable in boys and girls with some differences between the different studies (El-Said Badawi et al., 2013; Taha et al., 2015; Abdelkarim et al., 2017; Hadhood et al., 2017; Abd El-Fatah & Abu-Eleni, 2019). It must be noted that these studies also used different standards to categorise weight (WHO growth standards as well as IOTF standards, CDC standards, and national growth curves).

Overall, there has also been a rapid increase in the prevalence of overweight and obesity in the region during the last decade (WHO Health Observatory, 2016).

Accordingly, the Pakistan National Nutrition Survey 2018 found a prevalence of obesity of 10.2% in boys and of 11.4% in girls aged 10 to 19 years, and of obesity of 7.7% and 5.5% respectively (Ministry of National Health Services, Regulations and Coordinations, Government of Pakistan, 2018).

No current data are available for the State of Palestine as well as for Sudan since its separation into two countries. However, the Palestinian Micronutrient Survey 2013 included a sample of 15- to 18-year-old adolescents. In this collective, 14.9% of the boys and 17.7% of the girls were overweight and 7.2% and 5.4% respectively were obese, using the WHO BMI for age curve and cut-offs.

In a survey of 1320 younger children (6–12 years) that was conducted in Palestinian schools in the governorate of Nablus in 2017, the prevalence of overweight was 15.1% in girls and 14.1% in boys, and that of obesity was 13.8% in girls and 17.5% in boys. This study, however, used the CDC growth curve as reference (Al-Lahham et al., 2019).

In Sudan, a WHO Global School-Based Student Health Survey was conducted in 2012. Results have only been published for students aged 13 to 15 years of whom 7.8% were overweight (BMI >+1 SD but <+2 SD over the WHO reference median) and 3.6% obese (BMI >+2 SD over the

WHO reference median) (Sudan GSHS). Two more recent studies were conducted in the cities of Khartoum and Argo in Sudan and included younger children (5 to 12 years and 6 to 14 years, respectively). Both used the WHO reference to categorise body weight. In the sample from Khartoum (n=390), overweight showed a prevalence of 8.7%, 5.0% in boys and 12.8% in girls. Obesity was seen in 6.7% of the participants, 5.4% of the boys and 8.0% of the girls (Elrayah, 2018). The group from Argo consisted of 1223 children (613 girls). Overweight was found in 6.2% of the children and obesity in 1.6%. Overweight was more common in children aged >10 years than in those aged 10 years or less (8.6% vs. 4.0%), while the difference was less pronounced for obesity (1.8% vs. 1.3%). Again, more girls were overweight than boys (7.0% vs. 5.4%) but obesity was about equally common (1.6% of boys and 1.5% of girls) (Hussein, 2018).

In summary, this overview of the prevalence of underweight and overweight in the countries of the WHO Eastern Mediterranean Region shows that undernourishment is still a problem, as well as the increasing levels of overweight and obesity. However, malnutrition is not limited to an insufficient or excessive intake of dietary energy, but also includes micronutrient deficiencies, causing a triple burden of malnutrition.

2.3 Micronutrient Deficiencies

Although deficiencies can theoretically occur for any micronutrient, there are a number of particularly critical vitamins, minerals and trace elements that are often not supplied in sufficient amounts through the diet, especially in certain population groups. Globally, deficiencies of iron, vitamin A and iodine have long been recognized as common causes for health impairments and reduced wellbeing, particularly in young children, pregnant women and women of child-bearing age. However, more recently, other critical micronutrients have been added to the list, such as folic acid, zinc and vitamin D. While the supply of some critical micronutrients at the population level is regularly monitored, there is less data on others.

2.3.1 Prevalence of Anaemia

Anaemia is defined as an insufficient concentration of haemoglobin in the blood, either caused by a reduced level of haemoglobin in the red blood cells (erythrocytes) or a reduced number of red blood cells. Haemoglobin concentrations vary with age and sex, so that the thresholds to diagnose anaemia are age- and sex-specific, as shown in Table 10.

Anaemia can have a multitude of causes, which can be nutrition-related as well as non-nutrition-related. Among the nutrition-related causes, iron deficiency is certainly a major contributor, especially in menstruating women. However, insufficient supply of other micronutrients like folate, vitamins B_{12}, B_2, and B_6, vitamin A, zinc and copper as well as protein is also associated with anaemia.

Table 10 Haemoglobin concentrations in the blood at sea level to define and classify anaemia (g/dl). WHO VMNIS, 2011.

Population group	Anaemia			
	None	Mild	Moderate	Severe
Children				
<5 years	≥11.0	10.0–10.9	7.0–9.9	<7.0
5–11 years	≥11.5	11.0–11.4	8.0–10.9	<8.0
12–14 years	≥12.0	11.0–11.9	8.0–10.9	<8.0
Adults and adolescents ≥15 years				
Non-pregnant women	≥12.0	11.0–11.9	8.0–10.9	<8.0
Pregnant women	≥11.0	10.0–10.9	7.0–9.9	<7.0
Men	≥13.0	11.0–12.9	8.0–10.9	<8.0

Estimates on anaemia prevalence in children under the age of 5 years, non-pregnant and pregnant women of child-bearing age (15 to 49 years) are again available from the WHO Global Health Observatory (GHO), the most recent dating from 2019. The overall prevalence in the region was 42.7% for children under 5 years, 34.9% for non-pregnant women aged 15–49 years, and 36.8% for pregnant women of 15–49 years. In both groups, prevalence has decreased markedly since 2000, when it was 37% in women of reproductive age and 41.9% in pregnant women, but this trend has been ongoing only in pregnant women, while prevalence in women of reproductive age has shown a slight increase from 34.5% in 2014–2016. Results by country are presented in Table 11.

The highest prevalence of anaemia in all three population groups was seen in Yemen, the lowest in Kuwait and the United Arab Emirates. While high anaemia prevalence was mostly seen in some low-income countries like Afghanistan, Pakistan and Somalia, the richer countries also had significant proportions of the assessed population affected.

For the State of Palestine, the WHO GHO database has information on anaemia prevalence only for women of child-bearing age (15–49 years). Therefore, prevalence in pregnant women was taken from the Palestinian National Nutrition Surveillance System for 2018 (Ministry of Health Palestine, 2018). A cross-sectional study from 2012 in pre-school children from the Gaza Strip reported a prevalence of anaemia of 59.7%, with 46.5% of the children having mild and 13.2% moderate anaemia.

No severe cases were detected. This sample included children from a refugee camp in whom anaemia prevalence was higher than in the other children (70.0% compared to 52.5% and 40.0% in rural and urban settlements, respectively) (El Kishawi et al., 2015).

Table 11 Prevalence of anaemia in different population groups in the countries of the WHO Eastern Mediterranean Region. Al-Jawaldeh et al., 2021, based on the latest available estimates*.

Country	Anaemia prevalence (%)		
	Children under 5 years	Non-pregnant women of child-bearing age (15–49 years)	Pregnant women (15–49 years)
Afghanistan	44.9	43.2	36.5
Bahrain	23.4	35.5	33.5
Djibouti	52.0	32.1	37.0
Egypt	32.2	28.4	26.0
Iran	26.5	24.1	23.8
Iraq	29.4	28.4	30.9
Jordan	32.7	38.0	33.7
Kuwait	19.8	23.7	23.7
Lebanon	22.8	28.3	27.7
Libya	26.6	29.9	29.4
Morocco	30.4	29.8	32.6
Oman	24.3	29.1	30.2
Pakistan	53.0	41.1	44.0
Palestine	-	28.3[1]	30.5
Qatar	22.4	28.1	26.7
Saudi Arabia	21.8	27.5	27.3
Somalia	51.8	42.4	48.7
Sudan	50.8	36.5	36.8
Syria	32.9	32.8	33.2
Tunisia	30.4	32.1	30.5
UAE	20.4	24.3	23.7
Yemen	79.5	61.8	57.5

* Data are from the WHO Global Health Observatory 2019 unless otherwise indicated:

[1]for women of child-bearing age (15–49 years) regardless of pregnancy; [2]Ministry of Health-Palestine. National Nutrition Surveillance System; Public Health General Directorate. Nutrition Department: Ramallah, Palestine, 2018.

Anaemia prevalence was also assessed among Syrian refugees living in Jordan and Lebanon. The Jordanian study included refugees residing in one camp as well as in the community, whereas in Lebanon, only people living in the community were enrolled. In Za'atri camp in Jordan, 48.4% of children under the age of 5 years and 44.8% of non-pregnant women aged 15 to 49 years were anaemic. The prevalence was lower in refugees living outside camps in Jordan, with 26.1% of pre-school children and 31.1% of women of child-bearing age affected, as well as at four different locations in Lebanon, where it ranged from 13.9% to 25.8% in children and 18.4% to 29.3% in women. Most of the cases were mild or moderate with a low rate of severe cases (<0.5% in children and 0 to 1.1% in the women) (Moazzem-Hossain et al., 2016).

According to the classification by the WHO (WHO VMNIS, 2011), anaemia must be considered a public health problem of moderate (prevalence of 20.0 to 39.9%) or even serious (≥40%) significance in all countries of the region and all population groups studied.

A recent review looked at the progress that has been made in recent years in meeting the World Health Assembly target of reducing anaemia prevalence in women of child-bearing age by 50%, focussing also on children under 5 years and pregnant women. It was found that improvements have only been made in a few countries (such as Oman, Egypt, Iran among others) while most are not on track to reach the target as anaemia prevalence stagnated or even increased (Al-Jawaldeh et al., 2021a).

Reducing anaemia prevalence is complicated by its multifactorial aetiology. While anaemia is often considered mainly a symptom of iron deficiency, evidence from surveys with separate assessment of iron-deficiency anaemia suggests that the latter on average makes up less than half or even less than a third of total anaemia. This underlines the need for comprehensive multisectoral approaches to reduce anaemia prevalence (Al-Jawaldeh et al., 2021a).

2.3.2 Iodine

Iodine is another micronutrient that has often been found to be critical in many populations all over the world, mainly due to low amounts of this mineral in the soils of many regions worldwide. A very efficient approach to combat iodine deficiency is the iodization of table salt, which has been practised for almost one hundred years since its introduction in Switzerland and the USA during the 1920s. Currently, 145 countries have legislation for salt iodization; it is mandatory in 124 countries and voluntary in 21. In the WHO Eastern Mediterranean Region, 17 countries fortify table salt mandatorily. In Pakistan, it is voluntary, whereas no iodization is used in Djibouti, Iraq, Libya and Syria.

Iodine status is generally monitored by measuring urinary iodine excretion (UIC) in a nationally representative sample, in most cases, school children. Adequate iodine intake is assumed when the median UIC ranges from 100 to 299 µg/l. Values ≥300 µg/l are considered excessive.

As can be seen in Table 12, iodine intake is adequate in most countries in the Eastern Mediterranean Region. Only in Iraq and Lebanon was median UIC found to be below 100 µg/l, and no monitoring was done in Libya and Syria. Excessive levels were observed in Djibouti and Qatar (IGN, 2021). In Djibouti, this has been ascribed to high iodine concentrations in drinking water as an analysis of table salt samples showed that these were insufficiently iodized. However, in this study, median UIC in pregnant women did not exceed the reference range (Farebrother et al., 2018).

2.3.3 Status of Other Micronutrients: Zinc, Vitamin A, Vitamin D, Folate and Vitamin B_{12}

Deficiencies can occur for many micronutrients, but some have proved especially critical at least in some at-risk population groups. This is true for vitamin A, which, besides iron and iodine is one of the most frequently deficient micronutrients worldwide, as well as for zinc, folic acid and vitamin D. Chronic zinc deficiency is especially harmful to children, in whom it impairs growth and development, resulting in stunting. Folic acid is critical in early pregnancy when a deficiency increases the risk of neural defects in the developing foetus. Vitamin D stands out among vitamins in that it can be synthesized in the body under the influence of UV-B radiation. However, a large number of studies have shown that vitamin D status is too low in many populations all over the world,

Table 12 Median urinary iodine excretion and deduced iodine status by country of the WHO Eastern Mediterranean Region. Surveys were conducted in school-age children unless otherwise indicated (Source of data: Iodine Global Network, 2021).

Country	Salt iodization	Median urinary iodine excretion in µg/l	Iodine status	Year of survey
Afghanistan	M	171	Adequate	2013 (N)
Bahrain	M	247	Adequate	2012–2013 (N
Djibouti	-	335	Excessive	2015 (N)
Egypt	M	170	Adequate	2014–2015 (N)
Iran	M	161	Adequate	2013–2014 (N)
Iraq	-	84	Insufficient	2011–2012 (N)
Jordan	M	203	Adequate	2010 (N)
Kuwait	M	130	Adequate	2014 (N)
Lebanon	M	66	Insufficient	2013 (N)
Libya	-	n.d.	n.d.	n.d
Morocco	M	117	Adequate	2019 (N)
Oman	M	191	Adequate	2014 (N)
Pakistan	V	124	Adequate	2011 (N)
Palestine	M	193	Adequate	2013 (N)
Qatar	M	341	Excessive	2014 (N)
Saudi Arabia	M	133	Adequate	2012 (N)
Somalia	M	263	Adequate	2019 (N)*
Sudan	M	108	Adequate	2018 (N)*
Syria	-	n.d.	n.d.	n.d.
Tunisia	M	220	Adequate	2013 (N)
UAE	M	162	Adequate	2008–2009 (N)
Yemen	M	101	Adequate	2015 (N)

M mandatory; V voluntary; n.d. no data; (N) marks nationally representative surveys.

*survey conducted in women of child-bearing age (15–49 years).

even in regions with high sunlight intensity. Possible reasons include sun avoidance and an increase in the number of professions that are practised indoors, dark skin complexion, or wearing clothing that covers much of the skin. The latter is particularly relevant for women in the Middle Eastern Region wearing a veil.

Some nutritional surveys conducted in the region have measured the status of one or several of these micronutrients, mostly in groups at risk of deficiencies. The Pakistan National Nutrition Survey 2018 reported the status of zinc, vitamin A and vitamin D in children under 5 years and women of child-bearing age. In children, zinc deficiency was found in 18.6%, while 51.5% had insufficient vitamin A plasma levels, with 12.1% being severely deficient. The prevalence was comparable between sexes (51.7% in boys and 51.3% in girls). A high proportion of children showed insufficient vitamin D levels (62.7%) and severe deficiency was seen 13.2%. Girls were slightly more affected than boys (63.1 vs. 62.4%). Vitamin D insufficiency was also common in women of reproductive age (15–49 years) in whom it showed a prevalence of 79.7%. Severe deficiency (<8 ng/ml) was observed in 25.7%. Women from urban settings were more affected than those from rural environments (83.6% vs. 77.1%). Vitamin A deficiency was found in 27.3% of the women, with 4.9% being severely deficient, and low zinc levels were seen in 22.1%. Zinc deficiency was more common in women from rural environments (Ministry of National Health Services, Regulations and Coordinations, Government of Pakistan, 2018).

The Palestinian Micronutrient Survey 2013 reported on the micronutrient status of children under 5 years, adolescents aged 15 to 18 years and of pregnant and lactating women. In children under 5 years, zinc and vitamin A were most critical, with 55% of boys and 56% of girls suffering from zinc deficiency and 73% of both, boys and girls, with low or deficient plasma levels of vitamin A. Prevalence of deficiency was higher in the Gaza Strip than in the West Bank. In turn, the levels of folate and vitamin B_{12} were largely satisfactory. Zinc status was also critical in adolescents, with 70% of girls and 58.6% of boys aged 15 to 18 years being deficient (defined as serum zinc <11.5 μmol/l) while another 13.6 and 13.9%, respectively, had low zinc levels (i.e., serum zinc = 11.5–13.0 μmol/l). Vitamin A insufficiency was observed in 42.5% of the adolescent boys and in 33.2% of the girls. 10.8% and

5.2%, respectively, were markedly deficient (serum levels <0.7 µmol/l). Vitamin D insufficiency showed a strong difference between sexes, with 51.9% of the boys affected compared to 97.1% of the girls. The divergence was particularly striking for marked vitamin D deficiency (<25 nmol/l), which was very low in boys (0.6%) but affected almost a third (31.9%) of the girls. The status was only slightly better for folate, with 20.8% of the boys and 18.8% of the girls having insufficient plasma levels, and for vitamin B_{12}, which was present at insufficient levels in 29.8% of the boys and 24.9% of the girls. Among adolescents, the prevalence of deficiency was higher in the Gaza Strip for all micronutrients except for severe vitamin D in girls, which was more common in the West Bank. In turn, pregnant women (15–43 years) had a more satisfactory folate status, with 98.2% of women in their first trimester of pregnancy and 90.8% in the second and third trimesters having sufficient serum folate levels. Vitamin B_{12} insufficiency was found in 43.1% of the women in the first trimester and in 69% in the second and third trimesters. Deficiency was seen in 23.5% and 19.1%, respectively. Zinc deficiency was encountered in 58.9% of the women in the first trimester and in 74.9% in their second and third trimesters. Almost half of the pregnant women in the survey suffered from vitamin A insufficiency (47.2% of those in the first trimester and 57.8% in the second and third trimesters). However, vitamin A deficiency was seen in only 10% and 19.5%, respectively. A very high prevalence was seen for vitamin D, with all the women in the first trimester and 98.2% of those in the second and third trimesters having insufficient serum levels of 25-OH vitamin D (i.e., <50 nmol/l). Of these, 66.7% and 70.2% were deficient (25-OH vitamin D <25 nmol/l). Zinc deficiency was also very common in lactating women (18–48 years) in whom the prevalence was 82.6%. Folic acid levels were low in 17.5% of the women and deficient in 2.6%. Vitamin B_{12} insufficiency was found in 20.5%, of whom 7.7% were deficient. Vitamin levels were insufficient in 29% but only 4.8% were deficient. Vitamin D insufficiency and deficiency were again very common, with 68.7% and 30.0% of the women affected, respectively (Ministry of Health-Palestine & UNICEF, 2014).

In the Somalia Micronutrient Survey 2019, 5% of the included children under the age of 5 years old were found to have deficient zinc levels. Vitamin A deficiency was observed in 34.4%. Among women of child-bearing age, 10.7% were vitamin A-deficient, 35.1% had folate deficiency, and 36.9% had vitamin B_{12} deficiency (Ministry of Health FGS, FMS, Somaliland, UNICEF, Brandpro, GroundWork, 2020).

In Iran, the Second National Integrated Micronutrient Survey evaluated the levels of selected micronutrients in infants aged 15 to 23 months, in children of 6 years, in adolescents aged 14–20 years, and in pregnant women in their fifth month of gestation. Zinc deficiency (serum zinc <65 µg/l in pregnant women and <70 µg/l in the other groups) was observed in 19.1% of the infants, in 13.6% of the school-age children, in 11.4% of the adolescents (about 13% of the girls and 9.5% of the boys) and in 28% of the pregnant women. Vitamin A status was only assessed in the children aged 15 to 23 months and the pregnant women, of whom 18.3% and 14.1% were deficient (serum retinol <20 µg/dl), respectively. Prevalence of vitamin D deficiency (serum 25-OH vitamin D <20 ng/ml) was comparatively low in the infants (23.3%) while it affected 61.8% of the children aged 6 years old, 76% of the adolescents and 85.3% of the pregnant women. Among all age groups, the prevalence was higher in the female participants than in the male and was highest in the adolescent girls, of whom more than 90% were affected. Vitamin D was also measured in middle-aged adults (men aged 45 to 60 years and women aged 50 to 60 years). Deficiency was seen in 59.1% of both sexes, about 60% in women and about 58% in men (Pouraram et al., 2018).

For Oman, the National Nutrition Survey 2017 revealed a very low prevalence (0.2%) of vitamin A deficiency in non-pregnant women of child-bearing age (15 to 49 years). A higher prevalence (9.5%) was found in children under 5 years old. The youngest children (6 to 11 months) were particularly affected, with a prevalence of 23.5%. Vitamin D deficiency (25-OH-vitamin D<30 nmol/l) and insufficiency (25-OH-vitamin D >30 nmol/l but <50 nmol/l) were common in all groups, but more so in women of reproductive age, of whom 16.2% were vitamin D-deficient and 41.5% insufficient. In children under 5 years the prevalence of deficiency was slightly lower (10.6%) while that of insufficiency was higher (53.8). Deficiency was again highest in the youngest group, while older children suffered more from insufficiency. In women of reproductive age, the levels of vitamin B_{12} and folate were also measured, and it was found that 8.9% of the participants had insufficient vitamin B_{12} levels while folate was deficient in 11.6%. For both nutrients, the prevalence of deficiency was higher in younger women under 30 years of age (Ministry of Health, Sultanate of Oman, UNICEF, 2017).

The vitamin D status of adults (15 years and older) was evaluated in the Saudi Arabia Health Interview Survey. Insufficient levels (defined as 25-OH vitamin D <28 ng/ml) were found in 40.6% of the men and 62.6% of the women. The prevalence was higher in the younger participants (48.8% and 72.4%, respectively, in men and women aged 15 to 24 years, and 39.7% and 59.0% respectively in men and women aged 25 to 34 years) than in the older adults (20.5% and 38.9% in men and women, respectively, aged 65 years and older) (Ministry of Health, Kingdom of Saudi Arabia, Institute of Health Metrics and Evaluation, University of Washington, 2013).

The Afghanistan National Nutrition Report of 2013 reported the status of selected micronutrients in children under the age of 5 years, in adolescent girls (10–19 years) and in women of reproductive age (15–49 years). Vitamin A deficiency (retinol <0.7 µmol/l) was seen in 50.4% of the children under 5 years but was less common in women aged 15–49 years (prevalence of 11.3%). Zinc deficiency (<60 µg/dl) affected 23.4% of the children and 15.1% of the women. The prevalence of vitamin D deficiency (25-OH vitamin D <20 ng/ml) was observed in 95.5% of the women and 81% of the children. In 64.7% of the women deficiency was severe (25-OH vitamin D <8 ng/ml) while this was only the case in 16.8% of the children. In adolescent girls, folic acid status was assessed and 7.4% were found to be deficient (<3.0 ng/ml) (Ministry of Public Health of Afghanistan & UNICEF, 2013).

2.4 Young Children and Infant Feeding Practices

Rate of Exclusive Breastfeeding, Early Breastfeeding Initiation and Complementary Feeding

Healthy nutrition is important for young children and infants so that they can achieve their full growth and development, while at the same time avoiding overweight and obesity and acquiring healthy food habits for later in life.

Breastmilk is the best food for newborn infants, and up to the age of 5 to 6 months should be the only kind of food given to the infant (WHO, 1994). It allows adequate growth and healthy development, especially of the immune defence system, while at the same time preventing overweight. It is readily available without any need for payment, or for water, bottles or teats, which are potential sources of pathogenic microorganisms that cause diarrhoea (Walters et al., 2019).

Despite the clear advantages of breastmilk, the percentage of women exclusively breastfeeding their children during the first 5 to 6 months is low in many countries worldwide, regardless of income level. The Eastern Mediterranean Region is no exception to this. Based on the latest available national data on exclusive breastfeeding, only 4 countries, Afghanistan, Iran, Sudan and the United Arab Emirates, met the target of at least 50% of children under the age of 6 months being exclusively breastfed set by the World Health Assembly for 2025. This target has recently been raised to 70% until 2030, a level that was achieved by none of the EMR countries (see Table 13).

© 2023 Al-Jawaldeh and Meyer, CC BY-NC 4.0   https://doi.org/10.11647/OBP.0322.08

Table 13 Percentage of children exclusively breastfed during their first 5 to 6 months of life by country and year in the WHO Eastern Mediterranean Region.

Country	Prevalence (%)	Year of survey
Afghanistan	57.5	2018
Bahrain[1]	30.0	2014
Djibouti	12.4	2012
Egypt	39.5	2014
Iran	53.1	2010/2011
Iraq	25.8	2018
Jordan	25.4	2017/2018
Kuwait[2]	8.0	2017
Lebanon[3]	59.1	2022
Morocco	35.0	2017/2018
Oman	23.2	2016/2017
Pakistan	47.5	2018
Palestine	38.9	2020
Qatar	29.3	2012
Saudi Arabia[4]	47.8	2017
Somalia[5]	15.6	2019
Sudan[6]	61.5	2018
Syria	28.5	2019
Tunisia	13.6	2018
UAE[7]	59.7	2017–2018
Yemen	9.7	2013

Source of data unless otherwise indicated: UNICEF. Database on infant and young child feeding. Exclusive breastfeeding. 2021.

Other sources: [1]Nasreddine et al., 2018; [2]Vaz et al., 2021; [3]Hoteit et al., 2022a; [4]Saudi Arabia General Authority for Statistics. Household Health Survey 2017; [5]Somalia Micronutrient Survey, 2019; [6]Federal Ministry of Health-Sudan. Simple Spatial Survey Method (S3M II) Report. Federal Ministry of Health, General Directorate of Primary Health Care, National Nutrition Program: Khartoum, Sudan, 2020; [7]UAE National Health Survey 2018.

Exclusive breastfeeding rates are particularly low in Kuwait, Yemen, Djibouti, Tunisia and Somalia. The recent IPC Acute Malnutrition analysis in Yemen in 2020 revealed rates of exclusive breastfeeding below 35% in the northern zones assessed and below 25% in most of the southern zones (IPC, 2021).

Nevertheless, some progress has been made in some countries like Iran, Pakistan, Sudan (Abul-Fadl et al., 2019).

A recent survey from Lebanon among children under 5 years old revealed a prevalence of ever breastfeeding, exclusive breastfeeding, and bottle feeding at birth of 95.1%, 59.1% and 25.8%, respectively (Hoteit et al., 2022a). In turn, the National Nutrition SMART Survey from 2021 found that 32.4% of children under 6 months were exclusively breastfed in Lebanon when looking at the entire population, with higher rates among Syrian and Palestinian refugees (65.2% and 43.8% respectively) (Lebanon Nutrition Sector, 2021).

Breastfeeding should ideally begin immediately after birth or within an hour of giving birth in order to provide the newborn with the colostrum, the milk that is first secreted and that is particularly rich in bioactive proteins like enzymes, growth factors and immunoglobulins as well as in vitamins and minerals, thereby contributing to the child's health and development. Moreover, early initiation of breastfeeding increases the likelihood of exclusive breastfeeding during the first 6 months of the infant's life and the duration of breastfeeding (UNICEF, WHO 2018, Baby-friendly hospital initiative guideline).

The rate of early initiation of breastfeeding has been assessed in some recent health and nutrition surveys in the WHO Eastern Mediterranean Region.

The Afghanistan Health Survey 2018 reported that, of the infants ever breastfed, 63.7% received breastmilk within an hour after birth (KIT, 2019). This rate is comparable to that found in the Jordan Population and Family Health Survey 2017/2018, where 67% of the participating children were breastfed within an hour after birth and 83% within one day (Department of Statistics/DOS and ICF, 2019).

In Lebanon, 63.0% of newborns received breastmilk within one hour of birth, and comparable rates were also observed among Syrian and Palestinian refugees in the country (65.7% and 58.6%, respectively) (Lebanon Nutrition Sector, 2021).

A higher percentage was observed in Oman, where 82% of the enrolled children were breastfed within the first hour of life (Ministry of Health, Sultanate of Oman, UNICEF, 2017) as well as in the Somalia Micronutrient Survey 2019, which recorded that 86% of newborns received breastmilk within one hour and 9.1% within 23 hours (Ministry of Health FGS, FMS, Somaliland, UNICEF, Brandpro, GroundWork, 2020). In turn, a survey conducted in three governorates in Northern

Syria, Aleppo, Idlib and Hama, showed that only 37.8% of the children under 24 months were breastfed within one hour after birth (Nutrition Technical Rapid Response Team, 2017). In the Moroccan National Survey on Population and Family Health (ENPSF) 2018, early initiation of breastfeeding was reported for 49.4% of the children under 5 years (Ministère de la Santé, DPRF/DPE/SEIS, 2018). For Pakistan, a rate of 45.8% was reported in the National Nutrition Survey 2018 (Ministry of National Health Services, Regulations and Coordinations, Government of Pakistan, 2018).

After 6 months, breastmilk alone can no longer provide the infant's requirements for energy and nutrients so that other foods should be introduced in the child's diet in adequate amounts and variety. The quality of complementary feeding is a focus of many national nutrition and health reports. For its evaluation at population level, the WHO has developed a number of indicators for the diet of infants aged 6 to 23 months, such as minimum dietary diversity (MDD) and minimum meal frequency (MMF). The former is achieved if a child received at least 5 out of 8 selected food groups during the previous 24 hours, the latter if breastfed infants of 6–8 months are fed twice a day, breastfed children aged 9–23 months thrice a day, and non-breastfed children aged 6–23 months four times per day. Both indicators are combined to calculate the minimum acceptable diet that corresponds to the number of infants meeting the criteria of MDD and MMF divided by the total number of children of 6 to 23 months (WHO, 2008a; Global Nutrition Monitoring Framework, 2017).

The Afghan National Nutrition Survey 2013 included a sample of children under 5 years. The percentage of children receiving solid, semi-solid or soft food was lower in breastfed children (30.9% compared to 41.3% in the whole sample). Minimum dietary diversity was achieved in 27.6% of the children aged 6 to 23 months, minimum meal frequency in 52.1% and minimum acceptable diet in 12.2%. Again, the proportion was lower in breastfed children for minimum meal frequency (43.9%) but higher for minimum acceptable diet (16.3%). It was reported that most of the mothers participating in the survey introduced complementary feeding in their infants at the age of 3 to 4 months and therefore earlier than recommended. Solid or semi-solid complementary foods were introduced to 41.3% of infants aged 6 to 8 months.

The majority of children under 5 years consumed cereals and oil and fats (73% and 71% respectively), followed by dairy products and sugar or honey (67% and 62% respectively). Fruit and vegetables were eaten by fewer children (41.5% and 31.3%) as were meat, fish and eggs (29.5%). The percentage of children increased with age in all food groups, being low (3.2–11.9%) in the age group <6 months, but comparable to the pattern in women in the older children (aged 36 to 59 months) (Ministry of Public Health of Afghanistan & UNICEF, 2013).

The Jordan Population and Family Health Survey 2017 examined the feeding practices of infants and found that 22.5% of the children aged 6 to 23 months included in the sample received a minimum acceptable diet, the minimum dietary diversity was met in 51.4% and the minimum meal frequency in 62.2%. The percentages were higher in non-breastfed children, of whom 25.9% were fed a minimum acceptable diet, 57.9% with minimum dietary diversity and 81.4% with minimum meal frequency compared to 16.8% with minimum acceptable diet, 40.3% with minimum dietary diversity and 29.5% with minimum meal frequency in breastfed infants. In the whole sample as well as in both groups, the percentage of infants fed a minimum acceptable diet and with minimum dietary diversity increased with age, being highest in the group of 18 to 23 months. In turn, it decreased for minimum meal frequency among non-breastfed infants (Department of Statistics/DOS and ICF, 2019).

In Oman, the National Nutrition Survey 2017 found that while solid foods were introduced to 95.3% of infants aged 6 to 8 months, 80.7% of those aged 6 to 23 months received a diet with minimum diversity and 64.5% with minimum meal frequency. A minimum acceptable diet was given to 90.3% (Ministry of Health, Sultanate of Oman, UNICEF, 2017).

According to the Pakistan National Nutrition Survey 2018, only about a third (35.9%) of the infants aged 6 to 8 months were fed adequate complementary food. Among children aged 6 to 23 months, only 18.2% were fed with the minimum meal frequency, 14.2% with the minimum diet diversity, and just 3.6% received the minimum acceptable diet (Ministry of National Health Services, Regulations and Coordinations, Government of Pakistan, 2018).

In Sudan, a survey based on the Simple Spatial Survey Method found that only 24.1% of children received food with the adequate dietary diversity (Federal Ministry of Health, Sudan, 2020). In Somalia in 2019, 71.2% of the children aged 6 to 8 months were introduced to solid, semi-solid or soft complimentary foods, but at 6 to 23 months, only 17.2% received a diet with minimum diversity (Ministry of Health FGS, FMS, Somaliland, UNICEF, Brandpro, GroundWork, 2020).

Complementary feeding was also assessed in the Moroccan National Survey on Population and Family Health (ENPSF) 2018 and it was found that about 82% of the children aged between 6 and 23 months received solid or semi-solid complimentary food with no major differences between infants that were still breastfed and those that were not. Complementary feeding was adequate in 44.9% of the children (Ministère de la Santé, DPRF/DPE/SEIS, 2018).

In Northern Syria (Aleppo, Idlib and Hama), timely introduction of complementary feeding was found among 86.6% of the children and in 89% of those aged 6 to 7 months. However, minimum meal frequency was achieved in just 43.7% of the 6- to 23-month-old children and minimum dietary diversity in 57.3%. Cereal and dairy products were consumed by most of the children (81.9% and 84.1%, respectively), whereas lower proportions consumed fruits and vegetables (59.6% and 43.7% vitamin A-rich varieties) and protein-rich foods like meat, eggs and legumes and nuts (30.4%-56.4%) (Nutrition Technical Rapid Response Team, 2017).

While the Palestinian Micronutrient Survey 2013 did not report on complementary feeding practices based on the WHO indicators, it contains an assessment of the consumption of different food groups in children aged 6 to 59 months. Solid or semi-solid food was most often introduced at 6 months. Bread was the food consumed most often, being eaten at least once daily by 86.7% and by 92.6% of those aged 2 years or older. Of fruit and vegetables, potatoes, apples and bananas were introduced earliest and consumed most often (once a day in 32.2%, 30.8% and 26.3%, respectively) whereas other varieties were eaten less often. Milk was mostly consumed in its fermented form with 36.7% of the children receiving labneh daily. About a third (31.8%) of the children were fed meat 2 to 3 times a week and it was introduced at about 14 months. Tap or bottled water was the most consumed drink in this age group (Ministry of Health-Palestine & UNICEF, 2014).

In Lebanon, a recent nationally representative study showed that half of children started solid foods between 4 and 6 months. Using bottle feeding at hospital was more likely to induce early initiation of solid foods before 6 months of age (aOR = 0.5, 95% CI (0.32–0.77)) (Hoteit et al., 2022a). In addition, one out of three children (32%) living in Beirut and the governorate of Mount Lebanon (ages 6–59 months) had a low dietary diversity score (DDS) (Abi Khalil et al., 2022).

2.5 Dietary Intake and Consumption Patterns of Adults and Adolescents

Food consumption in the countries of the WHO Eastern Mediterranean Region is characterized by varying stages of a nutritional transition, from traditional to so-called Westernized dietary patterns and higher consumption of highly processed foods, fat, salt and sugar. High-income countries like the Gulf Cooperation Council member states that are advanced in this transition experience the associated high levels of overweight and obesity and associated metabolic diseases, whereas populations in countries with lower incomes or in states of political unrest or emergency are still threatened by hunger and micronutrient deficiencies (WHO EMRO, 2019 Nutrition strategy).

Generally, the supply of energy has increased over recent decades in almost all countries. This increase was mainly due to a higher fat supply and its contribution to energy intake while carbohydrate supply declined (Nasreddine et al., 2018).

Information on dietary consumption patterns can be obtained from recent nutrition surveys. A commonly assessed marker of a healthy diet is the intake of fruits and vegetables. Other factors are the consumption of processed foods with high contents of salt or sugar, of sweetened beverages, and of meat. Most of these data were obtained by using food frequency questionnaires or, to a lower extent, 24-hour diet recalls.

The Afghan National Nutrition Survey 2013 examined the dietary intake of women of reproductive age. Cereal products like bread, rice, wheat and maize were most frequently consumed, having been eaten by 98% in the last 24 hours and on average on 7 days per week. Oil and fats were also consumed regularly (95% of the respondents) and on almost all days of the week on average (6.6), followed by sugar and honey (78% and on 5.3 days per week) and dairy products (77% and on

4.4 days per week). Fruits and vegetables as well as meat, fish and eggs were consumed by about half of the participating women (56%, 50% and 45%, respectively) during the last 24 hours and on 2.9, 2.4 and 1.9 days per week on average. There were no major differences between the age groups.

The Bahrain National Health Survey found that about 15% of the participating adults aged 18 years and older ate adequate amounts of fruits and vegetables (i.e., five servings or 400 g per day). The percentage showed a steady increase with age, being highest in those aged ≥80 years (29.5%) and also higher in non-Bahraini than in Bahraini nationals (16.8% vs. 14.1%). It was also higher in people with higher education but was not consistently related to income (Ministry of Health, Kingdom of Bahrain et al., 2018).

A study from Lebanon using the data from two national dietary surveys found a significant decrease in fresh fruit consumption between 1997 and 2008/2009 in adults of both sexes aged ≥20 years. This decline was observable in all age groups studied and in men and women. In men, fresh fruit intake decreased by 40%, in women by about 34%. The decrease was most notable in the youngest group (20–39.9 years) (-53% in men and -42% in women) that also had the lowest intake of fresh fruits (as a contribution to total energy intake) while intake was highest in the oldest age group (≥60 years) in whom the decrease was also less (-14% in men and -28% in women).

The consumption of vegetables also tended to decrease in adult men and to increase slightly in women, but this was not statistically significant. Another food group that showed a strong decrease in all age groups and for both sexes was bread. In turn, consumption of chips and salty crackers as well as of added fats and oils increased significantly over the studied decade. Fast-food intake also showed a non-significant tendency to increase (Nasreddine et al., 2019). A recent study in Lebanon compared the intake frequency of different food groups before and during the COVID-19 pandemic and showed an increase in the consumption of legumes and pulses (3.2%, p-value=0.001) and whole-wheat foods in adults (2.8%, p-value=0.003). In contrast, a decrease of 5.4%, 6.9%, 5.8%, 5.1%, 3.1%, 3.4% and 2.8% was observed in the consumption of fruits (p-value<0.001), vegetables (p-value<0.001), processed meats, poultry and fish (p-value<0.001), other dairy products (p-value<0.001), sweet snacks (p-value=0.001), sugared beverages (p-value<0.001) and fats and oils (p-value=0.001) respectively. The Food Consumption Score (FCS) decreased by 4.6% (Hoteit et al., 2022b).

The Oman National Nutrition Survey 2017 examined the food consumption of non-pregnant and pregnant women aged 15–49 years. Fruits and vegetables were eaten 3 times or more per day by only about 14% and 6% of the pregnant women, respectively, and by about 9% of the non-pregnant women for both food groups. Pure fruit juice was also infrequently consumed, as more than 85% of the non-pregnant and pregnant women consumed it less than once a day. In turn, starchy foods were eaten at least 3 times a day by more than half of the respondents. The majority of the women stated that they did not consume processed meat, French fries, fast food and sugary foods daily (over 90% in the case of processed meat and fast food and 60–70% in the case of sugary foods and French fries). The same was also seen for sugared soft drinks. However, coffee or tea was mostly taken with sugar and at least once a day by 70% to 80% of the women. Unprocessed meat was also consumed rather frequently, with 66% of the non-pregnant and 77% of the pregnant women eating it once a day and 30% and 21%, respectively, 2 times or more (Ministry of Health, Sultanate of Oman, UNICEF, 2017).

The Palestinian Micronutrient Survey 2013 included a dietary assessment of adolescents aged 15 to 18 years and of pregnant and lactating women by food frequency questionnaires. Most of the participating adolescents consumed fresh fruits and vegetables once daily (about a third for fruits and around 40% for vegetables with only small differences between sexes). Consumption thrice or more per day was much less common, with only 3% to 4% of the respondents choosing this answer. White bread was the food that was most frequently consumed by the adolescent respondents and 58% of the boys and 43% of the girls consumed it at least 3 times per day. In turn, other cereal products like burghul or breakfast cereals were consumed less often. About a third of the respondents consumed potato crisps daily and about 39% of the boys and almost 25% of the girls drank soft drinks at least once daily. Poultry was the meat consumed most frequently, 2 to 3 times per week by 43% of the boys and 38% of the girls, while red meat and fish were eaten less often. Meat consumption was higher in boys than in girls and higher in the West Bank than in the Gaza Strip, where in turn fish was consumed more frequently. Yogurt and cheese were consumed once a day by about a third of the adolescents of both provinces.

Like the adolescents, the majority of the pregnant and lactating women in Palestine (84 to 96%) also consumed white bread at least once a day. Fresh vegetables and fruits were also consumed regularly by most respondents from these two population groups. Over 70% of the women ate vegetables daily, most often once a day. Fresh fruits were consumed more often in the West Bank, where 67% of the pregnant and 61% of the lactating women had them daily (most often once) but only 49% and 38%, respectively, in the Gaza Strip. Fermented milk products were also consumed daily by most women. Chicken was also the meat most often consumed by pregnant and lactating women, especially in the West Bank. Red meat was eaten more often in the Gaza Strip but consumption was overall lower than that of chicken. Fish consumption was rather low but again higher in the Gaza Strip, although the recommended 2 to 3 servings per week were only consumed by less than 20% of the sample. Less healthy foods like fast foods, potato crisps, sweets and cakes, or soft drinks were not regularly consumed and rather rarely on a daily basis (Ministry of Health-Palestine & UNICEF, 2014).

In the Saudi Arabian Household Health Survey 2017, consumption of fruits and vegetables was assessed in a sample of 24,012 households across the whole country, and it was found that 10.4% of the total population, including Saudi and non-Saudi nationals, ate 5 or more servings of fruits and vegetables per day. The percentages were comparable between women and men (10.5% vs. 10.4%) and also for participants of Saudi nationality (10.9%, 11.0% in Saudi women and 10.8% in Saudi men). The percentage was slightly higher in middle-aged people (aged 45 to 64 years) and lowest in the oldest group aged 65 years and above. More participants ate 5 or more daily servings of vegetables than of fruits (Saudi Arabia General Authority for Statistics, 2017).

In Tunisia, fruit and vegetable consumption in adults aged ≥15 years was assessed using the framework of the Tunisian Health Examination Survey 2016. It was found that almost half (48%) of the participants consumed vegetables daily and 25% did so 4 to 6 times a week, while only about 4% did not consume vegetables at all. The distribution shows little difference between men and women even though consumption of vegetables on 1 to 3 days per week only or not at all was slightly more frequent in women. A greater effect was seen for age, with younger people eating vegetables less frequently than older ones. Consumption was particularly low in young women, of whom 12.9% of the 15- to 18-year-olds and 9.7% of the 19- to 25-year-olds did not eat vegetables in the course of a week. In men, the respective frequencies were 8.5% and 7.2%. In turn, daily consumption was most frequent in men over 60 years and in women aged 50 to 69 years. Fruits were consumed less often, with 26.5% eating them daily, 21.5% 4 to 6 times per week and 45.4% 1–3 times per week. No consumption was reported by 6.6%. Differences between sexes were again small, despite a slightly higher frequency of absence of consumption in women than in men. The variability across age groups was less consistent, with zero consumption being lowest in the youngest age group of both sexes (15–18 years) whereas daily consumption was again highest in the older age groups. Five portions of fruits and vegetables were consumed daily by 20.2% of the participants, with a higher percentage among women than men (21.4% vs. 18.9%). The percentage was lowest in the youngest age groups of both sexes and highest in men ≥70 years and women aged 40 to 59 years. Moreover, consumption of adequate amounts of fruits and vegetables was more common in urban than in rural residents (République Tunisienne Ministère de la Santé, Institut National de la Santé, 2019).

Fruit and vegetable consumption was also assessed in the United Arab Emirates National Health Survey 2017–2018, based on data from 10,000 households of the 7 emirates. Of the adult respondents aged 18–69 years, 16.7% consumed at least 5 servings of fruits and/or vegetables per day. The percentage was slightly higher in women than in men of both Emirati and non-Emirati nationality (18.7% vs. 16.3% in Emirati and 18.1% vs. 16.2% in non-Emirati). The frequency with which adequate amounts of fruits and vegetables were consumed was higher in older adults (≥60 years). This survey also evaluated other dietary habits. About a quarter of the respondents always added salt or salty sauces to their food before or during eating and 16% did so often. Only about 30% rarely or never used additional salt or salty sauces. Foods with high salt content, such as salty snacks, fast food and pickles and preserves, were consumed regularly consumed by about 15% of the participants while a quarter never ate them. Salt use and consumption of salty foods was slightly higher in Emirati women than men and higher in non-Emirati than Emirati participants. The meat most frequently consumed was poultry, which was eaten by 46.3% of the respondents, while red meat was eaten by 21.9%. Fish and seafood were typically consumed by 25% and 6.9% stated that they do not eat meat or fish. No meat or fish consumption was more common in non-Emirati people, who also ate poultry more often and red meat less often than Emirati people (UAE Ministry of Health and Prevention, 2018).

A recent survey conducted in ten Arab countries (Bahrain, Egypt, Jordan, Kuwait, Lebanon, Oman, Qatar, Saudi Arabia, United Arab Emirates and Palestine) including 13,527 households in order to study food consumption before and during the COVID-19 pandemic, showed a change in the frequency of consumption of food products, with decreases for vegetables and dairy products excluding liquid milk. In turn, an increase in the consumption of legumes and pulses, nuts, unprocessed meats, poultry, fish, white bread, whole wheat bread, and milk occurred while no change in the consumption of fruits was observed (Hoteit et al., 2022c).

The shift towards more highly processed foods is accompanied by higher intakes of nutrients, with negative health effects. In light of the high prevalence of overweight and obesity in the region, particular attention is accorded to the intake of added and free sugars that are widely recognized as contributors to excessive body weight. A high consumption of soft drinks was reported for adolescents aged 13 to 17 years in the Global-School-based Health Survey. Data were available for 16 countries and the year in which the surveys were conducted ranged from 2007 to 2017. On average, more than a third of the adolescents had consumed carbonated soft drinks at least once per day during the 30 days preceding the survey. Intakes were particularly high in Egypt, Qatar, Iraq (only 13- to 15-year-olds were enrolled), and Kuwait, where 50 to 65% of the adolescents regularly drank soft drinks. Generally, consumption was more frequent among boys (GSHS).

Sodium intake, mostly in the form of table salt, was also found to be too high in most countries of the region in which intake had been assessed. Based on urinary sodium excretion data from nine countries from 2012 to 2020, salt intake ranged from 5.6 g/d to 11.9 g/d and thus exceeding the maximum level of 2 g sodium (corresponding to 5 g salt) per day recommended by the WHO (Al-Jawaldeh et al., 2018 & 2021). High sodium intake is a risk factor for hypertension, stroke and coronary heart disease as well as certain types of cancer (United Arab Emirates Ministry of Health and Prevention, 2018).

Trans-fatty acids (TFA) are another dietary risk factor that is associated with non-communicable diseases like those of the cardiovascular system. They are contained in partially hydrogenated fats and products made with these latter such as deep-fried foods, baked goods and salty snacks. Intake in the countries of the Eastern Mediterranean Region has been found to be comparatively high, exceeding the limit of 2 g of industrially produced TFA per 100 g of total fat in all foods recommended as a best-practice policy and even the less restrictive TFA limit of 5% of industrially produced TFA in oils and fats and in other foods (WHO, 2021b). An analysis by the Global Burden of Diseases Nutrition and Chronic Diseases Expert Group (NutriCoDE) found high intake levels of TFA at population level in the Eastern Mediterranean and North African Region, with a mean of 2.3% of total energy. The World Health Organization recommends that people limit the intake of industrially produced TFA to <1% of total energy intake to prevent negative health effects, especially with regard to cardiovascular health. According to the NutriCoDE study, 2 of the 3 countries with the highest mortality from coronary heart disease attributable to TFA in 2010 were located in the WHO Eastern Mediterranean Region (Egypt and Pakistan) (Wang et al., 2016).

In conclusion, the average diet in the countries of the WHO Eastern Mediterranean Region is characterized by inadequate consumption of vegetables and fruits and by excessive consumption of sugar, salt and trans-fatty acids. In the region, high rates of overweight and obesity coexist with malnutrition and undernourishment, particularly in young children, the latter being especially frequent in the countries with lower incomes. Improving the availability of a healthy nutritious diet and facilitating access to it by making food systems healthier, and at the same more sustainable, is crucial for the fight against malnutrition in all its forms and the non-communicable diseases associated with it that also place a heavy burden on the health systems of these countries.

Shifting to Sustainable and Healthy Consumption Patterns is the objective of Action Track 2 of the United Nations' Food Systems Summit, for which the WHO has identified 6 game-changing actions:

1. Fiscal policies for healthy and sustainable diets;
2. Public food procurement and service policies for a healthy diet sustainably produced;
3. Regulation of marketing of foods and non-alcoholic beverages, including breastmilk substitutes;
4. Food product reformulation;
5. Front-of-pack labelling; and
6. Food fortification.

These measures have also been proposed in the WHO EMRO's Regional Strategy on nutrition for the Eastern Mediterranean Region, 2020–2030 (WHO EMRO, 2019a). In the following chapters, these actions and some others will be presented in more detail and the progress of their implementation in the region will be examined.

PART 3

FOOD SYSTEM ACTIONS AS 'GAME CHANGERS' WITH A SPECIAL FOCUS ON REGIONAL ASPECTS AND EFFECTS

Goals and Objectives

Improving Food Environments and Empowering Consumers in their Food Demands to Make Diets Healthier and More Sustainable

The short overview given in Part 2 shows that the countries of the WHO Eastern Mediterranean Region are currently facing a multiple burden of malnutrition with severe undernourishment and micronutrient deficiencies coexisting with high prevalence of obesity, even in children, and unhealthy diet patterns rich in sugar, salt, saturated and trans fats. Notably, this co-occurrence is seen not only at the regional level but also at country level.

Changing food systems to facilitate the access to healthy food for of people of all ages in the Eastern Mediterranean Region is key to ensuring that people live longer lives in better health, and to controlling and preventing non-communicable diseases that also show a high prevalence in the region. At the same time, the region with its challenging environmental conditions is increasingly threatened by climate change that also endangers food security. Therefore, diets also have to become more sustainable and their ecological footprint must be reduced.

Considering the complexity of modern food systems, a successful approach to achieving these objectives requires a multi-sectoral strategy that is ideally embedded in a health-in-all policy (Leppo et al., 2013). With this in mind, the Food Systems Summit convened by the United Nations in September 2021 was intended to offer a platform for exchange and cooperation between countries and actors within the food system (https://www.un.org/en/food-systems-summit/).

© 2023 Al-Jawaldeh and Meyer, CC BY-NC 4.0   https://doi.org/10.11647/OBP.0322.10

As the anchor agency of Action Track 2: Shifting to Sustainable and Healthy Consumption Patterns, the WHO has proposed a package of six 'game changing' food systems actions:

1. Fiscal policies for healthy and sustainable diets;
2. Public food procurement and service policies for a healthy diet sustainably produced;
3. Regulation of marketing of foods and non-alcoholic beverages, including breastmilk substitutes;
4. Food product reformulation;
5. Front-of-pack labelling; and
6. Food fortification.

These actions have previously been identified as "best buys" to tackle the increasing threats of obesity and NCDs, as well as the ongoing serious issue of malnutrition, by creating healthier food environments that facilitate the access to nutritious food, minimize the exposure to unhealthy foods and empower consumers to make the right choices for their diets (WHO, 2017a; WHO EMRO 2019a). Taking into account the particular importance of a life-course approach to health and nutrition, one of the actions is dedicated to the significant role played by the protection of breastfeeding and healthy infant nutrition.

In the following chapters, these game-changing actions will be presented in more detail and the status and progress of their implementation in the Eastern Mediterranean Region will be assessed.

3.1 Fiscal Policies for Healthy and Sustainable Diets

Fiscal policies in the form of agricultural and food subsidies, incentives, price policies and taxes offer an effective way to change food systems and make consumption patterns healthier and more sustainable. As food prices are an important determinant of the range of food offered on the market on the one hand and consumers' choices on the other, agricultural and food subsidies as well as price policies and taxes can be used to promote the sustainable production of more nutritious commodities, increase the access to healthy foods and provide incentives for their purchase, while reducing the consumption of less healthy foods.

3.1.1 Repurposing Food Subsidies to Improve the Availability of and Access to Healthy Foods

Subsidies are widely used in all countries to support farmers, food producers, and consumers, ensure a sufficient production and supply of important food and feed crops and control the price of staples, thereby contributing to food security and reducing poverty. However, existing policies have been identified as obstacles to a sustainable and healthy food system, being harmful to the environment and promoting unhealthy consumption patterns (FAO, UNDP & UNEP, 2021).

This is particularly the case for agricultural subsidies that are coupled to certain commodities, production inputs or methods that have negative impacts on the environment and health. Over the period of 2018–2020, the 54 countries covered by the 2021 Agricultural Policy Monitoring and Evaluation report of the Organization for Economic Co-operation and Development (OECD) (including the 38 OECD member countries and 11 emerging countries) together spent on average 615 billion USD per year on agricultural support, the majority of which (71%) was paid directly to farmers (OECD, 2021).

For instance, a large proportion of subsidies is paid for the overproduction of cereals, meat, sugar and oilseeds mainly in monocultures, while the cultivation of vegetables and fruits is less supported in most countries. Such schemes are not only detrimental to health but also contribute to the environmental impact and climate footprint of agriculture by promoting the production and, subsequently, the consumption of foods of animal origin. This is not only the case for subsidies for livestock farming, but also for cereals and oil seeds like soybeans that are commonly used as animal feed and thus indirectly contribute to negative impacts on climate (FAO, UNDP & UNEP, 2021).

Repurposing agricultural subsidies towards more sustainable agricultural methods and healthier commodities intended for direct human consumption is considered a unique opportunity in the fight against climate change and environmental degradation on the one hand, and against inequity, food insecurity and unhealthy nutrition on the other (FAO, UNDP & UNEP, 2021).

In the last few years, the proportion of subsidies coupled to specific commodities has declined, while payments for cultivation methods that are more equitable and compatible with environmental protection and animal welfare has increased (OECD, 2021).

However, while agricultural subsidies have some degree of influence on the availability of different food commodities, their effect on food prices is much smaller. The reason for this is that the farm value of food, i.e., the cost that would have to be paid when directly purchasing at the farm, is relatively small, especially for highly processed foods, as the value for such foods increases during processing and a large margin is also added by the retailer (FAO, UNDP, UNEP 2021). Thus, with regards to healthier diets, policies directly affecting food prices have a stronger effect.

Historically and until the present day, fiscal policies have been used as a means to ensure adequate food supply to low-income population groups. This explains why it is predominantly inexpensive staple foods like sugar, oil and cereals that are subsidized. However, with the growing awareness of the significant health impact of a varied, nutritious diet, especially for the prevention of NCDs, it has become clear that new subsidy schemes are needed that include more nutrient-rich foods like fruits and vegetables while removing subsidies on less healthy foods, such as hydrogenized vegetable oils, sugar and sugar-rich or salt-rich foods. As the high prices of healthier foods have been shown to present a major obstacle to their purchase and consumption, especially among low-income population groups, lowering their price through governmental regulation can facilitate access to healthier diets.

A systematic review and meta-analysis found that both subsidies resulting in lower prices for healthier foods, mostly fruits and vegetables, and price increases for less healthy products had effects on consumption. However, the positive effects of subsidies were larger than the reduction of consumption caused by price increases (Afshin et al., 2017).

Another systematic review of field experiments showed that financial incentives like subsidies and vouchers increase the purchase of healthier foods. Some studies included in this review suggest a relationship between price reduction and the increase in purchases; however, this could not be examined further (An et al., 2012). Even though evidence on the cost-effectiveness of price incentives for the purchase of healthier foods at the national level is lacking, some countries in the region envisage modifications of their subsidy scheme as part of their national action plans in nutrition and NCD prevention.

To reduce fat intake and improve the fatty acid pattern of the diet, direct subsidies on fats and oils have been removed in Egypt, where palm oil was previously the main subsidized oil due to its low price. Subsidization of palm oil and shortening was also terminated in Iraq, and in Iran, subsidies on hydrogenized fats that are the main source of industrial trans-fatty acids have been removed to induce a shift to healthier fats and oils. In Kuwait and Qatar, subsidization has been restricted to edible oils with low content of saturated fatty acids. Kuwait also removed the subsidy on full-fat dairy products and full-fat cheeses (WHO EMRO 2015; WHO EMRO, 2021).

The removal of subsidies on unhealthy foods rich in sugar, salt and fat, and their application to healthy foods including mainly fruits and vegetables, are envisaged as strategies to strengthen and enforce legal frameworks that protect, promote and support healthy food in the United Arab Emirates' National Strategy Plan in Nutrition 2017, and its implementation is ongoing (Ministry of Health and Prevention, 2017).

On the other hand, the subsidization of fruits and vegetables to increase their consumption is listed among the recommended actions in the National Multisectoral Strategy for the Prevention and Control of Non-Communicable Diseases of Tunisia (Ministère de la Santé, République Tunésienne, 2018). In general, though, nutrient-rich foods like fruits and vegetables are not widely subsidized.

The need for changes in the food subsidy system has been highlighted in the case of Egypt, which has a long-standing system of subsidization of staple foods including bread, cooking oil and sugar. Introduced in the 1940s to improve food security by keeping prices for staple foods low and protecting the population from global price volatility, subsidies also provided a means to ensure political stability and to quench social unrest. In turn, nutritional objectives other than the supply of inexpensive food energy played no decisive role. Accordingly, by promoting the overconsumption of energy-dense but nutrient-poor foods, the subsidy system has contributed to the rising prevalence of overweight and obesity without eliminating micronutrient deficiencies, as suggested by high rates of anaemia and stunting in children. Furthermore, the distribution of food according to a fixed quota model does not correspond to the actual need, which promotes food wasting because unneeded products are thrown away or fed to animals. In 2014, the subsidy system was revised to allow for a more flexible allocation of food rations. The range of subsidized food was repeatedly expanded to include legumes, meat, fish and dairy products but fruits and vegetables were not selected. Considering the high costs of the subsidization borne by the government, further reform of the model should focus on the inclusion of more healthy, nutritious foods and, where possible, the promotion of local, sustainable food production (Ecker et al., 2016). More recently, a cash transfer system has been favoured, as experience from other countries showed that the money was spent on a higher-quality diet including meat and fruits (CGIAR PIM, 2021).

A simple representation of the effects of fiscal measures, including subsidies and taxation, is shown in Figure 5.

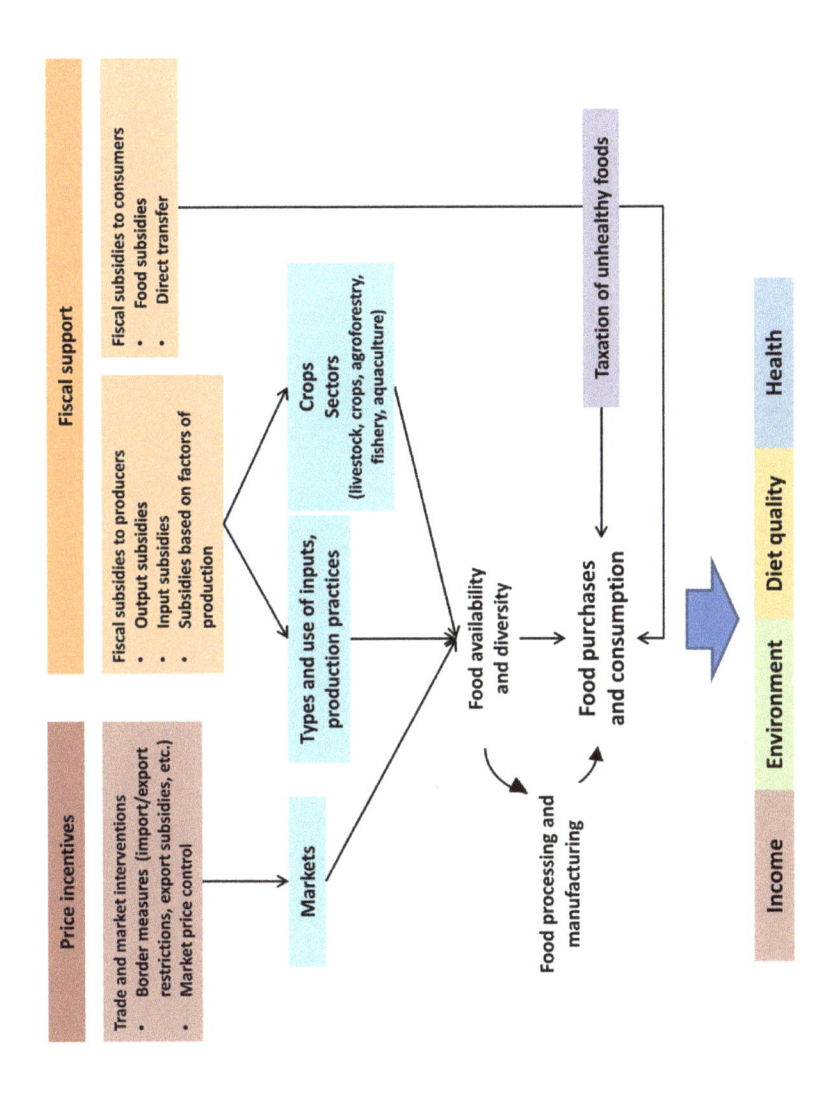

3.1 Fiscal Policies for Healthy and Sustainable Diets

Fig. 5 Effect of fiscal policies on the food system. Based on FAO, UNEP & UNDP, 2021.

3.1.2 Taxation of Unhealthy Foods

Taxation of foods high in sugar, salt, saturated and/or trans-fatty acids is another approach to promote healthier diets by decreasing the sales of these foods. This measure has so far been mostly used for sugar-sweetened beverages (SSBs) and sugar-rich foods. In 2019, 74 countries had some kind of 'sin tax' on SSBs in place, as did 8 regions and cities and the Navajo Nation in the USA (WHO GHO; Obesity Hub Evidence). Poland and Israel introduced a 'sin tax' on SSBs in 2021 and 2022 respectively (Obesity Hub Evidence), and a number of other countries are considering this measure including Kazakhstan (World Bank, 2021). In the WHO Eastern Mediterranean Region, this approach is practised in 7 countries, the Gulf Cooperation Council members Bahrain, Kuwait, Oman, Qatar, Saudi Arabia and the United Arab Emirates as well as in Morocco (Al-Jawaldeh & Megally, 2021; Belkhadir et al., 2020; Popkin & Ng, 2021).

Taxation of other nutrients and foods is less common. Mexico introduced an *ad valorem* tax of 8% on non-essential energy-dense foods with an energy content of ≥275 kcal/100 g together with a volumetric tax on sugar-sweetened beverages in 2014 (1 Peso per litre, which was increased to 1.4 Pesos per litre in 2019) (WCRF NOURISHING database; Congreso de los Estados Unidos Mexicanos, 2021). In the same year, the Navajo Nation in the USA passed the Healthy Diné Nation Act that imposes a 2% tax on unhealthy foods or foods with minimal-to-no nutritional value (Yazzie et al., 2020). A 5% tax has been imposed on fast food in the Sultanate of Oman since June 2019 (Al-Jawaldeh et al., 2020a). Energy drinks are also frequently subjected to higher taxation as in Mexico, where the rate is 25% (Congreso de los Estados Unidos Mexicanos, 2021) and the Gulf Cooperation Council member countries, where the rate is 100% (Al-Jawaldeh & Megally, 2021).

A tax on saturated fat (SF) was imposed in Denmark in 2011. Foods with SF content exceeding 2.3% were charged with 16 DKK (2.86 USD at the time) per kg of SF and a value-added tax of 25%. However, this tax was repealed in November 2012 for political reasons, even though it was shown retrospectively to have caused a small reduction of SF intake (Jensen et al., 2015; Vallgårda et al., 2015).

Different types of these so-called 'sin taxes' are used as shown in Table 14, and the type that should be chosen by a particular government depends on the local context. The majority of 'sin taxes' are imposed in the form of excise taxes. Excise taxes are indirect taxes, i.e., they are demanded from producers who recover them from the consumers by increasing the price, and they are charged on specific goods or services. A further distinction can be made depending on what is taxed. In general, taxation based on nutrient content has the most direct effect and does not depend on the product price. In turn, *ad valorem* taxes corresponding to a fixed percentage of the pre-tax price of a good are easier to levy, but unduly favour products that are cheaper but not healthier. Some countries also use custom taxes that are applied to imported foods and beverages only, but this may lead to disagreements with other countries if they are considered as protectionism and a barrier to free trade.

Table 14 Types of taxes on unhealthy foods. Based on WCRF, 2018.

Type of tax	Description
Excise tax	Levied from the producer of a good but generally passed on to consumers through higher prices.
Volumetric excise tax	Levied per amount or volume sold (e.g., per gram or litre).
Nutrient content-based excise tax	Levied per the nutrient content of the food (e.g., per gram of sugar).
Ad valorem excise tax	Corresponds to a percentage of the value of goods (e.g., 10% of the pre-tax product price).
Sales tax	Collected from consumers at the sales point as a percentage of the price.
Value-added tax	Charged on each production stage that adds value to the product.
Custom or import duty tax	Levied on imported products.

In the first place, taxes collected from the producer generally result in price increases that will decrease the sales volume of the taxed product. Additionally, such taxes also provide an incentive for manufacturers to reformulate their products to prevent them from being taxed.

Public health benefits from 'sin taxes' can be further enhanced if the revenues are used to fund health-promotion initiatives such as programmes to combat obesity in children or to subsidize healthy foods. This earmarking of revenues also makes 'sin taxes' more acceptable and increases public and political support for them (WCRF, 2018; Eykelenboom et al., 2019). A recent systematic review found that public acceptability of SSB taxation was highest when the raised revenue was to be used for societal health purposes. This study also underlined the need for transparency about the purposes of the tax, as it was found that some governments considered the tax income as a contribution to the general budget. An important factor contributing to the acceptability and efficacy of SSB taxes was the availability of healthy alternatives, especially safe drinking water (Eykelenboom et al., 2019).

Based on modelling studies, a taxation of 10–20% of the product price was found to be necessary to obtain a significant reduction of purchases and consumption and a significant impact on population health.

Evidence from countries that implemented taxes on sugar-sweetened beverages some years ago supports this measure as an effective approach to reduce purchases, and thereby the consumption of sugar-sweetened beverages (WCRF, 2018). A systematic review based on studies from 7 countries found that, for an increase in taxation by 10%, purchases and consumption of SSBs declined by about 10% on average (Teng et al., 2019). In Mexico the extent of the reduction of SSB purchases was inversely associated with socio-economic status and was also higher in people that were aware of the policy (Miracolo et al., 2021). Higher decreases were observed in Chile, where SSB consumption dropped by 21.6% after the introduction of taxation. In Portugal, the implementation of a tax on sweetened beverages in 2017 was associated with a decline in the consumption of these products by 11% based on market data, and by 21% based on tax data, and stimulated the reformulation of soft drinks resulting in an average reduction of energy density by 3.1 kcal/100 ml. It was estimated that these effects could prevent 40–78 new cases of obesity per year in Portugal, with the highest reduction projected among 10-<18-year-olds who have the highest energy intake from SSBs (Goiana-da-Silva et al., 2020). In the UK, a tiered taxation of sugar-sweetened drinks was introduced in 2018, charging 24 pence per litre on drinks with >8 g sugar per 100 ml and 18 pence per litre on drinks containing 5–8 g of sugar per 100 ml, while drinks with <5 g sugar per 100 ml are exempt from the tax. The sales volume of drinks subjected to the tax decreased by 50%, so sugar contents of soft drinks fell by 34% between 2015 and 2018, with the highest decline between 2017 and 2018 (Bandy et al., 2020).

A modelling study from Mexico suggested a 10% lower consumption of sugar-sweetened beverages due to taxation that in turn would prevent about 189,300 type 2 diabetes cases, 20,400 strokes and myocardial infarctions and 18,900 deaths in 35–94 year-old adults between 2013 and 2022, with the largest reduction among 35–44 year-olds. It was estimated that this could save 983 million international dollars of healthcare costs (Sánchez-Romero et al., 2016).

In the WHO Eastern Mediterranean, so far, 7 countries have introduced 'sin taxes' on sugar-sweetened beverages, including the Gulf Cooperation Council (GCC) members Bahrain, Kuwait, Oman, Qatar, Saudi Arabia and the United Arab Emirates (UAE) as well as in Morocco (Al-Jawaldeh & Megally, 2021; Belkhadir et al., 2020; Popkin & Ng, 2021). In the UAE, this tax was extended to all foods and beverages containing added sugars or artificial sweeteners on which a 50% *ad valorem* tax is charged since 2020. Moreover, taxation of sugar-sweetened beverages is also part of national nutrition policies and action plans in Egypt, Iran, Morocco, Palestine and Tunisia (WHO-GINA; Zargaraan et al., 2017). From 2021, Tunisia has levied a tax of 0.1 dinar (3.4 US cents) per kg of sugar (ITCEQ, 2020).

Table 15 provides an overview of the implemented taxation models in the countries of the region.

An evaluation of the impact of this measure has only been conducted in the GCC countries where decreases in the growth rate of sales volumes were observed after the introduction of the SSB taxes. In Saudi Arabia, the growth rate fell from 5.44% in 2016 to 1.33% in 2017, from 7.37% to 5.93% in the United Arab Emirates, and from 5.25% to 5.09% in Bahrain. In the other countries, the effect was delayed due to the introduction of the taxation in 2019 and 2020. Overall, taxation caused a reduction in the sales volume growth rate of 2.87% (Al-Jawaldeh & Megally, 2021).

In the Kingdom of Saudi Arabia, per-capita purchases of carbonated soft drinks and energy drinks decreased by 41% and 58% respectively between 2016 and 2018 (Alsukait et al., 2021).

Table 15 Taxation of foods and beverages containing added sugars in countries of the WHO Eastern Mediterranean Region. Source of data: Popkin & Ng, 2021; Zargaraan et al., 2017.

Country	Products taxed	Type of tax and amount	Year of introduction
Bahrain	Carbonated soft drinks, energy drinks	*Ad valorem* excise tax, 50% on SSBs and other soft drinks, 100% on energy drinks	2017
Iran	Soft drinks	*Ad valorem* excise tax, 15% on domestically produced and 20% on imported soft drinks	2013/2014
Kuwait	Carbonated soft drinks, energy drinks	*Ad valorem* excise tax, 50% on SSBs and other soft drinks, 100% on energy drinks	2020
Morocco	Carbonated and non-carbonated soft drinks with ≥5 g sugar/100 ml, energy drinks, nectars	VAT, 0.7 MAD (0.08 USD)/L on soft drinks; 20% higher excise tax on energy drinks; 50% higher excise tax on nectars	2019
Oman	Carbonated beverages except water, energy drinks	*Ad valorem* excise tax, 100% on energy drinks, 50% on other carbonated drinks	2019
Qatar	Sweetened carbonated beverages, energy drinks	*Ad valorem* excise tax, 100% on energy drinks, 50% on other SSBs	2019
Saudi Arabia	Sugar-sweetened beverages (SSBs), energy drinks	*Ad valorem* excise tax, 50% on SSBs and other soft drinks, 100% on energy drinks	2017

Country	Products taxed	Type of tax and amount	Year of introduction
United Arab Emirates	Sugar-sweetened beverages and beverages containing artificial sweeteners*, energy drinks	*Ad valorem* excise tax, 50% on SSBs and other soft drinks, 100% on energy drinks	2017
	Foods and beverages with added sugars or artificial sweeteners including SSBs*	*Ad valorem* excise tax, 50% on SSBs and other soft drinks, 100% on energy drinks	2020

* excluding beverages with >75% milk and milk substitutes, infant formula and food, foods and beverages for special dietary requirements and medical use.

MAD: Moroccan Dirham; VAT: value-added tax.

While an increasing number of countries worldwide are introducing 'sin taxes' on SSBs and/or foods with an unfavourable nutrition profile, Denmark charged a tax on soft drinks and sweets as early as 1922 but abolished this measure in 2014; the resulting financial burden on producers was considered too high, threatening jobs and stimulating people to buy cheaper products in neighbouring countries Sweden and Germany (www.fooddrinktax.eu). In Italy, the implementation of an SSB tax that was approved in 2019 has since been repeatedly postponed (www.reuters.com).

The taxation of SSBs and foods of low nutritional value has often met with significant resistance from the food and beverage industry and certain other stakeholders. The introduction of SSB taxes was blocked in a number of countries and in some US states (Backholer et al., 2018). Preventing industry interference requires strong engagement between civil society and governmental actors, and the involvement of all relevant government departments is advised. Moreover, it is crucial to base the implementation of taxes on strong evidence concerning the negative effects of unhealthy diet patterns, the national intake of critical nutrients and its drivers, as well as the expected positive outcomes based on experience from comparable approaches. The policy should be accompanied by public campaigns to inform the general population about the taxes and increase support for them (WCRF, 2018).

Fiscal policies in the form of food subsidies and taxation provide the government with a powerful tool to direct food purchases towards healthier diets. However, in the case of subsidization, there needs to be a shift away from traditionally price-supported staple foods toward more nutrient-dense, lower-energy foods. The earmarking of revenues from taxation, as well as from more efficient subsidy models for social health programmes, make the measures more acceptable and increase public support.

3.2 Regulation of Marketing of Foods and Non-Alcoholic Beverages as well as Breastmilk Substitutes through Traditional and Digital Media

The marketing of food and beverages has a significant influence on what people eat and thus on public health. Regulating the marketing of foods to prevent the promotion of energy-dense foods of low nutritional value that are rich in fat (especially saturated and trans fats), sugar and/or salt (HFSS foods, or High in Fat, Salt and Sugar) provides a strategy to reduce the consumption of unhealthy diets. Children are particularly vulnerable to advertisements, so such regulation has a particular impact on their health.

Besides HFSS foods, the marketing of breastmilk substitutes is another point of concern as it is intended to dissuade mothers from breastfeeding and contributes to low rates of breastfeeding.

3.2.1 Regulating the Marketing of Foods and Non-Alcoholic Beverages to Children and Adolescents

There is strong evidence that the exposure of children and adolescents to marketing of foods and beverages high in saturated fats, trans fats, sugars and salt (HFSS foods) is associated with a higher risk of obesity and associated NCDs. Surveys that were mostly conducted in industrialized countries between 2003 and 2013 revealed that food marketing to children and adolescents occurred predominantly through advertisements in TV and online channels, and the majority of promoted foods were high in energy, fats, sugars and/or salt but low in other, essential nutrients. A large proportion of these foods fell into the categories of sugar-sweetened breakfast cereals, confectionary, high-fat savoury snacks, soft drinks and fast food whereas fruits and vegetables were rarely or never advertised (FSA 2003; OfCom, 2004; IoM, 2006; Cairns et al., 2009; WHO EUR, 2013).

This was confirmed by a recent survey from Turkey, which found that 78.8% of foods advertised on television across all viewing time did not conform to the nutrient profiling model developed by the WHO Regional Office for Europe. Between the hours of 3pm to 7pm, considered children's peak viewing time, this applied to 46.2% of the advertised products. Compliance was even lower in foods marketed via the internet, of which only 25.6% met the criteria for healthy food. Most of the promoted foods belonged to the categories of confectionary, cakes, biscuits and sugar-sweetened beverages (WHO EURO, 2018).

Several studies have shown that children exposed to the marketing of unhealthy foods are more likely to develop a preference for such foods, and to pester for or purchase them, resulting in a higher consumption of unhealthier foods and a higher risk of childhood obesity and the associated damage to health. Such marketing can also compromise the development of nutrition knowledge (WHO-EMRO, 2018).

Controlling the marketing of foods and beverages to children to promote healthy diets is one of the strategies of the WHO Global Action Plans for the Prevention and Control of NCDs 2008–2013 and 2013–2020, and the implementation of policies aimed at reducing the impact on children of the marketing of HFSS foods and non-alcoholic beverages is one of the 25 indicators to monitor the progress towards attainment of the voluntary global targets suggested in the Action Plan 2013–2020 (WHO, 2008b; WHO, 2013). The contribution that marketing unhealthy food to children makes to childhood obesity, and the need for its control, were also emphasized by the Commission on Ending Childhood Obesity (ECHO) that was established by the WHO in 2014. Reducing the impact of marketing unhealthy foods to children, including cross-border marketing, was included in the recommendations by the Commission published in 2017 (ECHO, 2017).

To support Member States in the development of policies to reduce the marketing of HFSS foods to children, the WHO issued a set of recommendations in 2010 (WHO, 2010b) that were complemented in 2012 by an implementation framework as a guideline for policy development, implementation, monitoring and evaluation (WHO, 2012a) (see Table 16).

While broadcast, print and other traditional media are important channels for the marketing of food to children, others should not be neglected. For instance, direct marketing strategies such as promotions and product vouchers, product placement and branding, point-of-sale marketing, sponsoring of events, broadcasting programmes, school food campaigns and educational materials are common tactics. More recently, digital forms of marketing via social media, mobile apps, online games and similar channels are becoming more important as they are increasingly used by children and are superseding more traditional media like television (WHO EUR, 2013; Kelly et al., 2015; WHO EUR, 2016). Marketing can be disguised as entertainment in the form of games ("advergames") that are attractive to children and difficult to recognize as advertisements (WHO-EMRO, 2018).

Table 16 Recommendations on the marketing of foods and non-alcoholic beverages to children. Adapted from WHO, 2010 and WHO-EMRO, 2018.

Policy objective
Recommendation 1: The policy should aim to reduce the impact on children of the marketing of foods high in saturated fats, trans-fatty acids, free sugars or salt.
Recommendation 2: The policy should seek to reduce the exposure of children to, and the power of, the marketing of foods high in saturated fats, trans-fatty acids, free sugars or salt as both are determinants of the effectiveness of marketing.
Policy development
Recommendation 3: The policy should be as extensive and comprehensive as possible to account for the wide variety of media and marketing strategies that are used by the food industry for the marketing of unhealthy food and beverages to children. Such an approach will also prevent loopholes, limiting the ability of food producers to switch to other marketing techniques not covered by the policy. However, a step-wise policy that only covers certain age groups or settings or marketing techniques is still better than no measure at all, and can be extended gradually.

Recommendation 4: To prevent loopholes and limit evasive marketing tactics and standardize the implementation process, governments should clearly define the policy targets and criteria such as the targeted age group, the covered marketing techniques, channels and settings and the regulated foods, taking into account specific national challenges to ensure the effectiveness of the policy.
Recommendation 5: Marketing of foods high in saturated fats, trans-fatty acids, free sugars, or salt should be banned in settings where children gather such as among others nurseries, schools, school grounds and pre-school centres, playgrounds, family and child clinics and paediatric services and during any sporting and cultural activities that are held on these premises.
Recommendation 6: Development of the policy should lie in the hands of the Government that should also act as the leader of its implementation, monitoring and evaluation of the process but involve other stakeholders through a platform or working group. Assigning defined roles to other stakeholders can help to avoid conflicts of interest while protecting the public interest.
Policy implementation
Recommendation 7: Member States should cooperate to address the issue of cross-border marketing (in-flowing and out-flowing) of foods high in saturated fats, trans-fatty acids, free sugars or salt to children in order to achieve the highest possible impact of any national policy. Exposure of children to marketing from other countries with no or less stringent regulations should not undermine national measures.
Recommendation 8: The policy framework should specify enforcement mechanisms and establish systems for their implementation. In this respect, the framework should include clear definitions of sanctions and could include a system for reporting complaints.
Policy monitoring and evaluation
Recommendation 10: All policy frameworks should include a monitoring system to ensure compliance with the objectives set out in the national policy, using clearly defined indicators.
Recommendation 11: The policy frameworks should also include a system to evaluate the impact and effectiveness of the policy on the overall aim, using clearly defined indicators.

Accordingly, the WHO defines marketing broadly as "any form of commercial communication or message that is designed to, or has the effect of, increasing the recognition, appeal and/or consumption of particular products and services. It comprises anything that acts to advertise or otherwise promote a product or service" (WHO, 2010).

Nonetheless, exposure assessment and policies to control the marketing of food and beverages to children in many countries are focussed predominantly on traditional media, especially television. In light of the increasing use and the wider reach of new digital media, measures need to be extended on advertisements via these channels even though they are more difficult to recognize, and hence, much more difficult to monitor and control (WHO EUR, 2016; Kelly et al., 2015).

The impact of marketing depends on its power and the level of exposure to it. Marketing power is determined by creative contents, the design and execution, exposure by reach (the share of the target population exposed to the marketing) and frequency (WHO, 2012a) (Fig. 6).

Food producers and distributors
Food and beverage manufacturers
Food retailers
Restaurants and caterers
Trade associations and representative bodies

Marketing firms
In-company marketing resources

Power
(Creative content, design, execution of the marketing message)

Media organizations and broadcasters
TV stations
Film production companies
Newspapers
Radio stations
Video game producers

Content and access providers
Publishers
Internet search engines
Internet service providers
Billboard owners
Newsagents
Schools
Public authorities

Exposure
(Reach and frequency of the marketing message)

Impact
of the marketing message

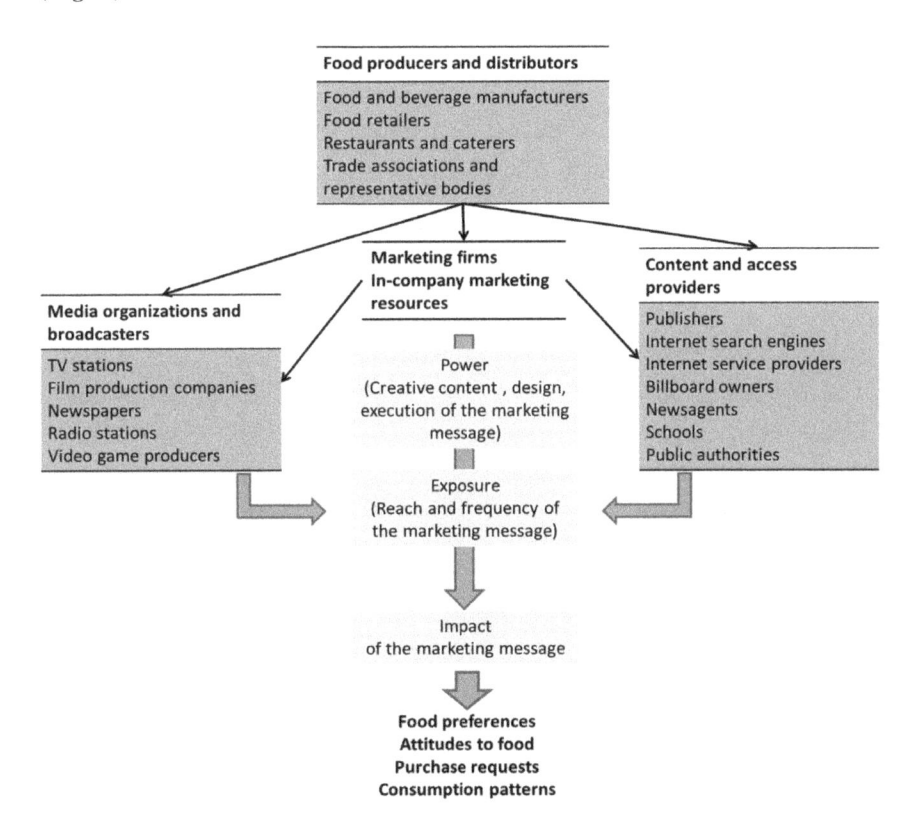

Food preferences
Attitudes to food
Purchase requests
Consumption patterns

Fig. 6 Stakeholders in the development and dissemination of marketing and determinants of its impact.

Policies to restrict the marketing of HFSS to children should ideally address all these determinants, calling for a multi-sectoral approach that involves government agencies and ministries in charge of business and industry, trade, commerce, consumer affairs, family affairs, child protection, media and communications besides those responsible for health affairs. The establishment of a working group to reconcile the different interests, responsibilities and points of view on the matter can help to achieve consensus among these actors, resolve disagreement and enhance the political support for the adoption of a policy. In general, the government should be the leading entity in developing policies, but other stakeholders, such as public health and consumer organizations, the private sector, academics and lawyers who are involved to counteract legal arguments raised by the food industry have to be included in their development and implementation (WHO EMRO, 2018).

Even though a comprehensive policy covering all forms of marketing across all media is the most effective measure to reduce the impact of HFSS foods on children, a step-wise approach focussing on a specific age group, certain product groups, types of media, forms of marketing and/or defined settings is more commonly chosen by countries. However, loopholes left by step-wise policies provide an opportunity for food companies to adapt their marketing strategy to take advantage of such gaps (WHO EMRO, 2018). A weakness of many actions lies in the lack of legally binding statutory regulations and the frequent reliance on voluntary self-regulation established by the food industry, for example the EU Pledge, the US Children Food and Beverage Advertising Initiative (CFBAI) and the Global Policy on Advertising and Marketing Communications to Children of the International Food and Beverage Association, among others. An issue common to those initiatives that are supported by some of the largest global food and beverage manufacturers and fast-food restaurants is the use of self-defined criteria for classifying foods that are not always based on scientific evidence, a focus on varying target groups and media and the lack of appropriate enforcement and monitoring mechanisms (EPHA, 2016; Boyland & Harris, 2017).

The implementation of policies to control the marketing of foods and beverages to children requires criteria according to which HFSS foods are defined. Nutrient profile models that are objective and based on scientific evidence provide the best approach. The categorization of foods should be based on nutrients that are associated with NCD risk or relevant for NCD prevention, and regional consumption habits and local food supply should be taken into account.

Currently, a number of systems are available presenting different advantages and disadvantages, and some have also served as a basis for front-of-pack labelling like the model developed by the UK Food Standards Agency for the Office of Communications (OfCom model, Department of Health, 2011) which uses a score of points given for nutrients that should be limited, and points for beneficial components.

Based on the nutrient profile model of the WHO Regional Office for Europe, the WHO Regional Office for the Eastern Mediterranean Region developed a regional model that was adapted to the characteristics of local diets of the Member States. The model distinguishes 18 food and beverage categories for which specific nutrient thresholds are applied (Table 17). It provides a uniform guideline to the countries of the region that is also meant to facilitate cooperation between the member states on the development and implementation of cross-border regulations to address the impact of global trading, and the propagation of media and internet content across borders (WHO EMRO, 2017a). This is important, as cultural and linguistic affinity in the region facilitates food marketing across borders through media channels that are broadcast in several countries, as well as through print media and even more so via the internet and social media platforms (WHO EMRO, 2018).

The status of the implementation of policies to control the marketing of food and beverages to children in the region was recently reported by the WHO Regional Office for the Eastern Mediterranean Region (EMR). It was found that the expenditure for the marketing of unhealthy food through mainstream broadcast, print and outdoor media by major multinational and regional food and beverage producers in the region increased significantly, almost doubling in the period between 2009 and 2012. This analysis did not include online and digital media and point-of-sale advertisements or sponsoring. Most of the promoted food did not comply with the criteria for healthy food, even though the study predated the release of the stricter nutrient profile model of the WHO Regional Office. Television was found to be the most important channel for the advertisement of unhealthy food (WHO-EMRO 2018).

Table 17 Nutrient profile model for the WHO Eastern Mediterranean Region (modified from WHO EMRO, 2017a).

Food category [a]	Marketing not permitted if exceeds, per 100 g [b]						
	Energy	Total sugars (g)	Added sugars (g)	Non-sugar sweeteners (g)	Total fat (g)	Saturated fat (g)	Trans fat (% of total fat)	Salt (g)
Chocolate and sugar confectionary, energy bars, sweet toppings and desserts	Not permitted							
Savoury snacks			0				1	0.1 [c]
Beverages								
Fruit juices (100%)	Not permitted [d]							
Vegetable juices (100%)			0					
Milk drinks (incl. sweetened and plant milk alternatives)			0	0	2.5		1	0.1
Energy drinks	Not permitted							
Other beverages (incl. soft aerated/carbonated beverages)			0	0			1	
Edible ices	Not permitted							

Food category [a]	Marketing not permitted if exceeds, per 100 g [b]							
	Energy	Total sugars (g)	Added sugars (g)	Non-sugar sweeteners (g)	Total fat (g)	Saturated fat (g)	Trans fat (% of total fat)	Salt (g)
Breakfast cereals, incl. chocolate breakfast cereals		15			10		1	
Cakes, sweet biscuits and pastries; other sweet baked goods, and dried mixes for making such goods	Not permitted							
Yoghurt, sour milk, cream and similar foods		10			2.5	2.0	1	0.1
Ready-made and convenience foods and composite dishes incl. pizza, filled pasta and pasta with sauce	225	10			10	4.0	1	1.0
Cheese					20		1	1.3
Butter, other fats and oils						20.0	1	1.3
Bread, bread products and crispbreads		10			10		1	1.0

Food category [a]	Marketing not permitted if exceeds, per 100 g [b]							
	Energy	Total sugars (g)	Added sugars (g)	Non-sugar sweeteners (g)	Total fat (g)	Saturated fat (g)	Trans fat (% of total fat)	Salt (g)
Fresh, dried or cooked pasta, rice and grains		10			10		1	1.0
Fresh and frozen meat, poultry, fish and similar incl. eggs							1	0.1
Processed meat, poultry and similar	Not permitted							
Processed fish						2	1	1.7
Fresh and frozen fruit, vegetables and legumes	Permitted							
Processed fruit, vegetables and legumes, incl. pickles, jams and marmalade		10	0		5		1	1
Sauces and dressings (incl. tahini and harissa)			0		10		1	1

[a] See (WHO-EMRO, 2017a) for details on and examples of included and excluded foods and beverages; [b] Products should, where possible, be assessed as sold or as reconstituted (if necessary) according to the manufacturer's instructions; [c] Salt equivalent; [d] In line with the WHO guidelines on sugars intake for children and adults, as fruits juices are a significant source of free sugars for children. However, marketing of 100% fruit juices in small portions may be permitted according to national context and national food-based dietary guidelines.

In addition, questionnaires were sent to the Member States in 2013, 2015 and 2017 containing a set of questions on the awareness of the Recommendations on marketing of food and beverages to children, the existence or planning of legislation contributing to their implementation and the content and shape of such laws. As of January 2017, only 3 countries in the EMR had adopted legislation contributing to the implementation of the Recommendations, none of which were comprehensive. It was revealed that awareness about the Recommendations was low in some countries, while others were planning or had already begun to integrate them into their national legislation. There was also often a lack of clear definitions of unhealthy food, and no sharp distinction between regulations of marketing of foods to children and regulations for the marketing of breastmilk substitutes, or standards for foods served in schools. However, improvements were found over the duration of the survey (WHO-EMRO, 2018). Measures to reduce the negative impact of food and beverage marketing on children are part of national nutrition policies and strategies in the member states of the Gulf Cooperation Council, as well as in Egypt, Iran, Jordan, Morocco and Pakistan (WHO-GINA).

The most complete legislation is in place in the Islamic Republic of Iran, where a ban on the advertisement of soft drinks on broadcast media was already imposed in 2004 (Omidvar et al., 2020). In 2010, the advertising of products and services posing a threat to health was completely prohibited by law. The ban, which was initially temporary, became permanent in 2016 and was extended to cover all types of advertising in all media. The list of banned products and services includes foods containing high levels of saturated fat, sugar, salt and trans-fatty acids, and since 2012 also high amounts of total fat and food additives, amounting to 24 food types in 2014. The selection of prohibited products and services is done by a task force established by the Ministry of Health and composed of representatives from the Ministry of Health, Ministry of Industry, National Standards Organization and Iran National Broadcasting. Clearer criteria for the definition were developed in 2017. For instance, products and services have to be commonly consumed, the decision to ban a product or service must be based on high quality evidence on the potential harm of their use and this harm must result from usual and common consumption, and there have to be alternative products or services posing no threats (Abachizadeh et al., 2020).

However, it was found that enforcement of the law was insufficient. While banning the advertisement of unhealthy products and services in public places such as on billboards as well as in print media was largely successful, this was not the case for national broadcasting, movies and the internet (Abachizadeh et al., 2020).

Moreover, there is limited focus on products and marketing addressing children. The depiction of children in the advertisement of goods is prohibited and the *Set of Production Criteria for Television and Radio Advertising* by the Business Council of Advertisements of the Iranian Broadcasting Organization forbids the promotion of food products during television and radio programs intended for children. However, this latter is an internal bylaw of the Broadcasting Organization without statutory power (Omidvar et al., 2021).

A recent review found that advertisements of foods targeting children and adolescents in Iranian media, mostly in television, were predominantly for salty snacks and sweets including sweet cakes, biscuits and cookies, candies and ice cream, chocolates and sugar-sweetened soft drinks with low nutritional value. Many included obese children as consumers or presenters and communicated misleading nutritional statements that were not covered by science (Omidvar et al., 2021).

In Egypt, the advertising of unhealthy food to children on public television and radio stations is prohibited by ministerial decree (WHO-EMRO, 2018).

A number of countries in the region have imposed bans on the marketing of specific food groups to children, like sugar-sweetened beverages, salty, fat-rich snacks and sweets and biscuits, but this selection is often not based on a comprehensive system for the classification of foods according to their nutritional quality [WHO EMRO, 2018].

In Saudi Arabia, the marketing of energy drinks is not allowed. Furthermore, official media have been requested by the Ministry of Health not to advertise unhealthy foods to children. A surveillance campaign in Saudi Arabia assessed 294 popular foods and beverages intended for children sold in 3 supermarkets in Riyadh that were advertised with cartoon characters for their compliance with the WHO guidelines for the intake of salt (1 g/100 g), total fat (30% of energy), SFAs and added sugar (10% of energy each). In 91% of the products, at least one nutrient exceeded the recommended limit. Most transgressions were observed in the case of sugar, the content of which was too high in all products from the sweets category and in all breakfast cereals. In turn, all chicken nuggets, potato crisps and popcorn products contained too much salt (Bin Sunaid et al., 2021).

A number of countries in the region are planning to incorporate the WHO Set of Recommendations on the Marketing of Foods and Non-Alcoholic Beverages to Children into national legislation, or are already doing so. It is part of the National Action Plan in Nutrition 2017 (Ministry of Health and Prevention, 2017) and the National Plan to Combat Childhood Obesity of the United Arab Emirates (Ministry of Health and Prevention, 2017), the National Nutrition and Physical Activity Action Plan of Qatar (Ministry of Public Health, 2017), the National Plan for the Prevention and Control of Chronic Non-Communicable Diseases 2016–2025 of the Sultanate of Oman (Ministry of Health, 2016), and the National Action Plan for Control and Prevention of NCDs 2019–2030 of the Kingdom of Bahrain (Ministry of Health, 2019).

In the United Arab Emirates, the implementation process started in 2018 and regular monitoring activities are planned. The national policy on the marketing and advertising of foods and non-alcoholic beverages to children is intended to impose restrictions on the advertising of unhealthy foods to children through media and advertising, free promotions, toys sold with unhealthy foods, brochures delivered to doors, activities and celebrations for children in catering businesses and to exclude companies selling unhealthy food and beverages from sponsoring sports events (Ministry of Health, National Action Plan in Nutrition 2017).

In the meantime, member companies of the International Food and Beverage Alliance (IFBA) operating in Saudi Arabia and the United Arab Emirates have vowed their full compliance with the Alliance's Pledge on Responsible Food and Beverage Marketing to Children. This implies that they will not market unhealthy food for children under the age of 12 years through all distribution channels. A survey conducted by the international market research firm Ipsos in 2019 showed that this pledge was kept (Ipsos, 2020). However, although some of the largest global food companies including Ferrero, Kellogg's, Mars, Mondelēz, Nestlé, PepsiCo and Unilever, are members of the IFBA, a large number of other producers (particularly local producers) are not covered by this measure. A comprehensive mandatory prohibition on marketing unhealthy food to children anchored in national law provides a more effective and uniform approach.

A recent survey in Lebanon evaluated the marketing of foods and beverages to children via local television channels, using data collected by Ipsos Lebanon and the nutrient profiling model by the WHO Office for the Eastern Mediterranean. On the 3 channels with the highest percentage of child viewers, almost a third (30.9%) of advertising was for food and beverages. This proportion was higher during programmes rated specifically for children (43.2%) compared to those for a general audience also suitable for children without or without adult supervision (32% and 28.8%, respectively). Most foods advertised during children's programs belonged to the chocolate and sugar confectionary category (33.3%), followed by cheeses (25%) and salty snacks (16.7%). Other beverages, including soft drinks, accounted for 11.1% of advertisements. In turn, there was no promotion of fruits and vegetables, neither fresh nor processed. During programmes for general audiences, chocolate and sugar confectionary as well as sweet bakery products were the most advertised (33.4% and 30.5% respectively) and 15.9% and 9.5% of advertisements were for alcoholic drinks and coffee respectively. Overall, only 16.3% of the promoted products met the criteria for healthy food given by the WHO-EMRO, and this proportion was even lower during the programmes for children, where no food complied with the nutrient profile. 17.9% of food advertisements were accompanied by nutrition and health claims, but of these only 20.7% met the nutrient profile criteria for healthy foods. On the other hand, only 3.9% of all advertisements, and 2.9% of those broadcast during children's programmes, included health disclaimers such as warnings to limit their consumption. These findings underline the need for regulation of the marketing of foods and beverages to children in Lebanon, where no national legislation existed at the time of the study (Nasreddine et al., 2019). However, the recommendations of the WHO on restricting the marketing of unhealthy foods and beverages to children have been discussed by representatives of the Ministries of Health and Education (Al-Jawaldeh & Jabbour, 2022).

In Oman, an assessment of five Pan-Arab satellite television stations that are mostly viewed by children, of six national radio stations and the most important print media showed that advertising was highest on television and between programmes intended for children (72.7% of advertisements). While the great majority of advertisements were for follow-up formula milk products (71.4%), the proportion of other foods was markedly smaller. Nevertheless, all sugar-sweetened foods, including those belonging to the categories of chocolate and sugar confectionary, sweet baked goods, breakfast cereals, ice creams and other beverages as well as savoury snacks were promoted during children's programmes, and the majority of these advertisements used cartoon characters, toys and other techniques considered attractive to children. Most foods promoted during radio programmes aimed at children were savoury snacks, but they included no sugar-sweetened foods or beverages. The marketing techniques that were used also specifically targeted children. In turn, advertisements for foods in print media were less commonly aimed at children, with the exception of those for chocolate and sugar confectionaries, even though these only made up a small part of the advertising (5.8%). None of the media included advertisements for fresh fruits and vegetables. The study also looked at marketing in grocery stores and food outlets in the proximity of schools, and it was found that bulk discounts, the distribution of free samples, gifts or games as well as the display of cartoon characters were techniques used to promote foods of which a large proportion fell within sugar-rich categories like chocolate and sweets, sweet baked goods, breakfast cereals and soft drinks (Al-Ghannami et al., 2019).

3.2.2 Regulating the Marketing of Breastmilk Substitutes: Implementation of the International Code of Marketing of Breastmilk Substitutes

Breastfeeding is widely acknowledged as the optimal nutrition for infants, supported by a large amount of evidence.

Consistent with the fundamental right of every child to health and adequate nutrition as stated in the "Convention on the Rights of the Child" (UNCRC, 1989), the Committee on the Rights of the Child urges the promotion and protection of exclusive breastfeeding during the first

6 months of life and its continuation until the age of 2 years or beyond, alongside appropriate complementary foods that are considered the optimal nutrition for young children (UNCRC, 2013a,b). Efforts to promote, support and protect breastfeeding were also endorsed in a Joint Statement by the UN Special Rapporteurs on the Right to Food, Right to Health, the Working Group on Discrimination Against Women in Law and in Practice and the Committee on the Rights of the Child in 2016, in which they considered the protection of infants and their mothers from harmful, inappropriate marketing of breastmilk substitutes and other commercial products undermining breastfeeding through the adoption of legal measures in accordance with International Code and the WHO Guidance, part of States' core obligations under the Convention on the Rights of the Child and other relevant UN human rights instruments (Joint Statement, 2016).

Nevertheless, the rate of breastfeeding in general and particularly of exclusive breastfeeding during the first 6 months of life is insufficient in many countries, with the availability and promotion of various industrial breastmilk substitutes (BMS) such as infant formula acting as major causes. While there is no doubt that BMS are needed in cases when mothers are unable to breastfeed, their aggressive promotion and advertisement as equal or even superior to breastmilk should not undermine breastfeeding. The use of BMS poses a particular threat in low-income countries and in emergency situations, where the costs for the products place a heavy burden on families, aggravating poverty. This leads to the use of expensive substitutes in a diluted form to save costs, promoting infant malnutrition. Moreover, inadequate supply of clean safe water that is needed for the preparation of the formula, and limited access to good healthcare increase the risk of infectious diseases like diarrhoea. Nevertheless, the market for BMS has been estimated at a value of more than 69 billion USD in 2020 and it is projected to grow further at an expected rate of 10% until 2027 (Global Market Insights, 2021).

Western Europe and Australasia have the highest consumption of infant formula, followed by the North American Region, but numbers are stagnating in these regions, while the largest increase is forecast for the Asia-Pacific and Middle Eastern-African Regions (Rollins et al., 2016; Changing Markets Foundation, 2017).

Notably, the increasing use of commercial dairy-based infant formula also has a significant negative effect on the environment, resulting from greenhouse gas emissions that have been estimated to be about twice as high as those associated with breastfeeding, and the use of water, land and fuel by the cattle sector as well as from packaging needed for the products (Pope et al., 2021).

Marketing strategies that are used by manufacturers and, to some degree, by importers, distributors and retailers to promote sales of BMS include direct marketing to consumers through media advertisements, the distribution of free samples and other brand-related gifts, as well as counselling and information material. In addition, healthcare workers in maternity wards and paediatric care units and even policy makers are recruited to promote BMS products by offering financial support, free training and other incentives. These strategies have been shown to influence infant feeding behaviour by changing attitudes and social norms about breastfeeding and BMS in favour of the latter. Marketing that presents BMS as equal or even superior to breastmilk in supporting healthy child growth and development offers a strong argument for choosing BMS over breastfeeding. Diminishing mothers' self-confidence in their ability to adequately breastfeed their children is another tactic used by BMS manufacturers. Adequate counselling and the offer of an environment encouraging breastfeeding have been shown to counteract these effects and to increase breastfeeding rates (Piwoz & Huffmann, 2015).

During the COVID-19 pandemic, some large manufacturers of BMS exploited the uncertainty and fears of mothers to promote their products as a safer alternative to breastfeeding to prevent transmission of the virus from mothers to infants, despite the absence of any solid evidence of a risk from breastfeeding and its importance for the infant's health and immune system (van Tulleken et al., 2020; Al-kuraishy et al., 2021).

The danger posed to breastfeeding by the aggressive marketing of BMS was recognized as early as the 1970s, highlighting the need for proper regulation of BMS marketing to protect breastfeeding and ensure the optimal nutrition of infants. In 1981, the World Health Assembly released the International Code of Marketing of Breast-milk Substitutes that covers the marketing of all breastmilk substitutes, including infant formula, other milk products and foods and beverages, as well as bottle-fed complementary foods that are marketed as a suitable, partial or total replacement of breastmilk. Moreover, the Code also regulates the quality and availability of BMS products and any information about their use. It should be noted that it is not intended to prohibit the use of BMS, or to restrict their availability or that of feeding bottles or teats, but only to regulate their marketing. According to the definition in Article 3 of the Code, BMS include "any food being marketed or otherwise presented as a partial or total replacement for breast milk, whether or not suitable for that purpose" (WHO, 1981). At the time of publishing, the Code gave no upper-age specification for the products. However, a distinction must be made between breastmilk substitutes in the narrow sense serving as a full replacement of breastmilk, and products intended for children older than 6 months to complement breastmilk when it is no longer sufficient on its own. Composition standards for the latter products, including follow-up formula and growing-up milk, as set by the Codex Alimentarius, slightly differ from the standards for infant formula to account for the changing nutritional requirements of infants and young children. As follow-up formulas were not defined as breastmilk substitutes in the original Codex standard, a revised version was proposed in 2018 and is still being further reviewed. A central issue concerns the appropriateness of a distinction between products for infants aged 6 to 12 months, and those for young children between 1 and 3 years. Considering that follow-up milk products are often cross-promoted with and labelled like infant formula, they also interfere with breastfeeding and their use is associated with a reduced frequency of daily breastmilk feedings or even its complete termination, which counteracts the WHO's recommendation to breastfeed for at least 24 months. Both types are therefore subject to regulation and labelling restrictions by the Code and the WHO Guidance (Helen Keller International, 2018; Joint FAO/WHO CAC, 2019).

To assist its Member States in protecting breastfeeding, preventing obesity and chronic diseases and promoting healthy diets for young children, the WHO published *Guidance on Ending the Inappropriate Promotion of Foods for Infants and Young Children* that was approved by the 69th World Health Assembly in 2016 (resolution WHA 69/9). It covers all commercially produced food or beverage products that are defined and specifically marketed as suitable for feeding infants and children from 6 months up to 36 months of age, including solid complementary foods and breastmilk substitutes that are defined as "milks (or products that could be used to replace milk, such as fortified soy milk), in either liquid or powdered form, that are specifically marketed for feeding infants and young children up to the age of three years (including follow-up formula and growing-up milks)". Marketing such products as suitable for the defined age group includes labelling with the words "baby/babe/infant/toddler/young child", recommendations of introduction to children aged less than 3 years; use of images of children of that age being bottle-fed. It advises not to promote such products to protect breastfeeding. Regarding complementary foods in particular, these should not be marketed as suitable for infants younger than 6 months, home-made complementary food prepared from fresh local products should be preferred and commercial products should not be marketed as superior to home-made food. The importance of continued breastfeeding for at least 24 months should be emphasized in messages promoting foods for infants and young children (WHO, 2017b).

Full compliance with the International Code of Marketing of Breastmilk Substitutes is also a central element of the "Ten Steps to Successful Breastfeeding" that were originally proposed by the WHO and UNICEF in 1989 as a set of policies and procedures to promote and protect breastfeeding and revised in 2018. Its implementation in care facilities is supported by the Baby-friendly Hospital Initiative (BFHI) that was introduced by the two organizations in 1991 to create an environment for mothers and their newborns that facilitates and protects breastfeeding (UNICEF/WHO, 2018).

Because the Code is not legally binding, Member States are responsible for its incorporation into national legislation, enforcement, control and monitoring of respective laws and are free to collaborate with other parties such as the WHO, NGOs and relevant institutions and professional groups as appropriate (WHO, 1981).

In 2014, the WHO and UNICEF in cooperation with the WHO Collaborating Centres, NGOs (Action Against Hunger, Emergency Nutrition Network, Helen Keller International, International Baby Food Action Network (IBFAN), World Alliance for Breastfeeding Action among others), and some Member States established a Network for Global Monitoring and Support for Implementation of the International

Code of Marketing of Breastmilk Substitutes and Subsequent Relevant World Health Assembly Resolutions (NetCode) to facilitate the adoption of the Code into national law and to build the capacities of Member States and civil society for its enforcement and monitoring. The vision of NetCode is that of "a world in which all sectors of society are protected from the inappropriate and unethical marketing of breastmilk substitutes and other products covered by the scope of the Code" (WHO/UNICEF, 2017a, b).

A protocol and a Monitoring Framework Toolkit were developed to support Member States in the monitoring and enforcement of the Code and the identification of and appropriate reaction to violations. The NetCode Toolkit contains two protocols to be used simultaneously or exclusively. The Ongoing Monitoring System Protocol applies to the continuous monitoring of compliance with the Code and the detection, reporting and treatment of violations of the Code and respective national laws. To this end, it contains a step-wise instruction for setting up a national monitoring system, including the establishment of an enforcement mechanism to stop and prevent violations and pursue any breaches of the Code and/or related national laws by manufacturers, distributors, retail outlets and healthcare workers (see Table 18) (WHO/UNICEF, 2017a).

Principal sites for ongoing monitoring include customs and borders, broadcast and print media channels and social networks, health facilities, points of sale and public areas where breastmilk substitutes can be promoted. In light of the ubiquity of marketing activities, Code monitoring is ideally integrated into existing control processes including product registration, customs and border control, food and drug inspection activities at points of sale, media monitoring, health facility assessments and the monitoring of health and nutrition programmes at community level (WHO/UNICEF, 2017a).

The Periodic Protocol, on the other hand, is intended to evaluate the level of compliance with the Code and the respective national laws in a quantitative manner, to study trends and changes over time, detect inadequacies of national laws and set priorities for the implementation and enforcement of the Code at a recommended interval of 3 to 5 years, focussing on 1) mothers of children under 24 months, 2) health facilities,

3) retail and product labelling and 4) the media (TV and internet) (WHO/UNICEF, 2017b).

The global implementation of the Code is regularly evaluated by the WHO and the results are published biennially.

While the need to promote and protect breastfeeding is generally recognized and 184 countries adopted the Code in 1981, the number of countries having fully integrated the Code into their national law is still insufficient. In 2020, 138 of the WHO's 195 Member states, including the Occupied Palestinian Territories, had transposed at least some provisions of the Code into national legislation, but substantial alignment was observed in only 26 (including the Occupied Palestinian Territories).

Table 18 Steps in setting up a national Code monitoring system. Based on WHO/UNICEF, 2017a.

Step	Procedures
1. Negotiating the political and bureaucratic environment	Obtaining high-level commitment
	Engaging relevant offices
	Identifying external supporters
	Anticipating and addressing opposition
2. Determining the coverage and extent of monitoring based on national laws	Establishing:
	what to monitor
	where to monitor
	when to monitor
3. Building a national monitoring team	Identifying existing monitoring mechanisms and processes
	Building a national monitoring team, designating a lead agency
	Team building and allocation of roles and responsibilities

Step	Procedures
4. Costing and budgeting for monitoring	Identifying available human and financial resources that can be allocated for monitoring the Code and/or national laws

Estimating resources that need to be requested and/or advocated for at national and/or sub-national levels

Reviewing systems and plans for their sustainability and efficiency |
| 5. Developing standard monitoring tools and a database | Using a standard monitoring form (provided in the protocol)

Developing data collection tools

Setting up a database for monitoring activities |
| 6. Capacity building of monitors | Training of the monitors

Awareness-raising on the importance of breastfeeding

Familiarization with the provisions of the national laws |
| 7. Monitoring and enforcing | Identifying violations

Reporting on violations

Verifying and acting on violations

Disseminating findings of the monitoring |
| 8. Evaluation of the system | Verifying the relevance, efficiency, effectiveness, impact and sustainability of the system

Qualitative and quantitative information collection

Every 3 to 5 years |

However, since the last report (2018), Code-related legislation was introduced or strengthened in 11 countries and stronger regulations were adopted by the European Commission. The majority of countries with national legislation substantially aligned with the Code was

3.2 Regulation of Marketing of Foods and Non-Alcoholic Beverages   117

located in the WHO Regions of Africa and the Eastern Mediterranean (9 and 7, respectively). EMR is therefore the region with the highest proportion of countries that have fully implemented the Code (31.8%) (Fig. 7) (WHO, 2020; WHO-GINA, 2012). The number of countries in the highest category of implementation increased from 7 in 2018 (including the Occupied Palestinian Territories) (Tables 19 and 20) (WHO, 2018a; WHO-GINA, 2012).

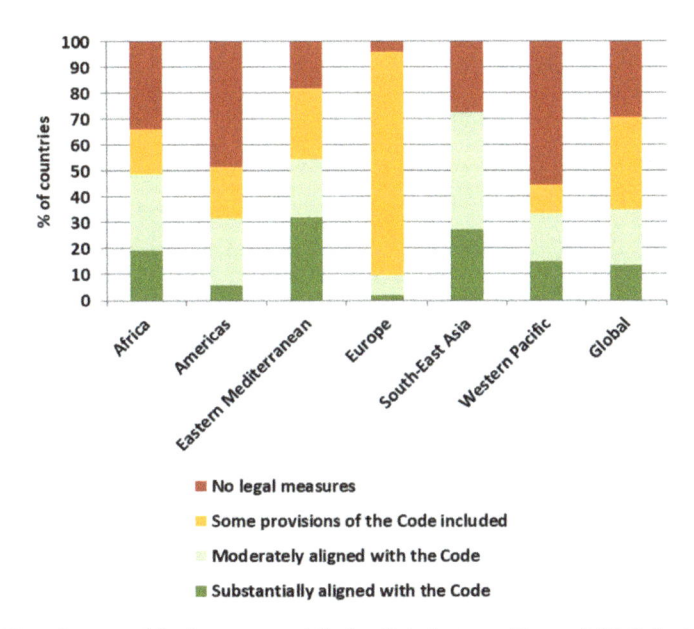

Fig. 7 Legal status of the International Code of Marketing of Breast-Milk Substitutes by WHO region in 2020. Source of data: WHO, 2020; WHO-GINA, 2012.

However, a recent study in Oman found that the large majority of foods advertised by 5 Pan-Arab satellite television stations that are frequently viewed by children was for follow-up milk formula (71.4% of advertisements, of which 41.0% were for milk formula, intended for children aged 1–3 years). Most of these advertisements (94–100%) included sounds or music, as well as pictures thought to attract children and featured child-friendly activities (Al-Ghannami et al., 2019).

Table 19 Status of implementation of the International Code on the marketing of breastmilk substitutes and products covered in countries of the WHO Eastern Mediterranean Region. Source of data: WHO, 2020.

Country	Legal status of the Code	BMS covered up to (months)	Other products
Afghanistan	Substantially aligned	Unspecified	Compl. foods Bottles, teats
Bahrain	Substantially aligned	36	Compl. foods Bottles, teats
Djibouti	Moderately aligned	Unspecified	Bottles, teats
Egypt	Some provisions	24	Compl. foods Bottles, teats
Iran	Some provisions	Unspecified	Compl. foods
Iraq	Some provisions	Unspecified	Compl. foods Bottles, teats
Jordan	Some provisions	6	Compl. foods
Kuwait	Substantially aligned	36	Compl. foods Bottles, teats
Lebanon	Substantially aligned	36	Compl. foods Bottles, teats
Libya	No legal measures	-	-
Morocco	No legal measures	-	-
Oman	Some provisions	4	Compl. foods
Qatar	No legal measures	-	-
Pakistan	Moderately aligned	12	Compl. foods Bottles, teats
Palestine	Substantially aligned		
Saudi Arabia	Substantially aligned	36	Compl. foods Bottles, teats

Country	Legal status of the Code	BMS covered up to (months)	Other products
Somalia	No legal measures	-	-
Sudan	Some provisions	4	Compl. foods
Syria	Moderately aligned	6	Bottles, teats
Tunisia	Moderately aligned	12	Compl. foods Bottles, teats
United Arab Emirates	Substantially aligned	24	Compl. foods Bottles, teats
Yemen	Moderately aligned	24	Compl. foods Bottles, teats
BMS: breastmilk substitutes. Compl. foods: complementary foods			

There is a growing awareness that children of all ages should be protected from marketing strategies that undermine their healthy nutrition, such as aggressive marketing of breast milk substitutes or of unhealthy foods and beverages for older children. However, there is a need for stronger and more comprehensive measures to control and reduce both types of marketing across all media that should be integrated in national legislation to ensure their implementation.

Moreover, marketing of unhealthy foods may also have negative effects on the food consumption patterns of adults—effects that are, however, much less considered (Boyland, 2019). The promotion of sustainably grown, local, healthy, nutritious foods, namely fruits and vegetables, is a particularly important part of campaigns to make diets in the Eastern Mediterranean Region healthier and more sustainable (Al-Jawaldeh et al., 2020a).

Table 20 Implementation of selected provisions of the International Code on marketing of breastmilk substitutes and products covered in countries of the WHO Eastern Mediterranean Region. Source of data: WHO, 2020.

Category	Provision	Countries with adoption into national law
Monitoring and enforcement	Identification of a responsible body for monitoring compliance	AFG, BHR, IRN, JOR, KWT, LBN, SAU, SYR, TUN, UAE,
	Definition of sanctions for violations	AFG; BHR, DJI, IRN, KWT, LBN, OMN, PAK, SAU, SDN, SYR, TUN, UAE, YEM
	Requirement that monitoring and enforcement should be independent, transparent and free from commercial influence	AFG, KWT
Promotion to the general public	Prohibition of advertising	AFG, BHR, DJI, EGY, IRN, JOR, KWT, LBN, PAK, SAU, SDN, SYR, TUN, UAE, YEM
	Prohibition of samples in public	AFG, BHR, DJI, IRN, JOR, KWT, LBN, OMN, PAK, SAU, SDN, SYR, TUN, UAE, YEM
	Prohibition of promotional devices at points of sale	AFG, BHR, DJI, JOR, KWT, LBN, PAK, SAU, SDN, SYR, TUN, UAE, YEM
	Prohibition of gifts to pregnant women and mothers	AFG, BHR, DJI, JOR, KWT, LBN, OMN, PAK, SAU, SYR, TUN, UAE, YEM
	Prohibition of contact with mothers	BHR, DJI, EGY, JOR, KWT, LBN, PAK, SAU, SYR, TUN

3.2 Regulation of Marketing of Foods and Non-Alcoholic Beverages

Category	Provision	Countries with adoption into national law
Promotion in healthcare facilities	Overall prohibition on use of healthcare facility for promotion	AFG, BHR, DJI, IRQ, JOR, KWT, LBN, OMN, PAK, SAU, SDN, SYR, TUN, UAE, YEM
	Prohibition of display of covered products	AFG, BHR, DJI, IRQ, JOR, KWT, LBN, OMN, PAK, SAU, SDN, SYR, TUN, UAE, YEM
	Prohibition of display of placards or posters concerning covered products	AFG, BHR, DJI, IRQ, JOR, KWT, LBN, OMN, PAK, SAU, SDN, SYR, TUN, UAE, YEM
	Prohibition of distribution of any material provided by manufacturer or distributor	AFG, BHR, DJI, IRQ, JOR, KWT, LBN, OMN, PAK, SAU, SDN, SYR, TUN, UAE, YEM
	Prohibition of use of health facility to host events, contests or campaigns	AFG, BHR, DJI, IRQ, JOR, KWT, LBN, OMN, PAK, SAU, SDN, SYR, TUN, UAE, YEM
	Prohibition of use of personnel provided or paid for by manufacturers or distributors	AFG, BHR, DJI, IRQ, JOR, KWT, LBN, OMN, PAK, SAU, SDN, SYR, TUN, UAE, YEM

Category	Provision	Countries with adoption into national law
Engagement with healthcare workers and health systems	Overall prohibition of all gifts or incentives to health workers and health systems	AFG, KWT, LBN, PAK, UAE
	Prohibition of financial or material inducements to promote products within scope	AFG, BHR, DJI, KWT, LBN, OMN, PAK, SAU, SYR, UAE
	Prohibition of provision of free or low-cost supplies in any part of the healthcare system	AFG, BHR, DJI, IRQ, KWT, LBN, OMN, PAK, SYR, UAE
	Prohibition of donations of equipment or services	AFG*, BHR*, DJI*, KWT*, LBN*, PAK*, SAU, UAE*
	Prohibition of product samples	AFG, BHR, DJI, IRN, JOR, KWT, LBN, PAK, SAU, SDN, SYR, UAE
	Restriction of product information to scientific and factual matters	AFG, BHR, DJI, IRN, JOR, KWT, LBN, PAK, SAU, SYR, UAE
	Prohibition of sponsorship of meetings of health professionals or scientific meetings	AFG, KWT, LBN, UAE
Labelling Infant formula	Prohibition of nutrition and health claims	AFG, UAE
	Required statement on superiority of breastfeeding	AFG, BHR, EGY, IRQ, JOR, LBN, OMN, PAK, SAU, SDN, SYR, TUN, UAE, YEM
	Required statement on use only on advice of a health worker	AFG, BHR, EGY, IRQ, JOR, KWT, LBN, OMN, SAU, SYR, UAE, YEM
	Prohibition of pictures that may idealize the use of infant formula	AFG, BHR, IRQ, LBN, PAK, SAU, SYR, TUN, UAE, YEM

3.2 Regulation of Marketing of Foods and Non-Alcoholic Beverages

Category	Provision	Countries with adoption into national law
Follow-up formula	Required information on recommended age of introduction	AFG, BHR, KWT, LBN, SAU, SDN, UAE
	Required note on importance of continued breastfeeding for 2+ years	AFG, EGY,
	Required information on importance of no complementary foods <6 months	AFG, KWT, SDN, YEM
	Prohibition of image/text suggesting use <6 months	AFG, LBN, PAK
	Prohibition of image/text undermining or discouraging breastfeeding or comparing to breastmilk	AFG, BHR, IRQ, KWT, LBN, PAK, SAU, TUN, UAE, YEM
	Prohibition of messages recommending bottle-feeding	LBN
	Prohibiton of professional endorsements	AFG

* Donations prohibited only if they refer to a proprietary product.

3.3 Food Labelling with Focus on Front-of-Pack Labelling

3.3.1 Front-of-Pack Labelling as a Tool to Facilitate Healthier Food Choices

Food labelling has been recommended as a tool to empower consumers to know more about the composition of the food they consume and to make healthier choices when buying food. To make diets healthier, particularly with regards to nutrients for which intake should be limited, like saturated fatty acids, trans-fatty acids, sodium and free sugars, consumers have to be aware of the main sources of these components in their diets. This is even more important considering the increasing consumption of industrially produced, highly processed foods and ready meals in in most parts of the world. Providing information on the nutritional composition of packaged foods has been recommended by the WHO as a tool to reduce the intake of energy, sugars, fats and sodium as part of a strategy to prevent and control non-communicable diseases (WHO, 2017a). This measure has been adopted by many countries worldwide and is often even mandated. However, so far, this is mostly done in the form of a table, panel or list containing the contents of energy, macronutrients, sugar, sodium/salt and (less commonly) dietary fibre and other nutrients, per 100 g or ml or per usual serving of the food on the back or side of the package. Levels of dietary fibre or micronutrients are most commonly included to support specific nutrition or health claims, as required for example in the European Union (Regulation EU No 1169/2011). Indicating this so-called back-of-pack (BOP) nutrition information on packaged foods is mandatory in over 60 countries worldwide, among which are the Gulf Cooperation Council member states and the Islamic Republic of Iran. Other countries provide at least a guideline for voluntary implementation (EUFIC, 2018).

Surveys have shown that information about the nutritional quality of food is desired by many consumers, but in a form that is easier to understand and faster to read than the format that is currently used (generally a list of the amounts of nutrients contained in 100 g of the food) (Gregori et al., 2015; Dana et al., 2019). Indeed, there is good evidence from a large number of studies that the detailed listing of the nutrient and energy content is hard to understand and use for a majority of consumers, particularly those with a low level of education. Moreover, they are often printed in small font size and therefore easily overlooked on the package, while studying them is perceived as too time-consuming during shopping. Consumers who use labels generally have a higher interest in nutrition and also some knowledge of the subject. Use and understanding of labels is higher among women, people from higher income classes, and those with higher education, so that the reliance on back-of-pack labels alone may further exacerbate health inequities (Cowburn & Stockley, 2005; Drichoutis et al., 2006; Grunert & Wills, 2007; Mhurchu & Gorton, 2007).

A solution is offered by additional nutrition labels that are displayed on the front of the food packaging, providing simplified information on the nutritional quality of a food in a salient form. There is now a wide variety of these front-of-pack labels (FOPLs) that are intended as a complement to rather than a replacement of the detailed BOP labels (WHO, 2019b).

3.3.2 Definition and Objectives of Front-of-Pack Labels

The use of FOPLs is also recommended by the WHO as an important contribution to making diets healthier and preventing obesity and non-communicable diseases. To support member states in the development and implementation as well as the monitoring and evaluation of an appropriate FOPL model, the WHO has issued *Guiding Principles and Framework Manual for Front-of Pack Labelling for Promoting Healthy Diets* (WHO, 2019b). In this document, FOPLs are defined as labels that:

- are presented on the front of food packages (in the principal field of vision) and can be applied across the packaged retail food supply;
- reflect an underpinning nutrient profile model that considers the overall nutrition quality of the product or the nutrients of concern for NCDs (or both); and
- present simple, often graphic information on the nutrient content or nutritional quality of products, to complement the more detailed nutrient declarations usually provided on the back of food packages (WHO, 2019b).

The recently revised draft of the Guidelines on front-of-pack nutrition labelling by the Codex Alimentarius Committee on Food Labelling defines front-of-pack labelling as a form of supplementary nutrition information that presents simplified nutrition information on the front of pre-packaged foods. It can include symbols or graphics, text or a combination thereof that provide information on the overall nutritional value of the food and/or on nutrients included in the FOPL at a national level. Nutrition and health claims are excluded from this definition (Codex Committee on Food Labelling, 2021).

In general, using FOPLs pursues 2 main objectives:

- Providing consumers with nutrition information in a more understandable format, empowering them to make healthier food choices;
- Prompting food producers to develop new products of higher nutritional quality and to reformulate their existing products to make them healthier (WHO, 2019b).

Besides these objectives, FOPLs can also contribute to:

- improve consumer understanding about the links between the nutrient content of foods and health, particularly for the prevention of NCDs;
- facilitate professional health advice on nutrition and healthy eating;

- reduce consumer confusion and deception about food products, particularly in relation to the misleading use of health and nutrition claims (WHO, 2019b).

While FOP labelling is most commonly used on pre-packaged foods, application could also be extended to unpackaged foods by offering information on retail shelves, or to foods served in restaurants, outlets or by caterers by including the information in the menu, for example.

Based on the objectives, FOP labelling is expected to affect:

- consumer understanding of the nutritional quality of foods;
- consumer food choices and purchasing behaviour;
- the nutritional composition of foods, especially regarding fat, saturated fat, sugars and salt levels (WHO, 2019b).

3.3.3 Types of FOPLs

A stocktake by the Codex Alimentarius Committee on Food Labelling in 2017 discerned 23 different FOP labelling systems used in 14 countries, 11 of which were developed and implemented by governments, 7 by industry, while the remaining 5 were developed in cooperation between government, industry and other actors. It was found that 23 countries had at least one of 16 systems implemented and 8 had 1 or more proposed. Three countries had simultaneously implemented one or more systems and proposed others. Implementation was voluntary in 17 countries and mandatory in 4. Two countries had several schemes in use, some of which were mandatory and others voluntary. (Codex Committee on Food Labelling, 2017). However, this stock-take only mentions the Nutri-Score system in France as proposed as it predates its final introduction on a voluntary basis in 2017 (Codex Committee on Food Labelling, 2017). This introduction was followed by other countries (Belgium 2018, Germany 2019, Netherlands 2019, Spain 2019, Switzerland 2019, and Luxembourg 2020, where it is recommended by the respective national governments) (Luxembourg Ministry of Consumer Protection, 2021). .

FOP labelling systems differ greatly from each other, but some general characteristics can be defined that serve to categorize the different systems. The information provided can be purely informative, indicating the amount of specific nutrients without any rating of the food, or it can be interpretive, offering some guidance to consumers on the nutritional quality of a food (Al-Jawaldeh et al., 2020b). The latter has also been termed 'directive' (Muller & Ruffieux, 2020). In this case, the tone of judgement can be negative, identifying foods with high levels of nutrients that should be limited; positive, identifying foods with relatively higher nutritional value; or indicating the relative healthiness of a food by a gradual score. Moreover, systems can provide information on different nutrients (nutrient-based systems) or combine a selection of nutrients and/or food components into one summary label (Al-Jawaldeh et al., 2020b). Nutrient-based FOPLs have also been classified as diet-directive, as they judge the contribution of a food to the entire diet, while summary labels are food-directive, judging the quality of the whole food (Muller & Ruffieux, 2020). An overview of classification criteria for FOP labels and examples are shown in Table 21.

Table 21 Classification of front-of-pack labelling systems.

Type of information	Form	Tone of judgement	Example(s)
Informative (non-directive)	Nutrient-based labels	Neutral	Guideline Daily Amount (GDA)
Interpretative (directive)	Nutrient-based labels (diet-directive)	Negative	Warning signals
		Positive	Healthier Choice Logo (Singapore)
		Gradual	Traffic light, Health Star Rating
	Summary labels (food directive): based on a summary evaluation of selected nutrients and food components	Negative	-
		Positive	Health seals: Keyhole, Healthier Choice, Weqaya (Abu Dhabi health logo "Prevention")
		Gradual	Nutri-Score, Health Star Rating

Some systems combine different characteristics like the Health Star Rating from Australia and New Zealand that includes information on the contents of energy, saturated fat, sodium and total sugars as well as one positive nutrient (protein, dietary fibre, certain micronutrients) per 100 g/ml or serving together with a summary indicator based on a nutrient profile (http://www.healthstarrating.gov.au). Other distinctions can be made depending on the nutrients or components of a food that are included in the profiling model, the reference amount for the calculation of nutrients (per 100 g/ml or per serving), and the legislative basis (mandatory or voluntary).

The most common FOPLs are the Guideline Daily Amount (GDA), Traffic light schemes, various health seals, warning symbols as well as the recently developed Nutri-Score system.

GDAs, or reference intakes (RI) as they were renamed in 2014, were developed by the food industry in the European Union. They present a summary of the most important nutritive values of a food, generally energy and critical macronutrients like sugar, salt and saturated fatty acids, usually per standard serving (http://www.referenceintakes.eu). A comparable scheme is known in the USA as Facts up Front (http://www.factsupfront.org). Besides the actual content, the contribution to the average daily recommended intake level is also indicated. These labels have been criticized in many ways. First, in their original version, they do not offer any interpretation of a food's nutritional composition and thus give no true help to consumers in their search for healthier foods. A revised version uses colour coding based on the traffic light model. Moreover, the reference values used do not apply to all population groups. The contribution of a food to the daily recommended intake level may be underrated, especially for children with lower absolute requirements for energy. Reference values for the European model have been considered as too high with regards to sugar contents, while serving sizes have been criticized as too small so that consumers are misled about the contribution of foods to their intake of critical nutrients. Another issue is the fact that there is no distinction between upper and lower limits of intake (Lobstein et al., 2007).

Health seals or logos are interpretive summary FOP labels, conveying a positive or endorsing judgement to indicate foods that comply with certain defined health criteria such as maximum allowable contents of salt, free sugars, total and saturated fat etc. They are sometimes regarded as health claims rather than as nutrition labels, even though they generally do not refer to specific health effects or body functions.

Often the criteria differ among food categories. Products carrying the health symbol are thus the healthier choice within their respective food groups. Examples include the Keyhole symbol widely used in Scandinavian countries, the Finnish Heart Symbol, and the Weqaya symbol used in Abu Dhabi (Al-Jawaldeh et al., 2020b).

On the other side of the spectrum are the nutrient-based warning symbols that signal foods with excessive levels of critical nutrients like salt or saturated fat. This type of label has become especially popular in Latin-American countries, where it was mandatorily introduced in Chile, Uruguay, Mexico and Peru, and it was also implemented in Israel (Jones et al., 2019). A positive version of this label type is used in Singapore with the Healthier Choice Logo in the form of a pyramid indicating foods with lower levels of critical nutrients like salt, sugar and saturated fatty acids. Into these classes fall two of the oldest FOPLs, the Nordic Keyhole as a positive endorsement that was established in Sweden in 1989, and the Finnish warning label for foods high in salt dating back to 1993.

A broader rating is provided by the gradual FOPLs like the traffic-light systems, the Health Star Rating or the Nutri-Score. These labels can be applied to a much wider range of foods, allowing comparisons within a food group as well as between foods from different categories. The nutrient-specific traffic light has the advantage of informing consumers about single critical nutrients. It was first developed by the UK Food Standards Agency (FSA) in 2004/2005 and implemented on a voluntary basis in 2013. Comparable systems were also introduced in Iran and Ecuador (Kanter et al., 2018). However, this scheme has sometimes been considered as too confusing for some consumers if they are faced with trade-offs between nutrients (e.g., one product rich in salt but low in saturated fatty acids vs. another high in saturated fatty acids but low in salt). Moreover, the traffic light is limited to less healthy nutrients and does not consider the positive aspects of a food. In turn, Nutri-Score rates foods with a single score that also includes positive aspects (protein, dietary fibre, and content of vegetables, fruits and nuts).

Nutri-Score is generally easier to use, especially by people with lower educational background, but gives no information on single nutrients. It is based on the same nutrient profiling model as the UK traffic-light system that was developed by UK FSA and the UK Office of Communications (Ofcom, 2004) as a model to restrict the marketing of foods with a high content of fats, sugars or salt to children (Julia & Hercberg, 2017). A combination is offered by the Health Star Rating used in Australia and New Zealand that includes both types of information. The main strengths and weaknesses of the most common systems are summed of in Table 22.

Regardless of the form, all FOPLs should be based on a nutrient profile that is founded on scientific and medical evidence.

Table 22 Major strengths and weaknesses of common front-of-pack nutrition labelling systems.

System	Strengths	Weaknesses
Health symbols	Simple and easy to understand.	No information on less healthy foods.
	Interpretive form facilitates healthier choices.	Only applicable to a rather small number of foods.
	Simple logo does not require knowledge about nutrients.	Does not allow comparisons between different food groups.
	Design can be based on already understood visual concepts (e.g., tick, heart).	Does not inform about nutrients of particular interest.
	Allows comparisons within a food group and one type of food.	Consumers may overrate the healthiness of foods carrying the symbol.
	As a positive symbol it may face less resistance than a system also or solely including negative aspects.	Producers may use the symbol as a pretext to increase the price of a product.
		Provides little incentives to reformulate less healthy products.
Warning symbols	Easy to understand concept.	Focus on a few negative aspects of a food.
	Provides information on specific nutrient(s).	May be met with more resistance from the food industry.
	Consumers are not faced with trade-offs.	

System	Strengths	Weaknesses
Traffic-light system	Colour codes are simple to understand (especially the colour red). Traffic light coding is already known to users. Interpretive form facilitates healthier choices. Allows comparisons within and between food groups as well as single food types. Informs about single nutrients of interest. Presents an incentive to reformulate products.	Information about several nutrients may complicate the overall rating of the food (trade-offs between nutrients). Focus only on negative aspects/critical nutrients The inclusion of informative elements (percentage of reference intake) in some systems may be confusing for some consumers.
Nutri-Score (interpretive summary label)	Colour codes are simple to understand (especially the colour red). Interpretive form facilitates healthier choices. Allows comparisons within and between food groups as well as single food types. Rates foods with a single score that does not require knowledge about single nutrients. Also includes positive aspects of foods. Presents an incentive to reformulate products.	No information on single nutrients of interest to many consumers.

3.3.4 Evidence Supporting the Use of Nutrition Labels and of FOPLs in Particular

A number of studies have been conducted to evaluate the effectiveness of nutrition labelling to improve consumers' food choices and their dietary habits. While it is difficult to draw a consistent conclusion from the results due to the large differences between the studies and the labelling systems studied, there is sufficient evidence that FOPL can promote healthier diets. A number of studies and study meta-analyses show that food labelling in general, and FOPL in particular, facilitate healthier food choices during shopping and enable consumers to rate foods according to their nutritional quality (Campos et al., 2011; Cecchini & Warin, 2016). While the effects differ between consumer groups, especially related to age and educational level as well as between countries, newer studies on FOPL give more consistent results and show that these simpler nutrition labels are preferred and better understood by consumers, including those with a lower level of education. This is particularly true for labels using colours to categorize food products and for summary labels allowing a fast and simple classification, even though no label has clearly emerged as the optimal type (Hieke & Wilczynski, 2011; Egnell et al., 2018; Machín et al., 2017; Goodman et al., 2018). In a meta-analysis, using FOP labels including GDA, traffic lights and various health logos increased the proportion of consumers making healthier food choices by 18% on average. In this study, the traffic-light model performed best with an increase of about 29% (Cecchini & Warin, 2016).

In a meta-analysis on the effects of FOPL (GDA, Traffic light, Health Star Rating, Nutri-Score, Warning symbols or respective similar systems) on healthiness of purchased food, including only studies conducted in April 2017 and afterwards (n=5), FOPL in general ensured a significant reduction in the contents of sugar and sodium of the purchased foods compared to unlabelled controls (-0.4 g/100 g and -24.5 mg/100 g, respectively) and a trend for lower contents of energy and saturated fat (-2 kcal/100 g and -0.154 g/100 g, respectively). An analysis by FOPL model revealed that a traffic-light approach reduced sodium contents by 34.9 mg/100g and warning symbols reduced sugar (-0.67 g/100 g), sodium (-33.8 mg/100 g) and energy (-4.4 kcal/100 g). The lack of significant effects for Nutri-Score is likely due to the fact that it was only included in one study. These findings were supported by the results of 3 more studies that were not included in the meta-analysis due to methodological differences. In turn, studies evaluating the effect of FOPL on food consumption did not show clear effects (Croker et al., 2020).

Research on the recently developed Nutri-Score label also shows promising results. In comparison to other FOPL systems like traffic lights, reference intakes and health logos, it was most effective in improving the food choices of the participants and their ability to rank foods according to their nutritional quality (Ducrot et al., 2016; Julia et al., 2016). It was also the system preferred by most participants and perceived as quick to process, easy to identify and easy to understand by about 20% of the collective (Julia et al., 2016). These findings were confirmed by a study in 12 countries suggesting that the Nutri-Score is best at empowering consumers to rank foods according to their nutritional quality and make healthier food choices (Egnell et al., 2018).

A recent analysis using data from the European Prospective Investigation into Cancer and Nutrition (EPIC, 1992–2014) found a significant association between diet quality, as assessed by the Nutrient Profiling System of the British Food Standards Agency that also underlies the Nutri-Score FOPL system, and cancer risk. A lower diet quality was associated with a higher risk of total cancer and with higher risks of cancers of the colon-rectum, upper aerodigestive tract and stomach, of lung for men, and of liver and postmenopausal breast for women (Deschasaux et al., 2018). In addition, FOPL, especially in the form of rating systems or health logos, was also shown to stimulate food manufacturers to reformulate their products to get better ratings (Vyth et al., 2010).

3.3.5 Developing and Establishing a FOPL System

The development and establishment of a FOPL system requires careful planning. To assist member countries in this endeavour, the WHO has compiled a framework manual, including guiding principles for the implementation of front-of-pack labelling to promote healthier diets (WHO, 2019b). The guidelines are based on experiences and lessons learned so far by various countries in the development and implementation of FOPL that were presented and discussed at a technical meeting in held in Lisbon, Portugal, on 9–11 December 2015, also taking into account the scientific evidence of the effects of FOPL on consumers' food choices and buying behaviour.

The proposed framework recommends a government-led iterative approach to the development and implementation of a FOPL system that also includes monitoring and evaluation of the model, based on the principles outlined in Figure 8.

Four steps should be taken:

- A country-specific contextual analysis needs to be undertaken to assess the population's dietary patterns and the prevalence of diet-related diseases, as well as the legal framework for the implementation of FOPL and to identify existing relevant national nutrition policies;

- The government should confirm or, if needed, extend the aims, scope and principles of the FOPL system so that national requirements are met, and it should provide the reference point for decisions throughout the development and implementation process;

- The development of the FOPL system should be government-led and in collaboration with stakeholders to warrant of the feasibility of the measure by the producers and retailers and its credibility to consumers;

- The selection of the FOPL system, its format and content should follow the agreed principles.

The early engagement of all stakeholders is a key factor to the successful implementation of the FOPL system. While the government, particularly those in charge of food regulations and health, should have ultimate responsibility for the process, other stakeholders, including the food industry, retailers, the scientific community, health organizations and consumer advocacy groups have to be actively involved in the development and implementation. The aims, scope and principles must be transparent and easily accessible and the system be based on a solid and transparent nutrient profile model, using 100 g / 100 ml as reference amounts (WHO, 2019b; Al-Jawaldeh et al., 2020b).

Having a regulation for back-of-pack nutrition labelling in place is a prerequisite for the establishment of FOPL as this information provides a basis for the FOP label. Mandatory implementation of FOPL ensures a high coverage of packaged food. However, careful monitoring and evaluation of the FOPL system is recommended to ensure that the measure is successful.

Please, can this be transcribed and offered as text?

Fig. 8 The WHO's Principles for the implementation of FOPL systems (WHO, 2019b).

3.3.6 Current State of Food and FOP Labelling in the WHO Eastern Mediterranean Region

Nutrition labelling on the back of packaging is mandatory in Iran, the member countries of the Gulf Cooperation Council and Tunisia, whereas it is voluntary in Lebanon, Jordan and Morocco, (EUFIC, 2018; Al-Jawaldeh et al., 2020b). In turn, FOPL systems have so far been established in just a few countries: Iran, Saudi Arabia and the United Arab Emirates. Furthermore, their introduction is being considered in Morocco and Tunisia where systems have been selected and tested. The systems currently used or considered in the WHO EMR are shown in Figure 9.

The first country to have implemented FOPL is Iran, starting with a traffic-light system in 2014 on a voluntary basis. In 2016, the display of the label became mandatory. The system is based on the UK model but was modified by substituting trans-fatty acids for saturated fatty acids, as the former are considered of greater relevance in the Iranian context (Edalati et al., 2019; Moslemi et al., 2020).

Saudi Arabia and the United Arab Emirates also introduced voluntary traffic-light labelling on packaged food products in 2018 and 2019 respectively, including the contents of sugars, salt, total and saturated fat, and in the Emirates this labelling became mandatory on 1 January 2022.[1]

In the Emirates, Abu Dhabi also uses a voluntary health symbol, the Weqaya logo (Arabic for prevention), which it has done since 2015. To display the logo, food manufacturers and caterers have to comply with the required food safety and hygiene concepts, and foods and meals that carry it have to meet the necessary nutritional criteria. Besides nutritional composition, a wide range of attributes is covered including the cooking method (deep-frying is not allowed), food additives, the serving size, marketing to children and meal composition. The nutritional criteria depend on the food category and include energy, total fat, saturated and trans fats, added sugars, salt/sodium, dietary fibre, and the amount of fruit, vegetables and legumes and wholegrains contained in the

---

[1] See: https://www.agriculture.gov.au/biosecurity-trade/export/controlled-goods/non-prescribed-goods/market-access-advice-notices/2020-03

product. Retailers wanting to use the logo on their products must apply specific marketing and health-promotion schemes (e.g., offering healthy recipes and cooking or shopping tips as well as educational materials on healthy nutrition) (Al-Jawaldeh et al., 2020b).

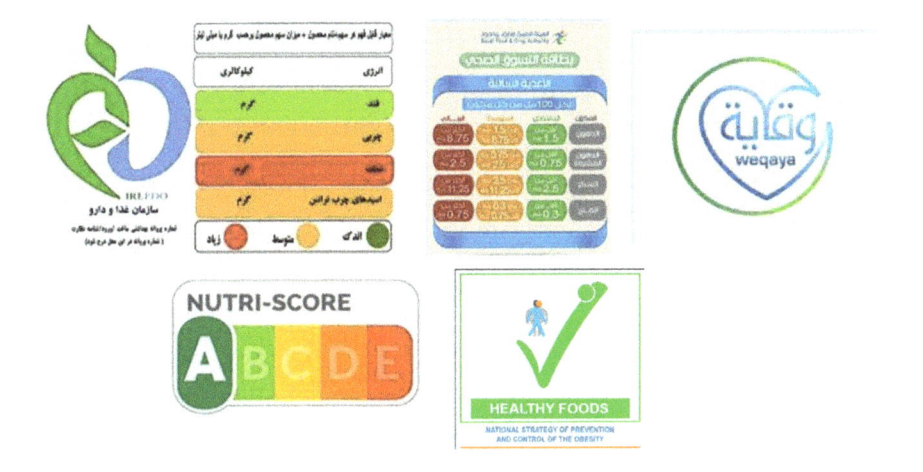

Fig. 9 FOPL systems currently used or planned to be used in the countries of the WHO Eastern Mediterranean Region. Clockwise from top left: traffic-light system from Iran; traffic-light system from Saudi Arabia; Weqaya health logo from Abu Dhabi; Healthy tick symbol currently tested and envisaged in Tunisia; Nutri-Score tested and envisaged in Morocco.

Morocco has tested various FOPL systems and it was found that the Nutri-Score system performed best as its display resulted in the greatest improvement of food choices by the participants in an experimental setting, including 3 different food categories. Participants were also better at rating the nutritional quality of products that carried the Nutri-Score compared to others (traffic light, Health Star Rating, warning symbols, and reference intakes) being considered as easy to spot and understand. Nutri-Score was also the label that most participants liked best with 65% wanting it on food packaging. In turn, warning symbols were perceived as triggering feelings of guilt. It has, however, to be considered that the participants were not very representative of the Moroccan population as 66.5% of them had a university degree while those with a lower educational level were underrepresented (Aguenaou et al., 2021).

Tunisia has developed its own health symbol in the form of a tick as part of its National Strategy of Prevention and Control of Obesity. The label contains a reference to this strategy, which is widely known and trusted. The tick was adopted as logo because in testing against other symbols it was the most accepted by consumers. Products carrying the health-tick symbol have to meet certain criteria for their contents of salt, sugar and fat that are derived from the WHO EMRO's Regional Nutrient Profile model, the WHO Nutritional Guidelines and the French SAIN LIM model.

Qatar have taken an alternative approach, with the implementation of a Food and Beverage Labelling and Calories Count Initiative at Restaurants and Coffee Shops in collaboration with the Ministry of Commerce and Industry. The initiative mandates the display of information about the content of energy and critical nutrients like salt, sugar and fat in all foods, meals and beverages in restaurants and cafes to facilitate the choice of healthier options for consumers (Ministry of Economy and Commerce, 2018; Al Tamimi, 2021).

Some studies have been conducted to evaluate the level and quality of implementation of FOP labelling and the compliance of the food industry.

A survey by the Saudi Food and Drug Administration (SFDA) between March 2019 and March 2020 revealed that, of 4335 of food producers whose products had been screened, only 80 (1.8%) displayed FOPL on 119 of their products. Most of these products were beverages (30%) followed by dairy products (23%) and confectionaries (13%). Traffic-light labelling was used by 36% while the majority used GDAs (63%) and 1% used the Health Star Rating. Most of the products with traffic-light labels were low in salt, total and saturated fat but had moderate or elevated contents of sugar (40% and 42% of products, respectively). The reference amount used was 100 g or 100 ml for 65% of the products carrying traffic-light labels as recommended (Bin Sunaid et al., 2021).

In Iran, a survey conducted by the Iranian Food and Drug Administration from September 2015 to September 2016 reported that 73% of locally produced and 61% of imported foods sold by retail chains in Tehran displayed traffic-light labels (Azizollaah et al., 2017). By May 2017, the number had increased to 80% of the sampled foods. Food manufacturers were supported by the Ministry of Health and Medical Education and training courses were offered. In addition, there is a "better-for-you" award for healthier choices within a given food category marked by the Green Apple symbol. In a study of shoppers recruited at a shopping centre in Isfahan, it was shown that use of the traffic light to guide food choices was rather low, with only 5.5% of the respondents stating that they chose food always or often according to labelling. However, this percentage increased to about 44% after an individual face-to-face lesson about the logo and how to interpret it. Participants were also better at answering questions about the nutrients covered by the label and their effects on health (Esfandiari et al., 2020). This shows the importance of education and media campaigns to facilitate the use of FOPL. The low level of public education and media campaigns to raise awareness about FOPL was also identified as a weakness of the labelling programme in a retrospective policy analysis based on interviews with stakeholders, which also pointed out a lack of cooperation between different sectors involved in the implementation process (e.g., the media and health sectors) and that no NGOs or consumer groups took part in the development and implementation of the strategy (Edalati et al., 2019).

Another study evaluated the accuracy of the Iranian traffic-light labelling with regards to trans-fatty acid (TFA) contents in 11 types of popular traditional sweets (9 samples of each were analysed by gas chromatography for their contents of TFAs). It was found that for 81.8% of the products, the information on the label differed from the actual content as measured, with 2 types of sweets having TFA contents over 7% of energy while the label indicated 2.7% and 0.2% of energy, respectively (Ghazavi et al., 2019). There was also a high proportion (61.6%) of non-compliant traffic-light labels with regards to salt content (Amini et al., 2021).

A study conducted in 2016–2017 in the region of Riyadh in Saudi Arabia to assess compliance with the National Food and Drug Authority's requirements to display energy, protein, carbohydrate, sugar, total fat, saturated fat, TFA and sodium on the back-of-pack labels showed that only 38% of the 1153 sampled pre-packaged products were labelled according to the standards, while 97% indicated only the contents of the "big four", i.e., energy, fat, protein and carbohydrates. The most frequently omitted nutrient were TFAs, followed by sodium, missing in 54.5% and 16% respectively. A higher compliance was observed for imported than for locally produced products with the latter only complying in 24.5% of cases (Jradi et al., 2020)

In light of the high intake of TFAs in the region, their declaration on nutrition labels on the back of the pack and as part of FOPLs is mandatory in many countries, including the Gulf Council member states, Iran, Jordan and the province of Punjab in Pakistan (Al-Jawaldeh et al., 2021).

In summary, food labelling provides an important tool to help consumers make healthier food choices and its effectiveness is markedly enhanced when it takes a simple and salient form that is easy to understand and interpret. Different FOPL schemes have so far shown promising results in studies in many countries worldwide. However, their use in the WHO Eastern Mediterranean Region remains limited to a few countries and should be extended together with other nutrition policies.

3.4 Reformulating Food Products

3.4.1 The Potential of Food Reformulation

Besides changing consumption behaviours through educational and fiscal measures the modification of food composition through recipe reformulation offers another possibility to make diets healthier. This approach is particularly promising with regards to food components like sodium, free sugars, saturated and trans-fatty acids that are known risk factors for the development of obesity, hypertension, cardiovascular diseases and other NCDs. Fiscal or labelling policies often present an incentive to food manufacturers to reformulate their products to avoid price increases or bad ratings. However, the marketing of the modified healthier products as well as nutritional education accompanying nutrition policies can in turn result in a higher demand for reformulated products as illustrated in Figure 10.

An advantage of reformulation is that it provides a means to improve diet without having to change consumers' eating behaviours. It may therefore be even more effective than consumer education in ensuring lasting improvements in diet quality, as suggested by an evaluation of the UK policy to reduce salt intake that showed that the reduction in average salt intake of the population over a time period of 5 years was almost entirely due to voluntary product reformulation by the food industry, while information campaigns had no major effect. Consumers even tended to switch to saltier products (Griffith et al., 2014).

Indeed, while it is widely acknowledged that the adoption of dietary patterns rich in unprocessed foods, including vegetables, fruits and whole-grain cereals, has a large number of beneficial effects, the wide availability and attractiveness of foods rich in unhealthy components make it difficult to reduce their consumption especially in population

© 2023 Al-Jawaldeh and Meyer, CC BY-NC 4.0   https://doi.org/10.11647/OBP.0322.14

groups with lower socio-economic status. The use of salt, sugars, SFAs and TFAs also has a number of advantages for food manufacturers by facilitating the processing, extending the shelf life and increasing the palatability of foods, making them very profitable. This effect is further magnified by the fact that regular consumers of highly processed fatty, salty and sweet foods very often develop a preference for these products, so that their intakes increase. In most processed foods, high levels of salt, sugars and fats are hardly perceptible, leaving consumers unaware of their excessive consumption (Monteiro et al., 2019).

Reducing the intake of unhealthy nutrients is clearly associated with reduced risks of obesity and NCDs. While food manufacturers, retailers, caterers and other private actors in the food business have to be actively involved in this process and cooperation has in recent years already been established in many countries, government-led approaches ensure the necessary compliance by setting the objectives and rules for enabling a healthy food and living environment (WHO-Euro, 2014).

Data from many countries supports the efficiency of food reformulation as a means to improve diet at population level, especially if embedded in a collaborative multifaceted approach (Federici et al., 2019). Most of the studies have evaluated the effect of the reduction of sodium contents in foods as this was also the target of most reformulation initiatives so far (Federici et al., 2019).

Early evidence came from the North Karelia Project started in 1972 in Eastern Finland, in response to the extremely high cardio-vascular disease (CVD) mortality rates that were due to the unhealthy lifestyle and nutrition in the region. Besides education of the population to modify food choices, reduce tobacco use and change other lifestyle factors, the intervention included the active involvement of the food industry to develop products with lower contents of salt and saturated fats. These modifications resulted in significant improvements to health, including decreased prevalence of hypertension and hypercholesterolaemia as well as a reduction of cardiovascular mortality, and they were later extended to the whole country (Vartiainen et al., 2018).

A number of factors determine the impact of food reformulation programmes on various health outcomes. For instance, whether it is implemented on a mandatory or voluntary basis has a strong effect on the adoption of the programme by food manufacturers and on their compliance with its terms. The extent of coverage with regards to food product categories also plays a role, as does the selection of nutrients the levels of which should be modified. If more foods of a given type are included in the reformulation programme, fewer unaltered and thus less healthy alternatives will be available on the market. This makes mandatory policies the approach of choice (Federici et al., 2019).

Especially small food manufacturers may be overstrained by the technological adaptations and knowledge required to reformulate their products and the subsequent costs. They also face a risk that the new product will not sell more, and might even sell less, so that the expenses of reformulation are not covered. Supporting food manufacturers in the reformulation process through knowledge transfer, technological assistance, training and capacity building contributes to the success of the policy. In addition, creating a demand for the reformulated foods makes their production more profitable and attractive for the food industry and ensures the pay-off of investments.

This can be achieved by a complementary public information campaign to raise awareness about the health risks arising from the consumption of foods high in salt, sugar, saturated and trans-fatty acids, and the benefits from adopting healthier consumption patterns. Food labelling or the use of nutritional claims can also contribute to higher demands for products with an improved nutritional profile, as long as it is understandable and usable by consumers.

Another approach is the use of fiscal instruments to steer consumer purchasing behaviour in the right direction, by subsidizing reformulated products or taxing unreformulated and less healthy ones (Gressier et al., 2020) (see also chapter 3.1).

3.4.2 Reduction of Salt Content

The reduction of salt and thereby sodium concentration is the most common goal of food reformulation, as the high intake of sodium or salt is directly correlated with hypertension, one of the most important risk factors to affect the cardiovascular system and currently the leading health risk factor worldwide. In addition, high dietary salt intake also increases the risk of certain types of cancer, particularly of the stomach (WCRF/AICR, 2018). In 2017, 10.4 million (95% UI 9.39–11.5) deaths, corresponding to about 19% of all cases worldwide were attributable

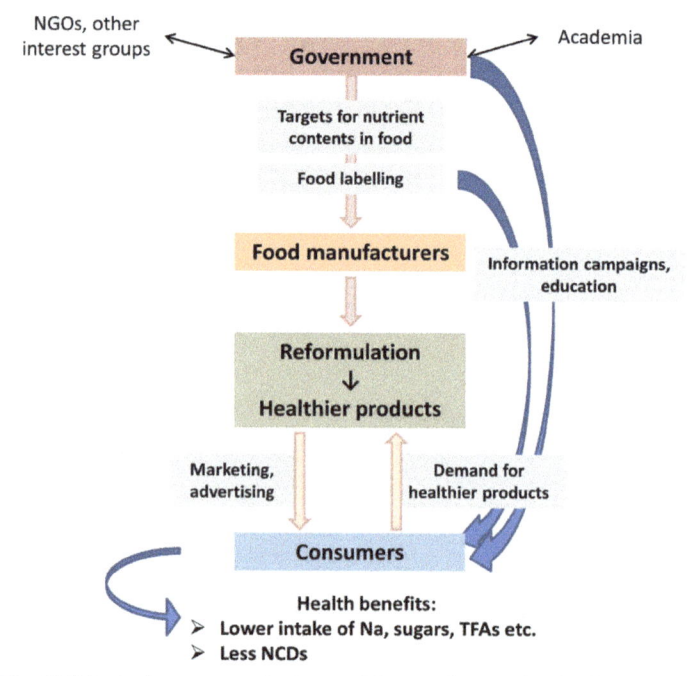

Fig. 10 Principal actors involved in and factors driving food reformulation.

to high blood pressure, and 218 million (198–237) disability-adjusted life years (DALYs) (GBD, 2018). The prevalence of hypertension is high all over the world and has been rising over the last decades. Based on data from 844 studies from 154 countries, the Global Burden of Disease, Injuries, and Risk Factor study 2015 (GBD 2015) found an increase in the prevalence of systolic hypertension, defined as systolic blood pressure (SBP) $\geq$ 140 mm Hg, from 17.3% to 20.5% between 1990 and 2015, corresponding to a projected number of 874 million people affected in 2015. In the same year, systolic hypertension caused an estimated 143 million DALYs and 14% of total global deaths, most of which were due to cardiovascular diseases including ischaemic heart disease and stroke. In this study, the Eastern Mediterranean and North African Region had a particularly high disease and death burden from hypertension, with Afghanistan showing the highest age-standardized rate of deaths related to SBP $\geq$ 140 mm Hg of all participating countries (456 per 100,000) (see Fig. 11) (Forounzafar et al., 2017). A subsequent study based on GBD

2019 found only a small reduction in deaths attributable to high sodium intake for the region (Chen et al., 2019).

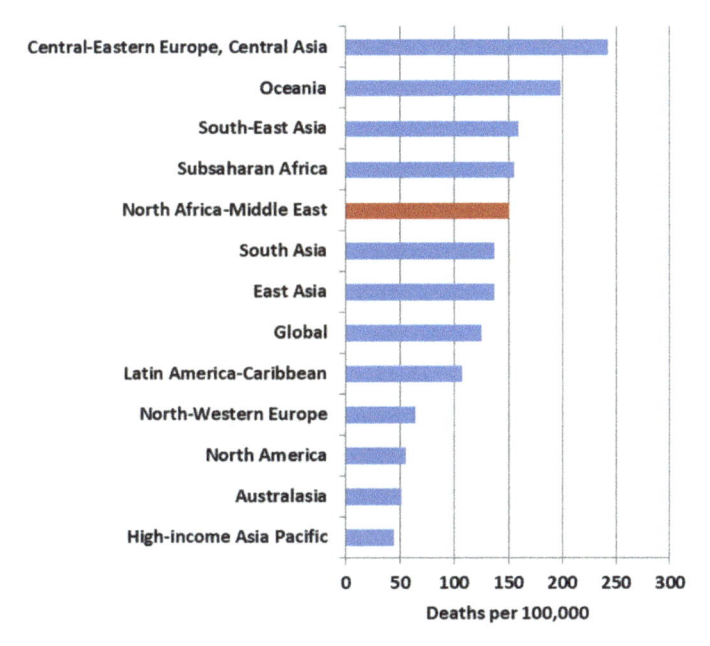

Fig. 11 Age-standardized death rates per 100,000 attributable to systolic blood pressure ≥140 mm Hg in 2015 by region. Source of data: Forounzafar et al., 2017.

High intake of sodium or table salt has been repeatedly associated with higher blood pressure and a higher risk for some cardiovascular diseases, particularly stroke. There is good evidence that limiting sodium intake to 2 g/d or even lower reduces blood pressure and results in less hypertension (WHO, 2012b). Reduced dietary intake of sodium has also been linked to lower risks for cardiovascular disease and death despite a weaker evidence base for this effect and a need for more high-quality research on this subject (Tuomilehto et al., 2001; WHO, 2012b; Cobb et al., 2014; He et al., 2014; Wong et al., 2016). The importance of preventive measures is underscored by the finding of the GBD 2015 that 29% of the DALYs related to SBP ≥ 110–115 mm Hg occurred in people with SBP between 110 mm and 140 mm Hg (Forounzafar et al., 2017).

High salt intake markedly exceeding the recommended amount is a global issue. Using data from 66 countries, global mean sodium intake in adults in 2010 was estimated at 3.95 g/d corresponding to about 10 g of table salt and ranging from 1.6 to 5.98 g/d (4 to 15 g of salt). Men had higher intakes than women across all regions (mean 4.14 g/d vs 3.77 g/d, respectively). Apart from the Sub-Saharan Region and some countries of Latin America, the Caribbean and Oceania, mean sodium intakes exceeded 3 g/d, with particularly high intakes (>4.5 g/d) observed in Central Asia, Eastern Asia, and high-income groups in the Asia Pacific. Intakes for the Eastern Mediterranean and North African Region were more variable, ranging from 2.1 to 5.4 g/d of sodium (5.2 to 13.5 g/d of salt). The lowest levels occurred in Sudan, Somalia and Djibouti, the highest in Bahrain and Tunisia (Powles et al., 2013).

More recent data based on urinary sodium excretion are available for 14 of the 22 countries of the WHO Eastern Mediterranean Region, of which six collected 24 h urine and 7 spot urine; Oman has both. Five of the countries had regional data only. Iran, Lebanon and Morocco also have recent estimates of salt intake in children and adolescents based on urinary sodium excretion, while Palestine has results only for school-age children but not for adults (Table 23) (Al-Jawaldeh et al., 2021b).

The reliability of data on sodium intake depends on the method used for assessment. As about 90% of the ingested sodium is excreted through the kidneys, measuring urinary sodium excretion is considered the best method to determine salt intake. In light of seasonal and diurnal fluctuations in sodium excretion, 24-hour urine samples are regarded as the gold standard to assess sodium intake, but assessment of spot urine samples presents a more convenient alternative both for investigators and study participants: it is applicable to larger samples, increases compliance with collection, and, at least at population level, shows a satisfactory level of accuracy (McLean, 2014).

Alternatively, salt intake can be estimated from dietary assessments, but the adequacy of this method depends on the availability of data on the salt content of foods that are often missing for regional dishes. Nevertheless, this method is required to identify the main dietary sources of sodium and salt. In this regard, it is important to ensure that data on the sodium contents of food, especially of processed foods and highly consumed dishes, is made available and kept up-to-date (WHO-EMRO, 2017b). Bahrain and Kuwait determined salt intake via dietary assessment only. For Bahrain, the survey that was conducted nationally and based on food frequency questionnaires (FFQs) and 24-hour recalls dates back to 1998–1999. Mean sodium intake was 5.3 g/d in men and 3.7 g/d in women, corresponding to 13.25 g and 9.25 g of salt respectively. The latest data from Kuwait, obtained through national surveys using questionnaires, are more recent, dating from 2014 and finding that the mean salt intakes in adults aged 18–69 years ranged from 9–15 g/d (Al-Jawaldeh et al., 2021b).

Table 23 Salt intake in adults, children, and adolescents in the countries of the WHO Eastern Mediterranean Region based on urinary Na excretion. Source: Al-Jawaldeh et al., 2021b unless otherwise indicated.

Country	Year	Method	Population	Salt intake (g/d)
Afghanistan[a]	2018	Spot urine analysis	Adults, 18–69 y	Total: 12.1 Men: 12.5 Women: 11.8
Egypt	2017–2018	Spot urine analysis	Adults, 15–69 y, national	Total: 8.9 Men: 9.5 Women: 8.1
Iran	2016	Spot urine analysis	Adults, ≥25 y, national	Total: 9.52 Men: 11.0 Women: 8.25
	2015	Spot urine analysis	Children, 9–15 y, regional (Shahroud)	Total: 9.7 Boys: 9.8 Girls: 9.3
Iraq	2015	24-hour urine analysis	Adults, ≥18 y, national	Total: 8.8* Men: 9.1* Women: 8.3*
Jordan	2019	Spot urine analysis	Adults, 18–69 y, regional (Amman)	Total: 11.0 Men: 12.5 Women: 9.6

Country	Year	Method	Population	Salt intake (g/d)
Lebanon	2014	24-hour urine analysis	Adults, regional (Beirut)	Total: 9.0 Men: 12.0 Women: 7.75
	2013–2014	Spot urine analysis	Children, 6–10 y, national	Total: 5.6
Morocco	2017–2018	Spot urine analysis	Adults, ≥18 y, national	Total: 10.6 Men: 11.9 Women: 9.3
	2015–2016	24-hour urine analysis	Children, 6–18 y, regional (Rabat region)	Total: 5.67 Boys: 5.55 Girls: 5.80
Oman	2017–2018	24-hour urine analysis	Adults, ≥18 y, national	Total: 9.0 Men: 9.6 Women: 8.7
	2017	Spot urine analysis	Adults, ≥18 y, national	Total: 8.6 Men: 9.5 Women: 7.4
Pakistan		24-hour urine analysis	Adults, ≥18 y, regional (Eastern Saudi Arabia)	Total: 8.64 Men: 9.24* Women: 6.55*
Palestine	2013	Spot urine analysis	Children, 7–12 y, national	Total: 7.0
Saudi Arabia	2009–2012	24-hour urine analysis	Adults, ≥14 y, regional	Total: 8.0 Men: 8.75 Women: 6.75

Country	Year	Method	Population	Salt intake (g/d)
Sudan	2016	Spot urine analysis	Adults, 18–69 y, national	Total: 8.2 Men: 8.2 Women: 8.2
Tunisia	2015	24-hour urine analysis	Adults, 24–64 y, regional (Bizerte)	Total: 8.1
United Arab Emirates	2015	24-hour urine analysis	Adults, 20–65 y, national	Total: 6.8

* Calculated (g salt/d = mmol Na per 24h/17.1).

Source: a) Ghimire et al., 2021.

Accordingly, reducing sodium and salt intake in the general population by 30% by the year 2025 is one of the targets of the WHO Global Action Plan for the Prevention and Control of NCDs 2013–2020 (WHO, 2013). The WHO strongly recommends a sodium intake of less than 2 g/d corresponding to less than 5 g/d of table salt from all sources. This level should be further reduced for children in accordance with their lower energy requirements compared to those of adults (WHO, 2012b). The reduction of salt intake is a highly efficient and cost-effective strategy in the fight against NCDs, particularly when the whole population is targeted. Mandatory reduction of salt content in processed foods, either by setting targets for the food manufacturers or by taxation of salty foods, has been found to be the most effective method and even more so when combined with other policies, such as information campaigns to raise public awareness about high salt intake and food labelling. A study modelling the effects and costs of 3 measures to reduce salt intake in 3 countries of the WHO Eastern Mediterranean Region (Palestine, Syria, and Tunisia) estimated that product reformulation could save 945 to 11,192 life years (Mason et al., 2014). Another modelling study from Bahrain found that interventions for salt reduction were most effective in fighting NCDs, with an estimated 44,023 healthy life-years gained and 5,467 premature deaths prevented over a 15-year period, in addition to economic and social gains from less absenteeism, higher work productivity and lower healthcare costs. In this model, salt reduction had the greatest return of investment with a factor of 7.15 even if only productivity was considered—it increased to 10.8 if social benefits were also included (Ministry of Health Bahrain et al., 2020).

Although leading to expenses for food producers, reformulation can be cost-saving due to benefits from lower healthcare expenditures and lower productivity losses exceeding the costs of the intervention. This is particularly true if it is part of a multifaceted approach. In turn, individual interventions targeting high-risk patients were found to be less cost-effective (Cobiac et al., 2013; Mason et al., 2014; Schorling et al., 2017).

With this in mind, the WHO issued the SHAKE Technical Package for salt reduction, providing a set of key measures to develop, implement and monitor salt reduction strategies, to assist member states in their efforts to reduce salt intake (Fig. 12). One of the 5 interventions proposed by the package focusses on the reformulation of industrially produced foods, providing assistance with the setting of targets for salt levels, the implementation of other strategies to prompt reformulation such as food labelling or taxations of foods not complying with the targets, as well as with the monitoring of the reformulation process (WHO, 2016b).

Evidence for the effectiveness of food reformulation to reduce salt intake comes from the United Kingdom, where a salt-reduction programme was started in 2003 following a report by the Committee on Medical Aspects on Food Policy (COMA) on Nutritional Aspects of Cardiovascular Disease in 1994 identifying excessive sodium and salt intake as a major contributor to hypertension.

To lower salt intake in the adult population from an average of 9 g/d to 6 g/d, voluntary reformulation of processed foods was targeted through close cooperation with the food industry to achieve a gradual reduction of salt content, with targets for around 80 different product categories to guide food producers (Public Health England, 2018). By 2008, salt content in pre-packaged bread had been reduced by over 30% and by 49% in breakfast cereals (Wyness et al., 2011). In 2014, salt intake measured by urinary analysis had declined by 11% to 8.0 g/d. An evaluation in 2017 still identified cereals and cereal products including bread as the main contributors to salt intake (29.5%) followed by meat

Surveillance	Measurement and monitoring of population salt consumption and salt content in foods, as well as monitoring and evaluation of the salt reduction programme.
Harness industry	Development of strategies to promote the reformulation of foods and meals to contain less salt, and setting of target levels for the salt content of foods.
Adopt standards for labelling and marketing	Implementation of standards for effective and accurate labelling by adopting interpretive front-of-pack labelling systems. Regulation of the marketing of food to prevent misleading advertising of foods high in salt.
Knowledge	Implementation of education and communication strategies to raise awareness about the health risks and dietary sources of salt to change dietary behaviour.
Environment	Implementation of strategies to promote healthy eating in community settings like schools, workplaces and hospitals.

Fig. 12 The SHAKE Technical Package for salt reduction. Based on WHO, 2016b.

products (27.3%) and found that across all product groups, retailers were more compliant with the targets than brand manufacturers (73% vs. 37% of average targets for salt levels met). Foods from the out-of-home sector were found to be saltier with maximum targets for salt level satisfied in 75% of the products compared to 89% of in-home products by retailers and 77% of in-home products by manufacturers (Public Health England, 2018).

The reduction of salt intake is also a high priority in the WHO Eastern Mediterranean Region. Eleven countries have set targets for salt intake at population level: Bahrain, Jordan, Kuwait, Oman, Qatar and Saudi Arabia have adopted a level of 5 g per day, as recommended by the WHO, while Egypt, Iran, Tunisia and the United Arab Emirates aim at a 30% relative reduction in salt intake, and Morocco a 10% reduction. The WHO Regional Office for the Eastern Mediterranean Region organized a series of multi-stakeholder technical meetings dedicated to population salt reduction strategies, leading to the development of policy guidance with actions for a progressive and sustainable reduction of national salt intake by 25% within 3–4 years, which was recommended to member states. They also set up a monitoring mechanism and a regional protocol on 24-hour urinary sodium measurements (Al-Jawaldeh et al., 2018a).

At the beginning of any food reformulation policy, it is necessary to identify major sources of salt in the diet and determine the baseline levels of salt in these foods. Assessment of salt content in food was done in 16 countries of the Eastern Mediterranean Region, Bahrain, Egypt, Iran, Iraq, Jordan, Kuwait, Lebanon, Morocco, Oman, Pakistan, Palestine, Qatar, the Kingdom of Saudi Arabia, Tunisia, the United Arab Emirates and Yemen. Bread was identified as a major source of salt intake. Salt content in bread varies across the region, having been found to range from 0.28 to 1.55 g per 100 g wet weight in diverse bread types with a mean of 0.76 g/100 (Al-Jawaldeh & Al-Khamaiseh, 2018). However, because its consumption is generally high in the region, bread can contribute significantly to salt intake even at lower salt concentrations. Processed foods also are a major source of sodium in the region as evidenced by data from Lebanon reporting a share of 67% (Almedawar et al., 2015). Despite some variation in the importance of single food groups between countries depending on cultural and dietary habits, bread and cereal products play a major role, followed by dairy foods including cheese and labneh (strained yogurt) and in some countries also sauces, condiments, salted fish and meat products (Almedawar et al., 2014; Al-Jawaldeh et al., 2018a). A study from Morocco also found high salt contents in common fast foods like pizza and sandwiches, especially per serving (El-Kardi et al., 2017).

As of 2021, salt reduction initiatives have been implemented or planned in 14 countries of the Eastern Mediterranean Region: Bahrain, Egypt, Iran, Iraq, Jordan, Kuwait, Lebanon, Morocco, Oman, Palestine, Qatar, the Kingdom of Saudi Arabia, Tunisia and the United Arab Emirates. It was mentioned that Djibouti and Sudan are planning strategies but clear evidence is lacking (Al-Jawaldeh et al., 2021). These initiatives generally include the setting of targets for salt content, or determining the extent of salt reduction for specific food groups that contribute markedly to the population's salt intake (see Table 24). All countries that have already implemented policies, or are planning to do so, have at least included bread in the list of affected foods, with some, such as Iran, Jordan, the Gulf Cooperation Council member states and Tunisia, also targeting other commonly consumed salt-rich foods. While the Government takes the leading role in all countries except Lebanon, partnerships have been established with the food industry and support is offered to food manufacturers—like in Egypt, where voluntary training for bakery personnel on a 20% reduction of salt content in bread is part of the programme, or in Bahrain where workshops have been held for bakers, caterers and other food suppliers (Al-Jawaldeh et al., 2021b). In 8 countries, the targets are mandatory.

Several countries that have implemented programmes on salt reduction in foods are pursuing monitoring activities. In Bahrain, Egypt, Iran, Jordan, Kuwait, Oman, Qatar, Tunisia and the United Arab Emirates, national multisectoral committees were charged with this task. In Bahrain, a monitoring system for bakery products is currently planned and an assessment of the nutritional profile of the 200 most commonly consumed products is envisaged, but is still in a pilot phase (Ministry of Health, Bahrain et al., 2020).

The results of surveillance programmes are available for some countries. Additionally, there are some smaller regional studies on the salt contents of bread and also other foods.

In Iran, a study assessed the salt content of the 5 most popular traditional bread types in 2018. A total of 925 samples were randomly collected in 5 Iranian cities and the analysed for their salt content. Mean salt content was 1.38 g/100 g and it was found that only 27.6% of the samples met the target level of the Iranian Institute of Standards and Industrial Research (ISIRI). Both findings suggest a lower compliance than in 2016, when the mean content was 1.02 g/100 g and 47.2% of samples met the ISIRI criteria (Hadian et al., 2021). However, a regional investigation in two Iranian provinces also dating from 2016 revealed a mean salt content of 1.95% in 5 bread varieties, higher than the allowed level of 1.8% at that time, and maximum levels as high as 4.17% (Aalipour, 2019). A low compliance rate with the latest national standard for salt in bread was also found in samples (n=59) taken in 95 bakeries in the county of Garmsar in Northern Iran, with only 16.3% containing <1% of salt. The mean salt content was 1.37% with variations between the four bread types analysed (Abolli et al., 2021).

Table 24 Policies on the reduction of salt in bread and other selected food sources in countries of the WHO Eastern Mediterranean Region.

Country	Food	Target(s) for salt content	Year	Leading institution	Legal basis
Bahrain	Traditional Arabic bread	20% annual reduction for 5 years until reaching 0.5% salt on a dry flour basis	2018	Government, Ministry of Health	Mandatory
Egypt	Subsidized Baladi bread	30% reduction	2017	Government (Ministry of Health and Population)	Mandatory
	All types of bread	1.8%	2015	Government	Mandatory
		1.0%	2018		
Iran	Common canned foods, salty snacks	Setting of maximum levels	2015		Mandatory
	Dairy products	Reduction from 4 to 3% in cheese, reduction from 1 to 0.8% in dough, ban of salt in probiotic yogurt			Mandatory
Iraq	Bread	Setting of maximum levels		Government	
	Arabic bread	<1% of dry weight	2019	Government	Mandatory
Jordan	Highly consumed foods (e.g., cheese)	Revise existing legislation to set targets for salt content		Government	
	Pita bread, other types of bread	20% reduction in 2 steps that was achieved until August 2013	2013		Voluntary
Kuwait	Cheese	Revision of salt standard			Voluntary
	Salty snacks	≤1.5%	2017	Government	Voluntary

3.4 Reformulating Food Products

Country	Food	Target(s) for salt content	Year	Leading institution	Legal basis
Lebanon	Bread	Standards to be proposed to the Parliament	2012	Academia and government	Voluntary
Morocco	Bread	Roadmap on the gradual reduction of salt content in bread issued in 2016	2015	Government, Ministry of Health	Voluntary
Oman	Bread	Gradual reduction of salt content by 20% starting in late 2015 in the main three bakeries supplying most of the bread in the country

Since May 2019: 0.5% for Arabic flat bread and of 1% for other bread types (e.g., sliced bread or French bread) | 2019 | Government, Ministry of Commerce and Industry | Mandatory since May 2019 (after a voluntary phase since late 2015) |
| | Other food products | 30% reduction of salt | planned | | |
| Palestine | Bread | Gradual reduction of salt content

Targets set by year: 2019: 0.9%,

2021: 0.8%,

2022: 0.7%

2023: 0.6% | 2019 | Government, Ministry of Health | Mandatory |

Country	Food	Target(s) for salt content	Year	Leading institution	Legal basis
Qatar	Bread	20% reduction of salt in bread already initiated in the main national and other bakeries of the country. Target: reduction to <0.8% of salt	2013	Government, Ministry of Public Health	Mandatory
	Other foods	Targets for salt levels to be set in meetings with the food industry	2019	Government, Ministry of Public Health	Voluntary
	Bread, all types	1.0%	2018	Government, Saudi Food and Drug Authority	Mandatory
	Yogurt drink	1.0 g/100 ml	2018	Government, Saudi Food and Drug Authority	Mandatory
Saudi Arabia	22 products incl. cheeses, butter and fat spreads, pasta, meats, canned fish, vegetables, beans, and soups, ready meals, pizza, cakes, biscuits, chips, table and cooking sauces, potato products, flavour enhancers and beverage powders[a]	Recommended limits for salt content[a)]	2018	Government, Saudi Food and Drug Authority	Voluntary

Country	Food	Target(s) for salt content	Year	Leading institution	Legal basis
Tunisia	Bread	Progressive reduction of salt by 30%	2015	Government, Ministry of Health	Voluntary
	Other foods	Proposal for reformulation of foods to reduce salt content	2018	Government, Ministry of Health	Planned
United Arab Emirates	Bread	<0.5%	2017	Government (Ministry of Health and Promotion)	Voluntary
	Other foods including pickles, cheeses, fast foods, snacks and other processed food	Task force on reducing salt contents	2017	Government (Ministry of Health and Promotion)	Voluntary

[a] Bin Sunaid et al., 2021.

In another study, the salt content of various industrially and non-industrially produced processed foods including tomato paste and sauces, canned vegetables, pickles and nuts were evaluated, with samples taken in 2016 and 2018 to compare the findings. Overall, compliance with the ISIRI standard—that is, 1.5–2.0% for canned vegetables, tomato paste and tomato sauce, 1.9% for nuts and seeds, and 4% for pickles—was higher in 2016 than in 2018. While all samples of canned vegetables met the target in 2016, this was true for 96% in 2018. The same percentage was found for pickles in 2018, when all industrial products complied but less than 80% of the artisanal ones did so. Salt content in nuts and seeds varied widely, and again compliance was higher in the industrial products than in the non-industrial products, of which 88% in 2016 and 72% in 2018 had salt levels according to the standards. The lowest compliance was observed for tomato paste and sauce, being 83% in 2016 but only 48% in 2018. Non-industrial products were only included in 2018 and their compliance was 40% (Zendeboodi et al., 2020).

Monitoring in Kuwait revealed that salt content in bread, most of which (80%) is produced locally by one large bakery, had been reduced by 12–16% only instead of the targeted 20% mostly because of technical issues with regards to texture and taste. Insufficient compliance was also found for corn and potato crisps, of which only 35% fulfilled the target of not more than 1.5% of salt (Al-Jawaldeh et al., 2021b).

Two studies in Morocco evaluated the knowledge of bakers about the national salt reduction strategy and their understanding of the measure. The first from 2018 included 432 bakeries all-over the country, of which more than half (59%) were artisanal, and found that only about a quarter (26.6%) of the bakers interviewed had heard about the initiative, mostly through the media. While all respondents knew of the negative health effects of high salt intake, the contribution of bread as a source of salt was underestimated, with most bakers thinking that fast food was the main source. No major differences were observed between artisanal and industrial bakeries. None of the bakers had been informed of the planned progressive reduction of salt content in bread by 10% per year started in 2015 and accordingly, none had adopted it. However, almost all (89.6%) expressed willingness to do so in the coming 2 years, even though some (7.2%) feared a loss of consumers. This fear was observed more among artisanal than in industrial bakers (11% vs. 1.7%, n.s.) whereas commitment was slightly higher among industrial companies (90.4% vs. 85.8% (Bouhamida et al., 2020).

Another study from Morocco showed that bread with a salt content reduced by 10% to 23% was actually preferred by the participants of the investigation, compared to the bread with a salt level of 17.42 g per kg of flour, corresponding to the average salt content of white bread in Morocco. The regular bread was rated as too salty by 75.6% of the study participants. Breads with their salt content reduced by 10%, 16% or 23% (corresponding to a salt content of 15.68 g, 14.63 g or 13.41 g per kg of flour, respectively) were each liked by over 70% of the respondents. The bread with 23% less salt was most frequently rated as just about right in terms of its saltiness (by 74.8% of the participants). Notably, bread with 30% less salt was liked by about half the respondents (51.7%) and found to have adequate saltiness by a third. Consumers' willingness to buy was highest for the bread with 16% and 23% less salt (Guennoun et al., 2019). This shows that a salt reduction of 30%, as intended in most countries of the EMR with salt reduction policies, is acceptable for consumers, especially if it is done gradually.

A study from 2018 conducted in Oman evaluated the salt content in 26 pre-packaged bread types sold in Muscat using the nutrition information on the labels. The mean sodium content was 318.15 mg per 100 g, corresponding to 0.79 g salt. Compared to the findings of an earlier study from 2015 analysing a total of 15 samples of 3vdifferent bread types that had a mean sodium content of 355.89 mg per 100 g (0.89 g of salt) this shows a reduction by 10.6%. However, the authors remarked that pre-packaged bread is not the most consumed bread in Oman, where fresh bread from bakeries is preferred. Moreover, not all pre-packaged bread bore nutrition labels, limiting the number of samples (Alhamad et al., 2015; AbuKhader et al., 2020).

In Lebanon, a study conducted in 2019 assessed salt content in 30 popular traditional dishes. The mean sodium content was 416.08 mg per 100 g, equivalent to 1.04 g salt. Thus, the majority (67%) of the dishes contained a high amount of salt. The percentage contribution of 100 g of each traditional dish to the mean daily requirement of salt in a 2000-kcal diet ranged between 12.8%-35.5% (Hoteit et al., 2020).

In Qatar, the Ministry of Public Health regularly collects bread samples that are analysed in its Central Food Laboratory for their salt content to detect deviations from the target of 0.8% (Al-Jawaldeh et al., 2021b). An earlier survey conducted in the city of Casablanca in 2011 and 2016 assessed the effect of the awareness campaigns on knowledge, attitudes and practice (KAP) regarding the amount of salt used by bakers in 418 bakeries, and analysed the salt content of samples of commercial white bread from 160 bakeries.

An evaluation in 2019 in Saudi Arabia, where monitoring falls under the responsibility of the Saudi Food and Drug Authority (SFDA), found that, based on the values indicated on the nutrition labels, 85% of 297 included bread products complied with the mandatory target for salt content of 1%. However, compliance with the voluntary targets for other food categories was lower, only reaching 47% on average. No ready meal met the recommended salt level and, in many other categories, the share of compliant products was less than 50% (Bin Sunaid et al., 2021).

In Tunisia, the feasibility of and consumer reaction to salt reduction in bread was tested in a pilot study in the city of Bizerte with the voluntary participation of 22 of the 42 bakeries of the town. Starting from an initial level of 1.7 g/100 g, mean salt content was reduced by 35% to 1.1 g/100 g after 3 months and remained at this concentration for the rest of the intervention, which lasted for 3 years. In parallel, 184 consumers participated in an evaluation of the perception of bread saltiness in the first 3 months of the study. Salt content was reduced up to 40%. The saltiness of bread with 30% less salt than the initial level was perceived as normal by 79% of the participants, however a 40% reduction was noticed by 97%. This shows that a 30% reduction is very feasible and acceptable to consumers (El Ati et al., 2021).

Potential obstacles to the implementation of the salt reduction policy were studied in an evaluation conducted in 2018 in Iran, using interviews with stakeholders such as bakers, a representative from Iran's Flour Industries Union, health inspectors, staff of the monitoring units, policy-makers, employees of the Ministry of Health and Education, the Ministry of Agriculture and the Iranian National Standards Organization as well as academic personnel. It was found that the top-down approach of the policy was perceived as a problem and that bakers would have appreciated greater involvement in the development and implementation of the initiative. This was augmented by the fact that bakers felt isolated in dealing with the technical issues arising from salt reduction with regards to dough structure and fermentation. For example, it was observed that salt content varied with the seasons, with a higher compliance with the salt standard of 1% in the second half of the year rather than in the first (71% vs. 52% of samples). Insufficient flour quality was another cause for non-compliance. This was seen as a serious issue, especially in combination with lack of technology and skilled personnel to implement the necessary changes, and fears were voiced by the Iranian National Standards Organization that unauthorized and potentially harmful salt substitutes might be used that are difficult to trace in the bread. Moreover, there was some confusion about the exact protocol for measuring the salt content in bread. It was concluded that, among other measures, better training of bakers and their involvement in the adaptation of the policy would contribute to its successful implementation (Loloei et al., 2019).

So far, there have been no evaluations of the health effects of salt reduction in foods in the Eastern Mediterranean Region. However, a regional study from Iran investigated the effects of salt reduction in bread on blood pressure in 2 cities in in South-Eastern Iran, of which one served as the intervention centre and the other as a control. Over a 4-week period, the salt content of bread was gradually reduced by 40% (from 1.5% to 0.9%) accompanied by educational measures including the placing of banners and posters in public places and the distribution of brochures informing selected households about the harmful effects of high salt intake. The latter was the only intervention in the control city. Urinary sodium excretion and blood pressure were measured at the beginning of the study and after twelve weeks. Salt intake decreased by about 10% in intervention city compared to about 5% in the control city. Mean systolic blood pressure declined by 6.2 mm Hg (about 5%) and this decrease was significantly greater than in the control city where only a slight reduction was observed (-1.1 mm Hg, about 1%). A small reduction was also observed for diastolic blood pressure in the intervention city, but the difference to the control group was not significant. When asked about the reasons for adding excessive salt to their bread, bakers mentioned the poor quality of flour as the main reason (Jafari et al., 2016).

Despite a number of achievements in many countries of the WHO Eastern Mediterranean Region, further efforts are needed to obtain a permanent reduction of salt intake and of salt content in processed foods. This is particularly the case in countries that have so far not taken any steps in this direction, including Afghanistan, Libya, Somalia, Sudan and Yemen. In Pakistan, the Provinces of Punjab and Sindh have regulations for maximum salt levels in some foods, including some biscuits and other fine bakery goods, canned meat, potato chips, and fat spreads, but not for bread. While these countries face a high level of malnutrition, the prevalence of NCDs is increasing as well. Despite a scarcity of data on salt intake, there is evidence of excessive levels from Afghanistan and Pakistan. Moreover, there is a need for increased monitoring and evaluation activities to ensure the correct implementation of salt standards in foods and to investigate the effects of the policies on population salt intake and health indicators like blood pressure and the prevalence of hypertension.

3.4.3 Eliminating Trans-Fatty Acids in Food

Trans fatty acids (TFAs) are another group of nutrients associated with negative health effects. TFAs are unsaturated fatty acids that differ from the commonly occurring cis-form in that they have one or more double bonds in the trans configuration, meaning that both adjacent carbon atoms are located on opposite sides of the molecules. In turn, the cis-configuration that is predominant in fatty acids in most plants and animals creates a kink in the molecule that is missing in TFAs (see Fig. 13). If TFAs are integrated in membranes, their straight structure causes a tighter packing, reducing the fluidity of the membrane. They also have higher melting points, a property that makes them attractive for industrial food production. For instance, the TFA elaidic acid is solid at room temperature, contrary to its cis-isomer oleic acid which is the major fatty acid in olive oil. There are two main food sources for TFAs: while they occur naturally in fat from ruminants including milk and meat fat, the greatest amount stems from industrial partially hydrogenated fats that are used in the production of processed foods. Both kinds of TFAs differ in their composition, with vaccenic acid dominating in ruminant TFAs and elaidic acid in industrial TFAs (Pfeuffer & Jahreis, 2018; Oteng

& Kersten, 2020). Unlike sodium and sugars that still have nutritional value when consumed in moderation, industrial TFAs are always detrimental to health. However, the effects of natural TFAs are less well known. Recent evidence suggests some positive effects. Moreover, their concentration in dairy and meat fat is small (Guillocheau et al., 2019).

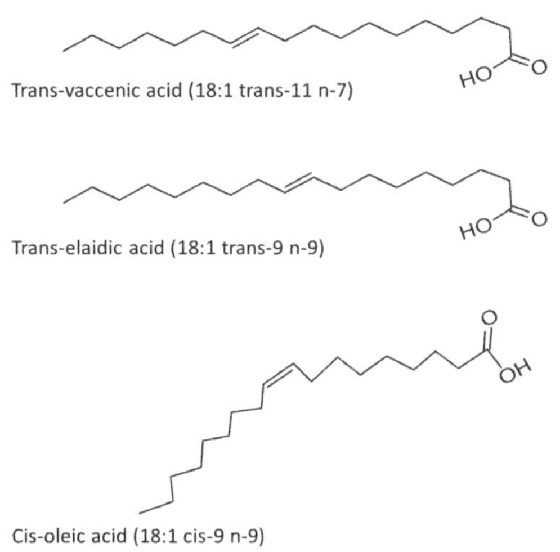

Trans-vaccenic acid (18:1 trans-11 n-7)

Trans-elaidic acid (18:1 trans-9 n-9)

Cis-oleic acid (18:1 cis-9 n-9)

Fig. 13 Structure of common trans-fatty acids compared to the cis-unsaturated oleic acid.

In turn, processed foods like fast foods, some bakery goods including biscuits, cakes and pastries, and deep-fried products were found to contain as much as 60% of their total fat as TFAs (Stender et al., 2008). Partial hydrogenation of liquid oils serves to generate solid or semi-solid fats that show increased oxidative stability, extended shelf-life, and specific sensoric properties. These attributes, together with their low cost, make them useful for the industrial processing of foods. In the 1950s to 1970s, the use of partially hydrogenated oils as a cheap replacement for animal fats increased after the negative health effects of saturated fatty acids (SFAs) had been discovered (Stender et al., 2008; WHO, 2021a). However, TFAs increase the risk of coronary heart disease and cause hyper- and dyslipidaemia to a higher degree than SFAs by raising total and LDL cholesterol and simultaneously lowering HDL cholesterol, making them more atherogenic than other fatty acids

(Oteng & Kersten, 2020). They were also associated with increased inflammatory reactions, endothelial dysfunction, insulin resistance, diabetes mellitus type II, steatohepatitis, and oxidative stress (Oteng & Kersten, 2020).

Increasing energy intake from TFAs by 2% (about 4g for 2000 kcal) was associated with a 29% higher risk for coronary heart disease (CHD) in a meta-analysis of 4 prospective cohort and 3 retrospective case-control studies (Micha & Mozaffarian, 2009). Based on the convincing evidence for the higher risk of CHD from TFAs in partially hydrogenated vegetable oils (PHO), the earlier recommendation to keep TFA intake as low as possible and preferably below 1% of total energy (corresponding to 2 g/d for a total energy intake of 2000 kcal) issued by the WHO/FAO in its technical report series 916 from 2003 (WHO/FAO, 2003, Uauy et al., 2009) was retained and has since been adopted by many other nutrition and public health entities.

In 2003, Denmark was the first country worldwide to impose a limit of 2 g industrially produced TFAs per 100 g of total fat for all foods, including those for out-of-home consumption, and to ban the production and use of partially hydrogenated oil. Other countries followed this example, with 10 doing so by 2018. In the same year, the elimination of TFAs in foods until 2023 was identified as one of the priority targets of the 13th General Programme of Work to guide the work of the World Health Organization over the period of 2019–2023. To assist member countries in this endeavour, the WHO released the REPLACE action framework, consisting of a set of 6 multisectoral strategic actions (Fig. 14) (WHO, 2021a).

The best practice policy is considered to be a combination of a mandatory national limit of industrially produced TFAs to 2 g per 100 g of total fat in all foods, with a mandatory national ban on the production or use of partially hydrogenated oil as an ingredient. However, many countries have less restrictive TFA limits, implementing the 2% limit only for industrially produced TFAs in oils and fats, with a higher limit of 5% for TFAs in other foods, or setting a limit of 5% for industrially produced TFAs in oils and fats only.

Other complementary measures include the mandatory declaration of TFAs on nutrition labels, the inclusion of TFAs on front-of-pack labelling

3.4 Reformulating Food Products

to facilitate healthier choices for consumers, as well as the reformulation of processed foods to reduce TFA content. The implementation of TFA limits can also be restricted to specific settings like school canteens. (WHO, 2021a).

Much progress has been made, especially since May 2020, so that in 2021, 57 countries worldwide had implemented or passed mandatory TFA policies of which 40 had adopted best-practice policies, protecting 3.2 billion people and 1.4 billion people respectively.

The introduction of these measures, even on a voluntary basis, was associated with a reduction of the contents of TFAs in foods and of their consumption level. In Denmark, the percentage of products with TFA contents exceeding 2% of total fat declined from 26% in 2002/2003 to 6% in 2012/2013. In 2012/2013, transgressions of the law occurred only in cookies and biscuits (Ministry of Food, Agriculture and Fisheries of Denmark, 2014).

Fig. 14 The REPLACE Action Package of the WHO. Based on WHO, 2021a.

The introduction of mandatory regulations against TFAs in Austria, New York, Canada and Argentina also entailed a decrease of TFA concentration in dietary fats and other major food sources, as did the voluntary approaches pursued in different European countries (Stender et al., 2012; Restrepo & Rieger, 2016a; Hyseni et al., 2017; Grabovac et al., 2018; Kakisu et al., 2018). In Denmark and New York City, TFA reductions in food were accompanied by decreases in cardiovascular mortality although this could not be confirmed for the Austrian population (Restrepo & Rieger, 2016a; Restrepo & Rieger, 2016b; Grabovac et al., 2018).

However, the implementation of best-practice policies has so far been concentrated in high-income or upper-middle-income countries. Thirty-one of the 40 (77.5%) belong to the European Union or the European Economic Area, where Regulation (EU) 2019/649 limiting industrially produced TFAs to 2% of total fat in all food products came into effect in April 2021 (European Commission, 2019). In turn, only 2 lower-middle-income countries (India and the Philippines) have passed policies for the elimination of TFAs and 3 others (Bangladesh, Nigeria and Sri Lanka) are expected to pass their policies soon. Just 3 low-income countries (Afghanistan, Chad and Ethiopia) have any measures or policy commitments in place to eliminate TFAs in food. In the African region, only South Africa has implemented a best-practice policy, but national plans on nutrition or to reduce NCDs that also focus on the elimination of industrially produced TFAs exist in 12 countries, and planning and discussion about strategies are currently underway in some other countries (Fig. 15) (WHO, 2021b).

In the WHO Eastern Mediterranean Region, the Kingdom of Saudi Arabia is the only country that has fully implemented a best-practice policy. The Gulf Cooperation Council (GCC) agreed on a limit of 2% of total fat for TFAs in vegetable oils and soft spreadable margarines, and of 5% of total fat in other foods in 2015. For this regulation to come into effect in a GCC member State, it must be approved by the relevant country. This has so far been done by Bahrain, Kuwait, Saudi Arabia and the United Arab Emirates in 2016 and 2017, while the implementation process has been initiated in Oman and Qatar.

Iran was the first country to address the issue of TFAs by assessing dietary TFA intake and content in foods within the frame of a national consumption survey in 2000, and by reducing the limit of TFA content in oils from less than 20% to less than 10% in 2005.

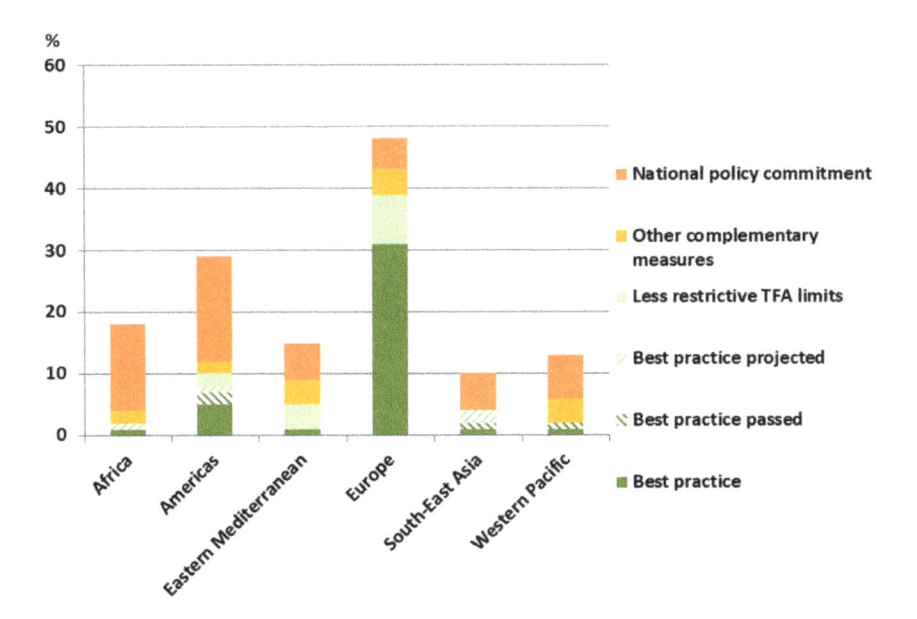

Fig. 15 Number of countries by WHO region with mandatory policies for the elimination of TFAs in food. Best practice: Legislative or regulatory measures limiting industrially produced TFAs to 2 g per 100 g of total fat in all foods and settings and imposing a ban on the production and use of PHO as an ingredient in all foods. Other complementary measures: legislative or other measures that facilitate healthier choices with regards to industrially produced TFAs for consumers (like mandatory declaration of TFA on nutrition labels, front-of-pack labelling systems including TFAs, or product reformulation) or impose mandatory limits on industrially produced TFAs in foods in specific settings like public schools only. National policy commitment: national policies, strategies or action plans expressing a commitment to reduce industrially produced TFAs in the food supply. Source of data: WHO, 2021b.

Other countries have mandatory limits for TFAs in certain foods: Morocco imposes a threshold of 2% in oils and fats, and of 5% of total fat in snacks, biscuits and cakes; Palestine sets it at 2 g/100 g in prepared foods. In Pakistan, vanaspati ghee, margarine, butter and oil products should not contain more than 5% of TFAs, while the province of Punjab has a stricter limit of 0.5% in vanaspati, margarines, fat spreads and shortening, and of 3% of total fat in milk formula. An overview of policies in the countries of the WHO EMR is shown in Table 25.

A number of countries mandate the labelling of TFAs on foods including the Gulf Council member states, Iran, Jordan and the province of Punjab in Pakistan (Al-Jawaldeh et al., 2021c).

Table 25 Mandatory limits, bans and labelling of trans-fats in foods in the countries of the WHO Eastern Mediterranean Region in 2021. Source of data: WHO, 2021b.

Policy category	Policy measures	Countries
Best practice	TFA limit of 2% of total fat in all foods. Ban on production and use of partially hydrogenated oils	Saudi Arabia
Less restrictive TFA limits	TFA limits of 2% in oils, fats and fat spreads, 2% of total fat in biscuits, 5% in shortening for bakery products	Iran
	TFA limits of 2% of total fat in vegetable oils and soft spreadable margarines, and 5% of total fat in other foods (GCC GSO standard)	Bahrain, Kuwait, United Arab Emirates
Other complementary measures	Mandatory labelling of TFAs on food packaging	Bahrain, Iran, Jordan, Kuwait, Oman, Pakistan (Punjab), Qatar, Saudi Arabia, UAE
	Mandatory limits of TFAs in certain settings and foods	Morocco, Pakistan
	Technical regulations for food reformulation	Jordan, Tunisia
National policy commitment to eliminate TFA	Implementation of GCC GSO standard initiated	Oman, Qatar
	Draft of a roadmap for action on industrial TFA elimination	Egypt
	Establishment of a working group for drafting a best-practice policy	Pakistan
	Advocacy for the implementation of a ban on the production and importation of industrial TFAs	Tunisia

Intakes of TFAs have been found to be very high in many countries of the Eastern Mediterranean Region, even though only 9 of the 22 countries (41%) had reliable estimates of TFA intake at population level based on dietary assessment or food consumption data, as established in a recent review of TFA reduction initiatives in the region (Al-Jawaldeh et al., 2021c). Intakes at the national level ranged from 0.34% of energy intake (EI) in Morocco to 6.5% EI in Egypt. High levels were also observed in Pakistan (5.7% EI) and Iran (4.2% EI) even though the latter value dates from the year 2007 and a more recent study from 2020 found a mean intake level of 0.7% EI. In Lebanon and Tunisia, intake was reported separately for genders, amounting to 2.4% EI in men and 2.3% EI in women and 0.1% in both sexes, respectively. For Jordan, a mean TFA intake of 0.2–0.4% EI was deduced from household budget surveys. For Sudan and the United Arab Emirates, only regional data was available. In North and South Sudan, mean TFA intake in adult women was 0.1% EI. Male and female students from the University of Sharjah, UAE, consumed 1.1% EI and 1.0% EI as TFAs. Few data were available for TFA intake in children and adolescents. Intakes of 2.2% EI in girls and about 2.3% in boys were reported from Iran, while in Jordan, 6–18-year-old children were estimated to consume between 0.8 and 1.3 g TFA per day. For Lebanese children aged 5–10 years an average TFA intake level of 0.16 g per day was observed (Al-Jawaldeh et al., 2021c).

High TFA intake in the region contributes to the significant death toll from CHD. According to estimates based on the Global Burden of Disease Study 2019, the contribution of high TFA intake to age-standardized deaths and DALYs is highest in the North Africa and Middle Eastern Region (Afshin et al., 2019). Based on this data, Egypt has the highest estimated proportion of CHD-related deaths attributable to TFA intake over 0.5% (8.4% of deaths) and Iran is third (7.0% of deaths) (WHO, 2021b). This underlines the importance of reducing TFAs in the food chain.

Regular monitoring is crucial to ensure the compliance of the food industry. So far, surveillance activities have been established in Iran and in 4 of the 6 GCC countries (Bahrain, Kuwait, Qatar and Saudi Arabia). In Iran, the Food and Drug Administration is in charge of post-marketing surveillance performed on an annual basis, comprising the analytical determination of TFAs in edible oils and fats, including consumer edible vegetable oil, frying oil, regular and fat-reduced margarine and shortening.

In addition, TFA content in bakery products, biscuits and confectionary products is controlled by the Iranian National Standards Organization (INSO) (Al-Jawaldeh et al., 2021c). An evaluation of traditional Iranian sweets showed that the TFA concentration in some products exceeded the permissible level of 2% of total fat, with 2 types of baked goods reaching 7.8% and 7.9%, respectively. In 81.8% of the samples, the TFA levels indicated on the nutrition labels differed from the actual TFA levels determined by chemical analysis (Ghazavi et al., 2020).

In Bahrain, TFA content is monitored in fats and oils and bakery goods through direct chemical analyses, and the correct listing and proper labelling of TFAs on locally produced and imported pre-packaged products is controlled (Al-Jawaldeh et al., 2021c).

In the Kingdom of Saudi Arabia, monitoring and inspection of locally produced and imported foods falls within the scope of the Saudi Food and Drug Authority (SFDA) in collaboration with the Ministry of Municipal and Rural Affairs. Samples are chemically analysed in SFDA laboratories (Al-Jawaldeh et al., 2021c).

In Kuwait, the National Technical Food Committee is responsible for monitoring the implementation of the national TFA standards and evaluating the compliance of food manufacturers. The latter is done through chemical analyses of TFA concentrations in randomly selected samples of potential food sources with typically high TFA contents, in collaboration with the food laboratory of the Ministry of Health. The accuracy of the declaration of TFA contents on the nutrition labels is also monitored. The Department of Standards and Inspection conducted a capacity-building program to train the inspectors and ensure the compliance of the food industry with the various GSO standards and technical regulations, including Trans-Fatty Acids (GSO 2483/2015), the Requirements of Nutritional Labelling (GSO 2233/2012 and the Nutritional and Health Claims Requirements (GSO 2333/2013) (Al-Jawaldeh et al., 2021c).

In Qatar, the Health Promotion and NCD Section of the Public Health Department at the Ministry of Public Health, having developed guidelines for school canteens, cafeterias and vending machines in all healthcare settings and workplaces as part of the Workplace Wellness Program, conducts annual evaluations in public settings that are implementing the guidelines (Al-Jawaldeh et al., 2021c).

In Iran, where action to reduce TFAs in oils was started early, the measures have already shown some effects. Following the reduction of the allowed amount of TFAs in edible oils from 20% to <10% in 2005, the average content of TFAs in oils declined from 27–29% in 2002–2003 and 31% in 2004–2005 to 5.6% in 2008 (Peymani et al., 2012). Analyses of fats and oils sampled by the Iranian Post Marketing Surveillance in households in 6 Iranian provinces showed that the TFA content of edible oils was below 5% (Esmaeili et al., 2014) and a decline in various oil and fat types was also observed by the Iranian Food and Drug Administration (Amerzadeh & Takian, 2020). The intake at population level decreased from 4.2% EI on average in 2001–2003 before the introduction of policies for TFA reduction to 0.7% EI in 2018 (Amerzadeh & Takian, 2020).

As policies to reduce TFAs in foods have been introduced more recently in other countries in the region, there is no data yet to evaluate the effects of these measures. However, in the United Arab Emirates, estimated TFA intake in female university students was found to have fallen from 1.7% EI in 2014 to 1% EI in 2017–2018 after the adoption of policies to reduce TFAs (Al-Jawaldeh et al., 2021c).

An inspection of the compliance of 1117 food manufacturers (37% local manufacturers) with the Saudi Food and Drug Authority's Technical Regulation on trans fats (SFDA.FD 2483) in July 2020 revealed that 7% had non-compliant products. In 20% of the 2,697 evaluated products, including margarine, cheese, various baked goods, chocolate, ice cream and others, TFA-containing ingredients were not listed in the product information. Additionally, the nutritional information on the nutrient labels of some of these products differed from the composition measured in the chemical analysis conducted during the study (Bin Sunaid et al., 2021). A survey in 2018 found that over 94% of the 400 tested food samples complied with the TFA limits of 2% in fats and oils and of 5% of fat in all other foods (NCD Alliance). An evaluation of the compliance with labelling requirements in Saudi Arabia in 2016–2017 reported that 2% of 1143 food products for which full ingredients were indicated listed partially hydrogenated fat, and less than 5% contained hydrogenated fat specified as trans-fat. However, this survey predates the enactment of the ban on partially hydrogenated oil in Saudi Arabia in December 2018 (Jradi et al., 2020).

3.4.4 Future Needs and Further Steps in Food Reformulation

Many countries in the WHO Eastern Mediterranean Region have identified the reformulation of frequently consumed foods that are major contributors to the intake of critical nutrients like salt, TFAs and sugar as an important tool to make diets healthier. Particular targets are salt and TFAs, for which the majority of the countries of the region already have defined targets for the permitted maximum levels in foods or intend to set them. Less progress has been made with regards to sugar despite a high intake level in the region (Al-Jawaldeh et al., 2018b). So far, most initiatives are based on voluntary pledges by the food industry. Such agreements are, for example, part of the Healthy Food Strategy launched by the Kingdom of Saudi Arabia and have been signed by a number of large international food companies, including Mars, Kellogg's and Nestlé (Food Navigator Asia).

Major barriers to successful food reformulation are technical issues and high expenses that may not be covered by the income generated by the product. Indeed, manufacturers often fear that reformulated products could be disliked by consumers so that they switch to another brand offering a conventional alternative. Setting mandatory standards that all producers have to comply with is seen as the best approach to address this issue and increase the compliance of the food industry.

Governments must also support manufacturers in the process of reformulation by offering workshops and financial incentives, as especially small and medium-sized companies may be overwhelmed by the associated technological and financial requirements. It has been suggested that rewards for compliant producers may be more effective than penalties (Loloei et al., 2019).

The active involvement of food producers in the development and implementation of food reformulation policies also contributes to the success of such measures and increases compliance. As discussed above (3.4.2), interviews with bakers in Iran revealed that the national salt policy was perceived as a top-down action with unrealistic targets that had been forced on them. There were even concerns that due to the low quality of the flour, food producers would have to use additives with potentially harmful health effects that would be difficult to detect in the bread (Loloei et al., 2019). The latter is a general matter that needs attention during reformulation to ensure that technological adaptations do not result in new health hazards. Effective food reformulation requires adequate alternatives to replace the reduced or eliminated components if these have a technological or sensory function. In the case of TFAs, the use of palm oil presents an option that is cheap and does not require elaborate technologies (Kaushik & Grewal, 2017). However, palm oil is rich in saturated fatty acids and therefore not a healthy alternative. Moreover, the intensive cultivation of oil palms is a major contributor to deforestation in tropical rainforests and hence to climate change, loss of biodiversity and damage to the livelihoods of local populations (EPHA, 2018).

While surveys in Canada showed that the elimination of TFAs was not associated with marked increases in the SFA content of foods but, on the contrary, with higher levels of cis-unsaturated fatty acids (Ratnayake et al., 2009), in Denmark and Argentina, SFAs were found to be the main replacements for TFAs in foods (Ministry of Food, Agriculture and Fisheries of Denmark, 2014; Kakisu et al., 2018). In Iran, the use of palm oil has been restricted by setting maximums for SFA in frying oils for household and industrial use. Oil producers have reacted by adapting the composition of their products to conform to the new standards (Moslemi et al., 2020). It is therefore important to guide food manufacturers through the reformulation process and to make available healthy alternatives to partially hydrogenated oils, such as high oleic canola oil, which is more stable than oils rich in polyunsaturated fatty acids. Besides technical support to producers, agricultural and trade policies can increase the availability of suitable oil alternatives at affordable prices (Skeaff, 2009; WHO, 2021a). In bread, salt, besides its sensory properties, plays an important role for the structure and rheology of the dough by slowing down yeast fermentation, interacting with gluten to increase dough strength and contributing to the formation of a good crust. A study in Iran found that lower use of salt in bread was associated with a higher use of baking soda to account for the consequent problems with bread texture and to compensate for the low quality of wheat flour. Baking soda has been found to reduce the absorption of minerals like calcium and iron, promote the uptake of heavy metals, and destroy vitamins like thiamine and riboflavin (Abolli et al., 2021). Bakers often lack awareness about the negative effects of high salt intake and the technical know-how to reduce salt content in bread without loss of quality. Ideally, a reformulation policy should therefore be accompanied by workshops and training for food producers. On the other hand, the feasibility of and commitment to the reformulation will be increased by the engagement of food manufacturers in the policy development, and by taking into account their practical experience with the production process.

Cooperation is also required between all government agencies concerned by the policy and consumer organizations. This is best ensured by a multisectoral approach and through the establishment of a working group composed of representatives of all stakeholders to facilitate the exchange of views and needs. Educating consumers about healthy nutrition and raising their awareness of the negative effects of unhealthy eating habits increases the acceptability of and the demand for healthier foods, providing an incentive for food manufacturers to reformulate their products.

An important point to consider is that processed foods for at-home consumption, while contributing significantly to the intake of salt, TFAs and other nutrients that should be consumed less, are not the only source. Modern living and work conditions lead to a higher reliance on restaurant and take-away foods; however, these are not always included in food reformulation policies. A recent study from Iran revealed high contents of salt, saturated and trans-fatty acids in 5 popular foods sampled in restaurants in Tehran. Notably, with one exception, all meal portions exceeded the limit for salt of 5 g/d recommended by the WHO by at least double, and supplied about half the recommended daily intake level of total fat. Average TFA content was above 1% of total fat in 2 meal types. This shows the importance of extending policies aiming at making diets healthier to restaurant foods (Mohammadi-Nasrabadi et al., 2021).

Studies also show a need for more and better monitoring to increase compliance with targets. Since, in most countries, reformulation programmes have only recently begun, there is still a lack of evaluation surveys to investigate their impact on the intake of salt, TFAs and other nutrients that should be reduced and to show their potential effects on health indicators including blood pressure, NCD and obesity prevalence.

The evaluation of reformulation initiatives is required to ensure that the intended outcomes are achieved and to make adjustments as needed, to provide a basis for the accountability of the government and for transparency. Evidence about the effectiveness of a policy helps to gain public support and can provide incentives to food manufacturers to reformulate their products and to consumers to buy them. Moreover, it also contributes to the exchange of knowledge at the local, national, regional and even global level and can help other countries in the developing and implementation of their own policies (WHO, 2021b). Indeed, a number of countries in the WHO Eastern Mediterranean Region have so far not taken steps to reduce the amount of salt and TFAs in their population's diet, even though the consumption of processed foods with high contents of these components is increasing among their populations. These countries would benefit from the shared knowledge and experience of other members of the region.

3.5 Public Food Procurement and Service Policies to Support Healthy Sustainable Diets

3.5.1 The Role of the Government as Food Provider

All over the world, governments do not only influence the food system by setting the legal and regulatory frameworks but also by acting directly as food providers in public settings, including government offices, public schools and universities, public hospitals and care homes, day-care centres, military institutions, prisons etc., as well as through social and emergency food programmes. This role offers the government a unique opportunity to take action to contribute to a healthy and sustainable diet for a large proportion of the population, covering the whole food value chain. In this way, the government's requirements for food can be linked to socioeconomic, developmental and environmental objectives (McCrudden, 2004; Kelly & Swensson, 2017).

Accordingly, "Promot[ing] public procurement practices that are sustainable, in accordance with national policies and priorities" is a target of Sustainable Development Goal 12 *Responsible Consumption and Production* (https://www.un.org/sustainabledevelopment).

On average, OECD countries spend 29% of their total expenditure and 12% of their GDP on total public procurement (including food provision). This share is even higher (18%) in the countries of the MENA Region that are members of the OECD members and include many of the countries of the WHO Eastern Mediterranean Region[1] (OECD, 2016).

---

[1] The MENA-OECD Initiative comprises Algeria, Bahrain, Djibouti, Egypt, Iraq, Jordan, Kuwait, Lebanon, Libya, Mauritania, Morocco, Oman, Palestinian Authority, Qatar, Saudi Arabia, Syria, Tunisia, United Arab Emirates and Yemen.

© 2023 Al-Jawaldeh and Meyer, CC BY-NC 4.0   https://doi.org/10.11647/OBP.0322.15

The large amounts of food bought by governments give them a strong purchasing power that enables them

- to reduce the cost of healthy food and increase its availability;
- to support local food producers especially smallholders;
- to promote sustainable agriculture and food production;
- to reduce inequities by providing healthy food to disadvantaged and vulnerable population groups and facilitating market access to small local food producers.

Public food procurement provides governments with a unique opportunity to make food systems healthier and more sustainable, as it covers the entire food value chain. Governments could start by increasing the production of healthier food crops using more sustainable agricultural techniques, through healthier and sustainable food processing and product reformulation, to actual food consumption, the reduction of food loss and waste and raising awareness of healthy nutrition.

By setting criteria for the composition of healthy foods, governments can also stimulate food manufacturers to reformulate their products to meet these specifications, increasing the availability of healthier food options on the market. Public food procurement is thus an important tool to make food systems healthier and more sustainable (Fig. 16).

3.5.2 Principles of a Healthy Diet in the Context of Public Food Procurement

Serving healthy food does not only benefit consumers but also the government, thanks to its positive public health effects and the prevention of diseases associated with malnutrition and unhealthy diets, which alleviate the burden on health systems. Serving healthy, sustainable food in public settings also serves as an example. It can contribute to the development of a liking and even a preference for healthy food, particularly among children.

Nutrition criteria are required to ensure that the food served in public institutions conforms to the principles of a healthy diet. While such criteria have to be harmonized with already existing national

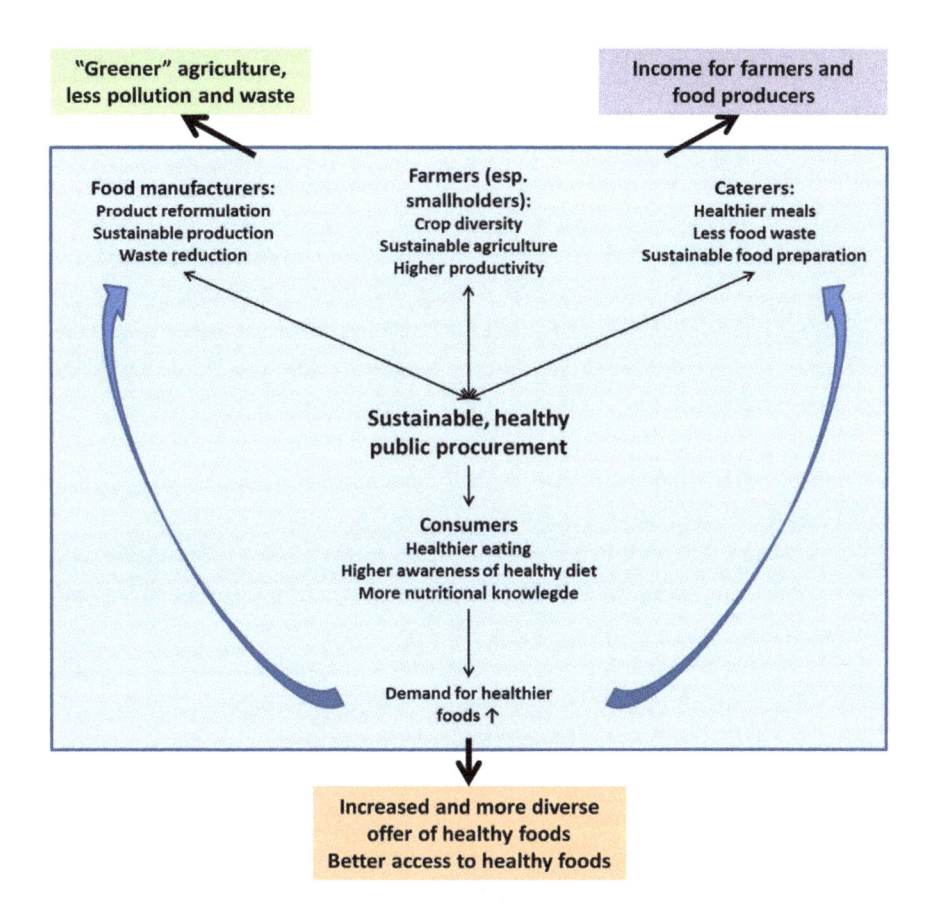

Fig. 16 Public food procurement as part of a sustainable healthy food system.

dietary guidelines as well as the local dietary customs to make the food culturally acceptable, general principles apply:

- intake of free sugars should be reduced;
- saturated fats should be replaced by unsaturated fats and industrially produced trans fats eliminated from the diet;
- salt content should be lowered and only iodized salt be used;
- consumption of whole grains, vegetables, fruits, nuts and pulses should be increased;
- safe drinking water should be freely available.

Nutritional criteria that define which foods should be encouraged, limited or prohibited in public settings can be nutrient-based or food-based.

Nutrient-based criteria focus on the contents of certain critical nutrients in a specific food category, in most cases by setting maximum permissible amounts of nutrients that should be limited like sodium, sugars or saturated and trans-fatty acids. They should be based on national (if available) or regional dietary recommendations. A starting point for the development of nutrient-based criteria for healthy public food procurement and service policies is provided by the WHO Healthy Diet Fact Sheet and the WHO regional nutrient profile models, such as the Nutrient Profile Model for the Marketing of Food and Non-Alcoholic Beverages to Children in the WHO Eastern Mediterranean Region (WHO EMRO, 2017a) (see Chapter 3.3 for more detail). The nutrient-based criteria that the latter has developed to regulate the marketing of food to children can be adapted by countries for school food policies and guidelines.

Food-based criteria apply to specific food categories for which consumption should be limited or encouraged, like sweetened beverages, sweets and foods rich in fat or salt. Such criteria can be based on existing national or regional food-based dietary guidelines.

Additional criteria pertain to the handling, preparation or service of food, defining how food should be prepared or offered for sale so as to promote safe healthy diets. This includes, for example, the prohibition of cooking methods like deep-frying, the setting of serving sizes to prevent the overconsumption of energy and of nutrients of concern, and the use of food or menu labelling to support healthier food choices. Criteria for the sustainable purchasing of local or seasonal food also fall in this category (WHO, 2021c).

3.5.3 Sustainable Public Food Procurement

In the context of the food system, the sustainability of public food procurement is determined by social, economic and environmental aspects.

On the socioeconomic side, sustainable public food procurement creates social benefits and promotes equity on two counts. School feeding and food aid programmes, in particular, improve the access of vulnerable population groups to healthy food.

On the other hand, public food procurement can provide a source of income to local smallholders, small manufacturers and vulnerable producer groups like women's cooperatives, thereby contributing to the fight against poverty and food insecurity. Nowadays, most public food procurement programmes include initiatives to purchase from local producers, favouring smallholders and small and medium enterprises. With better incomes, households have more money to spend on food, resulting in more diverse diets of higher nutritional quality. The latter is also promoted by a more diverse crop production by smallholders, which increases their own diet diversity as well as the availability of more diverse foods in local markets where surpluses are sold.

Higher incomes also allow smallholders to invest in production equipment, making them more resilient to crop failure and livestock diseases and increasing productivity, which further increases food security. Public demand for more sustainable foods creates incentives to invest in more sustainable cultivation techniques with positive ecological effects on biodiversity, CO_2 footprint, water and soil quality.

However, public procurement is highly regulated to prevent corruption and the misuse of public funding and warrant integrity. Besides laws and regulation, open tendering is the usual approach to awarding contracts. While this is justified, it places a high bureaucratic burden on applicants and is characterized by high levels of competition that are often not manageable for smallholders and other small producers. Public food procurement programmes have to include approaches to eliminate or reduce barriers to entry into public food markets for small producers. This is generally done by preferential treatment or reservation schemes, conferring competitive advantages to qualified suppliers. Reservations or set-asides allocate a certain quota of purchases to tenderers fulfilling specific criteria, so that competition between bidders only occurs on equal terms. On the other hand, targeted suppliers can also be preferred by reducing their bid price by a defined percentage to make their offers more attractive, or by increasing the bid price of non-qualified tenders. Eligibility criteria include the sustainability of foods and production methods, regionality and gender among other criteria. Preferential treatment bears the risk of market distortions and disproportionate price increases resulting from the absence of competition. Governments can minimize this risk by pre-setting prices (FAO, 2018).

An increasing number of countries are relying on digital technologies for public procurement to facilitate access to public markets and the bidding procedure, while at the same time making the process more transparent and reducing the administrative burden and associated costs. This process, commonly termed e-procurement, can offer a particular opportunity to small suppliers, as

- online tendering increases the visibility of business opportunities;
- small-value procurement opportunities are made available to a wider supplier audience;
- no physical attendance is required from suppliers, facilitating bidding for providers from remote areas of the country;
- costs and efforts are reduced through paper-free submission;
- information on suppliers responding to a bid is more accessible to public buyers;
- contracts can be tracked more easily and policy decisions can be based on evidence generated by the system.

Food requirements for public procurement will result in an overall increase in the demand for healthy, sustainable foods, providing incentives for the higher production of these foods that in turn will make them more available and accessible. It is, however, crucial to make sure that domestic production can keep pace with the increased demand, to prevent price increases and shortages that would make healthy foods less available and accessible to poorer population groups.

Public e-procurement as a tool to facilitate access to public markets for small suppliers — the case of Tunisia

Tunisia introduced a comprehensive digital procurement system in 2013. In the course of the reform, the e-procurement platform TUNEPS was established in co-operation with the Korean International Co-operation

Agency (KOICA), building on the South Korean expertise in digitalizing procurement and the Korean e-procurement system KONEPS. After a pilot phase, e-procurement became mandatory for all entities, including municipalities in September 2019.

The system comprises four main components, e-bidding, e-contracting, an e-catalogue and the e-shopping mall. Both public buyers and suppliers are required to register and to receive approval of their registration and then have to request an electronic certificate from the National Agency for Electronic Certification to use TUNEPS. In this way, transparency is enhanced as the e-bidding also involves the disclosure of the results of the selection process, the registration of objections and bid guarantee information. Document encryption and the requirement to adhere the procurement plan ensure consistency between procurement planning and execution. For the preparation and finalization of an electronic contract, the public buyer and the winning bidder are supported by the e-contracting function. The e-catalogue enables the classification, registration and management of information related to products according to the United Nations Standard Products and Services (UNSPSC), a standard international classification system, so that buyers can obtain information on products and their technical characteristics. A virtual market place for small-value procurement is offered by the e-shopping mall function, where requests for goods and services can be sent by public buyers and registered suppliers can respond.

These functionalities, together with the mandatory implementation, make the Tunisian e-procurement system an advanced model by international standards and attest to the country's leadership in e-procurement in the Middle East and North Africa (MENA) Region as well as globally.

The main objectives of the reform were to increase transparency and efficiency and improve overall access to procurement opportunities. The electronic platform enhances traceability and accessibility and provides a tool for rapid exchange between suppliers and buyers, resulting in an acceleration of procedures and lower costs compared to a paper-based system. By increasing transparency as well as the confidentiality and security of transactions, e-procurement encourages good governance and strengthens economic development.

OECD, 2020

Public food procurement also offers a means for environmental leveraging and climate-smart action.

Steps to make public food procurement more environmentally friendly include:

- purchasing local and seasonal food to limit the CO_2 footprint;
- setting criteria for sustainable farming methods;
- increasing the proportion of products from organic agriculture as far as they are available;
- reducing the use of water for farming and food processing;
- reducing the use of packaging, especially plastic packaging;
- recycling of waste materials used for packaging and preparation;
- using energy-saving food preparation, cooking and cooling techniques;
- on-site preparation of meals reduces transport and need for cooling and reheating;
- reducing food waste in canteens;
- reducing the serving size and frequency of animal food (esp. meat), e.g., by declaring a vegetarian day per week.

3.5.4 Implementing Healthy and Sustainable Public Food Procurement

The development of a policy for healthy and sustainable public procurement should be preceded by a situation analysis to assess the state of nutrition and health in the country and thereby identify the priorities for public health, and establish how public procurement can be used to tackle existing problems and shortcomings. The landscape of public food procurement has to be carefully assessed to understand the activities, settings and actors involved.

A situation analysis should take into account the different aspects of healthy public procurement policy as shown in Table 26.

Table 26 Aspects of healthy public procurement to be considered in the situation analysis.

Aspects	Points to address (examples)
Nutritional aspects	Characterization of the current nutritional and health situation;
	Identification of the main problems to be addressed by the policy (e.g., nutrient deficiencies, high prevalence of obesity and NCDs) and of causative factors (high intake of sodium, TFAs and sugar, low consumption of fruits and vegetables).
Economic aspects	Selection of potential suppliers of food esp. smallholders and small catering firms;
	Finding ways to improve/facilitate their access to markets and bids;
	Determining who the public buyers of foods are.
Environmental/ sustainability aspects	Assessment of the sustainability of food production and the availability of local and seasonal (organic) food, as well as the extent of food waste and how this latter can be minimized.

In the WHO's Action Framework for developing and implementing public food procurement and service policies for a healthy diet, 4 guiding principles are proposed to "promote healthy diets, are based on evidence and human rights, safeguard public health interest, and ensure policy coherence" (Table 27).

The composition of food baskets purchased by the government needs to take into account:

- national or regional food-based dietary guidelines that define the targets for nutrient and calorie intake;
- aims and objectives of public procurement with regards to environmental, social and equity targets;
- agro-ecological aspects and seasonality;
- agricultural productivity (especially of smallholders);
- local culture and food preferences.

Table 27 Guiding principles for healthy public food procurement and service policies. Source: Adapted from WHO, 2021c. This is an adaptation of an original work, "Action framework for developing and implementing public food procurement and service policies for a healthy diet. Geneva: World Health Organization; 2021. Licence: CC BY-NC-SA 3.0 IGO." This adaptation was not created by the WHO. The WHO is not responsible for the content or accuracy of this adaptation. The original edition shall be the binding and authentic edition.

Guiding principle	Description
Evidence-informed development and implementation	The development and implementation of public food procurement and service policies should take into account the best available evidence and be aligned with evidence-informed concepts of healthy diets. Points to consider are the quality of the evidence, priority of the problem addressed, acceptability and feasibility of the policy, values and preferences of those affected by the policy, the balance of benefits and harms, resource implications and equity and human rights.
Human-rights-based approach	Healthy public food procurement and service policies should conform to the principles of international human rights, particularly the rights to adequate food and the highest attainable standard of health. This implies the availability of sufficient quantities of culturally acceptable food of adequate nutritional quality and safety and the accessibility of such food in sustainable ways that do not infringe other human rights. Transparency, responsibility, accountability, participation, and responsiveness to the needs of the people in the sense of good governance are important attributes of a human-rights-based approach to policy development.
Safeguarding public interest	To ensure the coherence of a healthy public food procurement and service policy and to create a supportive and synergistic policy environment, commitment and coherent actions by various sectors (health and non-health) is needed. While governments act as leaders of the policy process, active partnerships beyond government authorities are required, with (among others) civil society organizations and the private sector. To avoid and manage conflicts of interest, governments have to determine clear rules of engagement and to establish good governance practices.

Guiding principle	Description
Health in all policies (HiAP)	HiAP is an approach to public policies across sectors that systematically takes into account the health implications of decisions, seeks synergies and avoids harmful health impacts, to improve population health and health equity.[1] The HiAP approach contributes to policy coherence that is critical for improved nutrition.
Safe, healthy and sustainable diets	A sustainably produced and consumed, safe and healthy diet serves both people's health and planetary health. The Guiding principles for sustainable healthy diets by the Food and Agriculture Organization of the United Nations (FAO) and the WHO take a holistic approach to diets, considering nutrition recommendations, environmental costs of food production and consumption, and adaptability to local social, cultural and economic contexts (FAO & WHO, 2019).

[1] The Helsinki Statement on Health in All Policies at the 8th Global Conference on Health Promotion, Helsinki, Finland, 10–14 June 2013.

As with other policies, regular monitoring and evaluation are essential to assess whether and to what extent policies achieve the desired outcomes, and to identify reasons for failure and develop strategies for improvement. Monitoring and evaluation methods should be conceived and planned during the development of the policy. This also enables the gathering of baseline data to evaluate the policy's impact. Academic or research institutions may be involved in the evaluation.

Besides the outcomes of the policy, its process should also be evaluated to investigate its implementation and identify challenges, barriers, successes and enabling elements. This allows the policy leaders to gain information on the feasibility, acceptability and potential unintended consequences of the policy, providing a basis for its revision and improvement. In turn, the impact of the policy on the intended objectives is measured by an outcome evaluation. Different indicators have to be defined to measure short-, medium- and long-term outcomes. However, some ultimate outcomes such as changes in health status may take time to appear and can be influenced by other factors that are not related to public food procurement and service. The detection of an impact is facilitated by the inclusion of short-term objectives with immediate outcomes. Some examples of process and outcome indicators for policy evaluation are given in Table 28.

Table 28 Examples of process and outcome indicators for policy evaluation. Adapted from WHO, 2021c. This is an adaptation of an original work, "Action framework for developing and implementing public food procurement and service policies for a healthy diet. Geneva: World Health Organization; 2021. Licence: CC BY-NC-SA 3.0 IGO." This adaptation was not created by the WHO. The WHO is not responsible for the content or accuracy of this adaptation. The original edition shall be the binding and authentic edition.

Effect	Process indicators	Outcome indicators
Communication	Awareness of the policy	
	Knowledge about the policy content	
	Dissemination of information about the policy	
Training of staff	Proportion of settings offering training for staff	
	Amount of training offered	
	Increases in knowledge, alterations of attitudes and practices among actors	
Management of funds	Policy-related investments	
	Costs of food procurement	
Reach	Rate of adoption of the policy	
	Number of beneficiaries	
Nutrition	Selection of foods purchased, served or sold	
	Menu composition	
	Nutrient content of food served and sold	
	Altered portion size of meals	
	Proportion of healthier meals served or sold	

Effect	Process indicators	Outcome indicators
Health aspects		Changes in food consumption
		Dietary behaviour
		Changes in intake of critical nutrients
		Prevalence of overweight and obesity
		Incidence of NCDs
Socioeconomic aspects	Number of contracts with suppliers, processors and caterers	Poverty rate
		Food security of smallholders
		Employment rate
		Contracting of SMEs
		Productivity
		School and working performance
Environmental aspects		Proportion of organic farming
		Amount of food waste
		CO_2 footprint of procured food

The existence of sanctions against violations of the policy generally promotes its implementation. Therefore, actions to be taken in the case of non-compliance should be defined, as well as to whom they should be addressed. Sanctions can range from mere admonitions to administrative letters, reduction of funds for the non-compliant parties or fines. In turn, rewards for good compliance with the policies, e.g., in the form of awards and accreditation models offer incentives for implementation (WHO, 2021c).

3.5.5 Public Food Procurement for Healthy Sustainable Diets in Practice — Focus on School Feeding with Emphasis on the Eastern Mediterranean Region

As in other parts of the world, by far the most policies related to public procurement of healthy food in the Eastern Mediterranean Region are focused on school feeding and school meals. Policies on school health and nutrition have been implemented in at least 15 countries of the region, and school meals are provided in 9 countries, of which 4 do so free of charge to all school children (Egypt, Jordan, Kuwait and Morocco) and 1 to children from disadvantaged families (Tunisia). Regulations for food and beverages offered in schools exist in 11 countries and bans on vending machines for snacks, sweets and soft drinks in school buildings and grounds have been imposed in 5 countries. In turn, according to the Global Nutrition Policy Review 2016–2017, school fruit and vegetable programmes were only implemented in 3 countries (WHO, 2018b; Al-Jawaldeh et al., 2020c).

School meals make up a large part of public spending for food. Estimates from the UK showed that school dinners alone accounted for almost a third (29%) of the total expenditure for food procurement. The same percentage was spent for institutions of higher education and 25% for the health and care sector, corresponding to 83% of total spending (Neto et al., 2016).

The scope of school meal programmes and services varies widely, ranging from the provision of hot meals or snacks in school canteens, take-home food rations, to the distribution of food vouchers and cash transfers to households on the condition that children are enrolled into and attend school. Moreover, programmes can also involve policy advice and technical capacity development activities and services, as well as nutritional education as part of the school curriculum.

School feeding has a long tradition and the first national standards date back to the mid-19th century when they were introduced in the United Kingdom (Evans & Harper, 2009). Since then, an increasing number of countries have established national school feeding programmes alongside initiatives led by international and private actors (WFP, 2020).

The benefits of school feeding are widely recognized and go far beyond nutritional status alone. Besides its contribution to nutritional supply, the provision of school meals also presents an additional incentive to parents to send their children to school. It has been shown to increase school attendance, improve learning achievements and support social equity, setting the foundations for a successful adult life. It has been estimated that the gain from the efficient implementation of school feeding programmes can reach up to US$9 for every US$1 invested by creating value across multiple sectors such as education, health and nutrition, local agriculture and social protection (see Fig. 17).

The recent survey on the *State of World School Feeding 2020* by the World Food Programme (WFP) found that 161 of 163 countries evaluated (98.8%) have school feeding programmes, providing meals to an estimated 388 million children across all grades, corresponding to about 50%. At the global level, this number has increased by 9% since the last survey in 2013 and especially in low-income and lower-middle-income countries (by 36% and 86%, respectively). Nevertheless, coverage is still significantly lower than in upper-middle and high-income countries (20% in low-income countries and 45% in lower-middle-income countries vs. 58% in upper-middle and 78% in high-income countries). Moreover, 75% of countries have national policies regulating school feeding and on average, over 90% of the costs of programmes are paid from state funds (WFP, 2020). This underlines the potential of public food procurement for schools as a starting point for changing food systems.

Coverage by school feeding programmes also increased in the 11 countries of the Middle East and North Africa included in the survey (from 28% to 35% between 2013 and 2020), even though it is still below the average (48%). Among the countries of the WHO Eastern Mediterranean Region, it ranged from under 10% in Lebanon to almost 80% in Egypt. In Egypt alone, about 11 million children receive school meals (WFP, 2020).

An example of a long-standing national school feeding scheme is Tunisia, where a fully government-funded programme was established in 1958 after the country became independent and reformed its education system. The objective was to ameliorate the nutrition status of primary schoolchildren, targeting the most vulnerable groups in rural areas in particular. In 2020, 260,000 schoolchildren (48% girls and

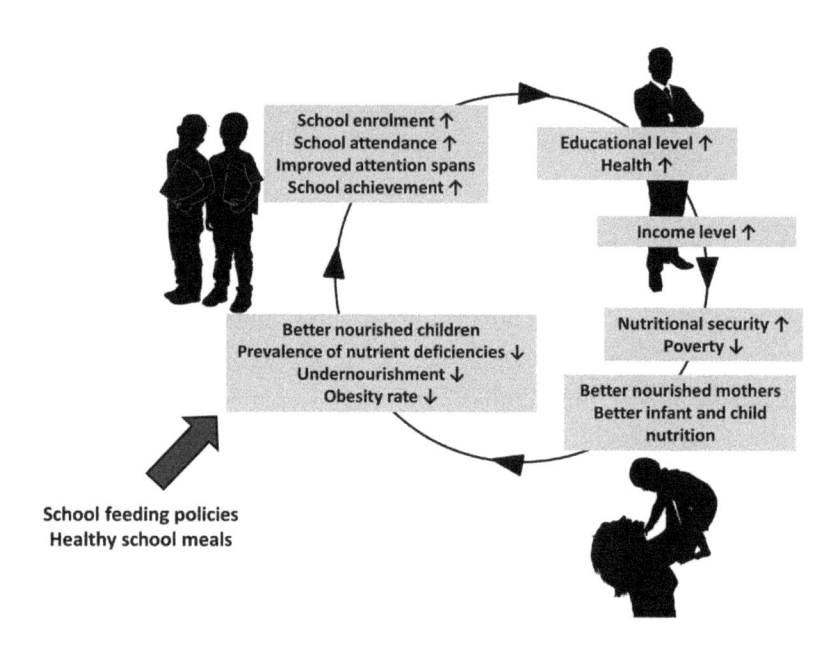

Fig. 17 Long-term benefits from school feeding. By the authors using free vectors from OpenClipart-Vectors, AnnaliseArt and Tumisu on Pixabay, https://pixabay.com/de/

52% boys, corresponding to 25% of children) in 2,500 primary schools (50%) benefitted from the programme. It is stewarded by the Ministry of Education and implemented in a highly decentralized way, with food procurement and management being conducted at the school level. In 2019, the budget of the national school feeding programme was doubled and reached US$16 million annually. US$1.7 million was invested by the Tunisian government in the construction and equipment of a pilot central kitchen and development of a School Food Bank. The WFP helped with the development of an innovative sustainable school feeding strategy in 2014 that started in several pilot programmes. Central features were the use of locally sourced foods for school meals, and meal preparation in a central kitchen according to nutrition and hygiene guidelines. To address the double burden of malnutrition, the National Nutrition Institute, Ministry of Health and WFP cooperated in the development of nutritious, balanced meals to increase diet diversity. A home-grown school feeding approach was implemented in partnership with the Ministry of Agriculture that included the establishment of school gardens as part of nutritional and environmental education and to increase the availability of vegetables and fruits for school lunches.

The lessons learned and best practices resulting from the pilot experiences provide a guideline for the nationwide expansion of the programme across schools in participating in the National School Feeding Programme (PNAS).

During the COVID-19 pandemic, the programme was suspended due to the closure of all schools, presenting a serious threat to children from low-income groups. This was addressed by the provision of flexible cash-based transfers (CBT) to households with school-age children as an innovative and rapid solution to limit the physical and social distress entailed by the COVID-19 pandemic (WFP, 2020).

A recent survey by the Global Child Nutrition Foundation from 2019, including 85 countries all over the world that reported having school feeding programmes, found that the majority of programmes (82%) obtained food from domestic purchases. Of the 7 participating countries from the Eastern Mediterranean Region (Egypt, Iraq, Libya, Syria, Tunisia, the United Arab Emirates and Yemen), this applied to about 70%. Moreover, 76% of all countries purchasing any food obtained at least some of it from local sources. Preferential treatment of small farmers or producers was reported for 34.5% of the programmes that purchased food locally through open bidding. Procurement from domestic sources was associated with higher food basket diversity, containing more vegetables, fruits, fish, meat, poultry, and dairy products (GCNF, 2019).

The great majority of the programmes (94%) were managed by governmental institutions, either at national, regional or local level. In the Eastern Mediterranean countries, this share was 67% while 33% were managed by international donor agencies or other partner organizations.

While many programmes actively involved farmers, this was not reported by the countries of the MENA Region. In turn, over 80% of the programmes from Eastern Mediterranean countries accorded a high priority to limiting food waste (GCNF, 2019).

Improving the nutritional quality of children's diet was considered an important goal of school feeding programmes by the majority (87%) of countries participating in the GCNF survey and by all of the countries from the MENA Region. Nutritionists were involved in 71% of the school meal programmes in the MENA countries, and the interest in reducing obesity was higher than the survey average (43% vs. 23% of programmes). This objective was more common in countries with high obesity rates. Half of the programmes reported that they involved training in nutrition for cooks and caterers (GCNF, 2019).

While most countries of the region have national dietary guidelines for educational settings, these consist mostly of lists of permitted and non-permitted foods, while only few countries have issued more comprehensive nutrient or food-based guidelines for school settings like the United Arab Emirates and Saudi Arabia. In turn, Bahrain, Iran, Iraq, Lebanon, Oman and Qatar have nutritional guidelines for the general public not considering age (Garemo et al., 2019).

A number of surveys have shown the weaknesses of many programmes, including those in countries with high income levels. In 2014, Iran issued its national guidelines for Healthy School Canteens (HSC) in a cooperation between the Ministry of Health and Medical Education (MoHME) and the Ministry of Education (MoE). A survey conducted in 64 primary schools in Tehran from November 2018 to March 2019 highlighted a number of issues in its implementation. It was found that, overall, 54.7% of the foods offered in school canteens did not comply with the national HSC guidelines. Taking the WHO's Nutrient Profile Model for the Marketing of Food and Non-Alcoholic Beverages to Children in the WHO Eastern Mediterranean Region as a reference, this proportion was even higher, reaching 85.6%. The great majority of the available foods fell into the category of cakes, sweet biscuits and pastries, and this was also the case for most non-permitted foods that were available (45.2% based on the WHO profiling model, and 28.8% based on the national HSC guideline). However, 54.6% of the allowed foods according to the HSC guidelines that were available also belonged to this group, whereas none of the products permitted by the WHO profile did (Babashahi et al., 2021).

One reason for the high rate of non-compliance with the guidelines was seen in the lack of clear criteria and references according to which foods are to be rated. Another reason was a lack of funding for the more expensive, healthier food. Indeed, serving unhealthy foods was considered more profitable (Babashahi et al., 2021).

In Saudi Arabia, *Regulations of Health Conditions for School Canteens* were issued in 2004 and revised in 2013. The regulations comprise a list of foods that are banned from school canteens including 8 categories: confectioneries, chocolates, chips, soft drinks, energy drinks, sweetened drinks, processed meat products and fried foods. Compliance with the policy was evaluated in 76 public schools from Riyadh, using a 4-level score to measure alignment with the regulations. It was found that around 95% of the school canteens reached the 2 middle categories, corresponding to an alignment of 25 to 75%, but only about 5% showed the highest compliance (75–100%). Energy-dense foods like cakes, biscuits and confectionary were frequently offered. A problem that was identified is the lack of clear guidance on healthy foods with high nutritional quality to be offered preferentially (Aldubayan & Murimi, 2019).

In Qatar, School Canteen Guidelines are developed by the Health Promotion and NCD Section of the Public Health Department at the Ministry of Public Health in cooperation with the Ministry of Education and Higher Education. It includes a categorization of foods into those items that can be served daily, those that should only be served weekly and those that should not be served at all. Among the latter are soft drinks, candies, sweets and chocolates, deep-fried foods, products with a high salt content and processed meats (Ministry of Education and Higher Education, Emirate of Qatar, 2016). As part of the Workplace Wellness Program, the Health Promotion and NCD Section of the Public Health Department also issued the Food & Beverage Guidelines in Cafeterias and Vending Machines that are implemented in all healthcare settings and workplaces (Al-Jawaldeh et al., 2021b).

The situation of school feeding in Lebanon is marked by crisis, with the country suffering from the ongoing state of emergency affecting the country. The accommodation of an estimated 1.5 million Syrian refugees puts high burdens on infrastructure and basic services, causing an aggravating economic and social crisis that exacerbates vulnerability and poverty in Lebanon as well as among refugee communities. Against this background, Lebanon is one of 4 countries besides the Democratic Republic of Congo, Niger and Syria that have been targeted by an Evaluation Series on School Feeding in Emergency or Fragile Contexts (2016–2019), commissioned by WFP and funded by Canada, aimed at improving learning at the strategic and operational levels, nationally and globally. Data collected by a quantitative and qualitative survey, combined with interviews with key informants, revealed the contribution of school feeding to higher diet diversity and reductions in food insecurity and short-term hunger among Lebanese and Syrian children alike. The differing needs of both groups were adequately addressed by the design of the school feeding programme, allowing for adjustments to respond to contextual factors and the nutritional requirements of beneficiaries. The impact on food security was greater in Syrian children that were more affected by food insecurity. School feeding and the provision of school snacks enhanced school attendance and increased the enrolment rate of Syrian refugee children. While educational efforts were coordinated and information was shared within the education sector working group, there were few direct synergies or concomitant actions between school feeding and other interventions by UN agencies and NGOs. Some positive effects of school snack distribution on social cohesion between Lebanese and Syrian children were also observed (WFP, 2020).

In the Emirate of Abu Dhabi, School Canteen Guidelines were jointly issued by the Abu Dhabi Education Council, Abu Dhabi Food Control Authority and the Health Authority in 2011. Besides instructions regarding food safety and hygiene, the regularly-updated guidelines contain recommendations on meal composition and on foods that should be regularly included in the diet and those to limit, and they give some examples of menus. They also indicate the requirements of energy, protein and some micronutrients for different age groups, but do not include nutrient-based criteria to categorize foods as healthy or less healthy (Abu Dhabi Education Council, Abu Dhabi Food Control Authority and Health Authority (2011).

Some common challenges to the successful implementation of healthy school feeding programmes are given in Table 29.

Many countries use public food settings as action sites to address key priorities in nutrition, such as the reduction of salt, sugar, and trans-fatty-acid intake. With regard to the latter, Iran has required government institutions involved in public food procurement to use oils complying with the limit of <10% of TFA content since 2005 and with stricter limits introduced over the following years (see chapter 3-4-3) (WHO,

2021c). Bahrain, Kuwait, Oman and Qatar have implemented or plan to implement policies to reduce TFAs in meals served in schools. Jordan and Qatar have programmes focusing on food in hospitals, and Saudi Arabia have similar programmes in hospitals, academic and military institutions and public places (Al-Jawaldeh et al., 2021c).

Table 29 Challenges to the implementation of healthy school feeding programmes.

Challange	Description
Lack of funding	Healthy foods that are generally more expensive than less healthy highly-processed products.
	Selling the latter has been reported to be a considerable source of income to canteen operators.
Lack of staff	Staff with nutritional knowledge and training in healthy diets are often not available in schools to implement and monitor school feeding programmes. Even authorities have reported problems with the monitoring of policies.
Low awareness about the importance of healthy diets for children	Healthy nutrition has often been a low priority for school operators and even government workers.
	The results of programme evaluations and outcomes that would support their implementation are often not published.
Lack of intersectoral coordination	Cooperation between various government institutions with responsibilities for school nutrition (e.g., Ministry of Health and Ministry of Education) as well as other stakeholders (parents, private sector) is often inadequate.
Lack of sanctions for violations of mandatory regulations	Weak implementation and monitoring of programmes as well as absent or marginal sanctions for non-compliance with mandatory regulations reduce commitment of canteen operators.

Challange	Description
Unclear or missing criteria	Guidelines do not always include clear criteria on which the selection of foods and composition of meals are to be based, such as the thresholds of certain critical nutrients, serving size and frequency of specific foods or food groups.
Inadequate equipment, furniture and/or facilities	Schools may not have the technical equipment or facilities to adequately store, handle and prepare fresh healthy foods in a way to ensure food safety.
Low availability of healthy foods	Fresh vegetables and fruits may not be available in sufficient quantities in some regions or seasons.

In Qatar, a traffic-light system was introduced in 2017 to categorize foods served in healthcare facilities. Foods labelled green should be sold and served most, those labelled yellow sometimes, and those labelled red only in limited amounts (Qatar-Tribune, 2017). Salt reduction is also included in many of the programmes (Al-Jawaldeh et al., 2021b).

Table 30 gives an overview of policies in public settings in some countries of the region.

A general problem is that most guidelines do not contain criteria and thresholds to clearly identify foods that are allowed and those that are forbidden. Indications are rather vague, stating that foods rich in fat, salt and/or sugar should be restricted or completely banned. However, studies have shown that caterers find it difficult to act on these guidelines because they are confusing to them (Aldubayan & Murimi, 2019; Babashahi et al., 2021).

Their purchasing power as public food procurers provides governments with a unique way to modify the food system to make it healthier. This applies particularly to school feeding, which makes up the greatest part of public food procurement in most countries; however, initiatives for healthy public procurement should not be limited this setting but also focus on the health sector, the military and penal institutions among others. The development of clear regulations and guidelines for food served in public settings is a key to the successful implementation of food procurement policies, as is regular monitoring and evaluation.

Table 30 Policies relating to public food procurement in different settings in countries of the WHO Eastern Mediterranean Region.

Country	Setting	Measures	Leading institution	Year
Bahrain	School canteens	Eliminating TFAs by prohibiting certain foods and modifying food preparation and cooking methods; workshops for canteen staff	Government, MOH, MOE	2017
	School canteens	Ban on carbonated soft drinks List of healthy foods to be offered	Government, MOH, MOE	1997
Iran	Healthy school canteen policy: providing of healthy foods and snacks including those with lower salt and TFA contents (<5% of TFA), ban on unhealthy foods.	School canteens	Government, Ministry of Health and Medical Education and Ministry of Education	2014
Jordan	Ban of TFAs and increased use of olive and sesame oil.	Canteens of public sector hospitals and royal medical service hospitals for inpatients and employees	Multi-sectoral committee and the WHO	2019
	Ban on soft drinks, potato crisps and sweets.	Schools	Government, Ministry of Education	2012

Country	Setting	Measures	Leading institution	Year
Kuwait	Mandatory display of the traffic-light system on food items sold in cafeterias and canteens; revision of hospital menus to reduce the salt content.	Governmental hospitals	Government, FNA on behalf of the Kuwait MOH in cooperation with PHFS	2021
	Kuwait Action Plan for SFA Intake Reduction and TFA Elimination, ban on the use of TFAs.	Governmental institutions (MOH hospitals, Ministry of Defense, Ministry of Interior, public authorities, schools and universities	Kuwait's Salt and Fat Intake Reduction Task Force and the Public FNA	2012 (not yet adopted)
Lebanon	Ban on vending machines in schools.	Schools		1980
	Standards for offered foods and beverages.	Schools		1980
Morocco	List of foods that are allowed or restricted. The latter include soft drinks, sweets, foods rich in fat, sugar and salt, fried foods.	Schools	Government, MOH	2013
Oman	National plan for the prevention and control of chronic NCDs 2016–2025. Limits to the availability of foods high in TFAs.	Schools	Government, MOH	2016 (not yet adopted)
	Limiting the availability of foods high in salt and sugar.	Schools	Government, MOH	2016 (not yet implemented)

3.5 Public Food Procurement and Service Policies 203

Country	Setting	Measures	Leading institution	Year
Palestine	Ban on sale provision of soft drinks, sugar- salt- and fat-rich snack foods and sweets.	Schools	Government, MOH, MOE	2010
Qatar	Food & Beverage Guidelines; School Canteen Guidelines for Cafeterias and Vending Machines that are mandatory for public schools; educational sessions in schools and workplaces.	Schools, hospitals, workplaces, and public places including grocery stores and shopping malls	Government, Ministry of Public Health	Ongoing
	Labelling of foods served in healthcare facilities with a traffic-light system.	Healthcare facilities	Government, Ministry of Public Health	2017
	Lists of foods that are allowed, restricted or banned. The latter include soft drinks, sweets, foods rich in sugar and salt, fried potato products, processed meat.	School canteens	Government	2016

Country	Setting	Measures	Leading institution	Year
Saudi Arabia	Ban.	Schools		
	Healthy Food Strategy: Education about healthier nutrition.	Schools, hospitals and the workplace	Government, SFDA	2015
	Healthy Food Strategy, vision 2030: Voluntary procurement policy and education to promote healthy life style in work environment.	Workplaces, schools, and public hospitals	Government, SFDA	2018
	Guidelines for the government nutritional subsistence purchase contract: replacement of SFAs by canola and corn oil as source of unsaturated fatty acids, ban on the use of PHO in foods.	Public hospitals, universities, military or social places	Government, SFDA	2019
Tunisia	Create supportive environments by offering low-salt options.	Public places, schools, workplaces	Government, MOH	2018 (not yet adopted)
United Arab Emirates, Abu Dhabi	School canteen guideline: limits for fats (≤30 E% total fat, ≤10 E% SFAs) and sugar (≤35 %) in foods, ban on hydrogenated fat, caffeine-containing beverages, MSG etc.	Schools	Government, Education Council, Food Control Authority, Health Authority	2011–2012, regularly updated

FNA: Food and Nutrition Administration, MOH: Ministry of Health, MSG: monosodium glutamate, PHFS: Patient Helping Fund Society, PHO: partially hydrogenated oil, SFAs: saturated fatty acids, SFDA: Saudi Food and Drug Authority, TFAs: trans-fatty acids.

3.6 Food Fortification, Including Biofortification

Micronutrient deficiencies are ideally addressed by increasing diet diversity, particularly through a higher intake of fresh vegetables and fruits, legumes, wholegrain cereals, and nuts and seeds together with moderate amounts of animal foods. However, this approach, although sustainable and also beneficial to the supply of energy, macronutrients and non-nutritive health-promoting components, does not provide a rapid solution to micronutrient deficiencies and is not always feasible as it requires the availability of and access to adequate amounts of nutritious high-quality foods, and sufficient purchasing power and behavioural changes among the target population. The latter can be particularly challenging in populations with a low level of education, making accompanying nutritional education necessary (Lopez Villar, 2015).

On the other hand, supplementation of isolated micronutrients is difficult to maintain over a longer period, especially in remote areas, and it has to be closely monitored. Compliance of recipients often tends to be low. It is most suitable for specific at-risk groups like infants and pregnant women under regular medical care, for severe cases of micronutrient deficiencies and for emergency situations. Both approaches are thus of limited applicability for large populations in low-income countries.

In turn, food fortification, defined by the WHO/FAO Codex Alimentarius as "the addition of one or more essential nutrients to a food whether or not it is normally contained in the food", is particularly indicated for populations with a low dietary diversity and diets that are mainly based on a few staple foods of plant origin (especially cereals). Such diets are often deficient in essential micronutrients like iron, zinc and vitamins of the B group, for instance, especially if the cereal component is refined by removing the nutrient-rich bran part. Fortification serves to prevent, reduce the risk of, or correct a demonstrated deficiency of one or more essential nutrients in the population; to reduce the risk of, or correct, inadequate nutritional status or intakes of one or more essential nutrients in the population; to meet requirements and/or recommended intakes of one or more essential nutrients; to maintain or improve health; and/or to maintain or improve the nutritional quality of foods (FAO/WHO, 2015). It is a widely-used and well-established practice to efficiently, conveniently and cost-effectively improve the intake of one or several micronutrients at population level (Allen et al., 2006). Originally meant to restore nutrients that were lost during food storage and processing or to assimilate the nutrient content of foods serving as a replacement for others (such as margarine for butter), fortification has since been acknowledged as a means to improve the nutritional status at population level by preventing or alleviating nutrient deficiencies (Nilson & Piza, 1998; Allen et al., 2006). Nowadays, a large number of countries use fortification for this purpose.

3.6.1 Types and Principles of Food Fortification

Fortification approaches differ with regards to the target groups, the food vehicles, the extent of the fortification measures and the legal context. The universal fortification of a widely-consumed staple with micronutrients makes it possible to reach large parts of the general population including low-income groups. This type of fortification is most suitable to address widespread micronutrient deficiencies in populations with a predominant consumption of staple foods, as is the case in many low-income countries. In another approach, fortification is targeted to foods intended for specific population groups like complementary foods for infants, foods distributed in emergencies or supplementary foods for athletes.

Legislation that covers fortification can be mandatory or voluntary; the former confers a higher level of certainty about the sustained fortification of a given food or food category over time (Allen et al., 2006).

Mass fortification of staple foods is generally government-led and regulated with clearly defined standards and should ideally be mandatory. It is most effective when the food vehicle, such as flour, grain or salt, for instance, is predominantly processed in a few large-scale production units that possess the necessary technical and financial means. Voluntary fortification, on the other hand, leaves it to food manufacturers to fortify their products. This market-driven fortification can complement government-led mandatory fortification as long as it is driven by corporate social responsibility commitments, but it may also serve commercial purposes and does not always address the nutritional needs of the target population. An appropriate regulatory framework to support all government-led fortification measures is required to prevent health risks and achieve the intended benefits. Technical standards for the addition of micronutrients and for the monitoring of the fortified products, as well as rules for labelling, should be provided to guide the manufacturers through the fortification process. Foods that are required or permitted to be fortified, as well as the nutrients to be added and the forms of these fortificants should be clearly defined. The choice of fortificants depends on their suitability for the vehicle food, their bioavailability and their interactions with the food matrix to avoid, or at least limit, sensory and negative physical effects like oxidation or taste deterioration.

The preparation and implementation of any fortification programme should be preceded by a comprehensive assessment of the nutritional situation in the target population, its dietary patterns and nutritional requirements. Moreover, the food vehicle must be made with care to assure that the target population consumes sufficient amounts of the fortified food (Allen et al., 2006).

Fortication of staple foods is widely practised in many countries. The most commonly used food vehicles include cereal products like wheat and maize flour and rice, plant oils, table salt and to a lesser degree sugar and milk.

An important determinant of the effectiveness and safety of food fortification is the dosage of nutrients added. It must be sufficiently high to ensure an intake in the target population that lowers the risk of deficiency to an acceptable level, particularly in those population groups most at risk of deficiencies, while at the same time avoiding excessive intake levels. In this way, any potential health risks can be prevented to make sure that the fortification programme achieves the intended positive health outcomes.

The dosage of a given fortificant is best based on the estimated average requirement (EAR) of the target population as recommended in the WHO's Guidelines on Food Fortification with Micronutrients (Allen et al., 2006). The EAR is defined as "the median usual intake value that is estimated to meet the requirement of half the healthy individuals in a life stage and gender group" based on a specific adequacy criterion derived from the scientific literature, taking into account various health parameters. According to this definition, the EAR intake level does not meet the nutrient requirements of the other half of the specified group. Provided that the distributions of the intake and the requirements are symmetrical, the proportion of individuals consuming less than the EAR is equal to the prevalence of inadequacy, so that the EAR can be used to assess the adequacy of a population's intake of a given nutrient (IOM, 2000). On this basis, the EAR cut-point method is the approach recommended by the FAO for setting the target intake level and the amount of nutrients added to the fortified food for nutrients. The acceptable prevalence of inadequate and excessive intakes is generally considered to be 2–3%, so that 97–98% of the population have adequate intakes. Only a few nutrients require more specific approaches. For instance, in the case of iron, the requirements of menstruating women, adolescents and young children are not normally distributed, so that the probability of inadequacy has to be fully calculated. The same applies to iodine, folic acid, niacin and vitamin D. For iodine and folic acid, the recommended amounts to be added are based on epidemiological field experience, while for for niacin and vitamin D the extent to which these two micronutrients are biosynthesized has to be taken into account. The level of fortificant that needs to be added to reach the intended adequacy can be determined based on the range of usual intakes and the average consumption amount of the vehicle food (Allen et al., 2006).

3.6.2 Quality and Safety of Food Fortification

The effectiveness of a food fortification programme depends not only on the preparation but also on a careful evaluation and regular monitoring of the implementation and compliance with the standards. These steps have to be included in the planning of the programme. Monitoring involves the ongoing collection and review of data on programme implementation activities to control the quality of the fortified products and their availability and accessibility to consumers, allowing the identification of problems and non-compliance and providing the basis for corrective actions.

An evaluation of the food fortification programme should be done after it has been fully implemented and is operating as planned, to assess its effectiveness and the impact on the target population to ascertain whether measure meets its objectives (e.g., improvement of nutrient intake and nutritional status as well as health or functional outcomes).

Monitoring has to take place at different levels (see Fig. 18). Regulatory monitoring at production sites, retail stores and customs warehouses for imported foods is performed by external regulatory authorities as well as by the producers themselves (internal monitoring) to ensure that food vehicles are fortified according to quality and safety standards and regulations. Monitoring at household level allows the programme managers to verify how easily households and targeted individuals can access fortified food of the intended quality (service provision), the actual purchase and consumption of the fortified food by the target population (service utilization), and the appropriateness of the amounts and frequency of consumption (coverage). Data obtained through household monitoring also allows the evaluation of the programme's impact and effectiveness. The frequency and intensity of monitoring depends on the compliance and technical performance of the production unit as determined by previous monitoring. They should be increased when problems are discovered until these issues are solved (Allen et al., 2006).

The risk of excessive intakes above the tolerable upper level of intake (UL) of the specific micronutrient should be minimized. Even though excessive intakes of certain micronutrients do not necessarily result in toxicity, they can have subtle negative effects on health and interfere with the absorption, activity and metabolism of other micronutrients leading to an imbalance (Meltzer et al., 2003). This risk is particularly high for nutrients with a narrow safety range, that is, a small difference between the recommended daily nutrient intake and the UL, such as vitamin A and all minerals and trace elements. High consumers of the fortified

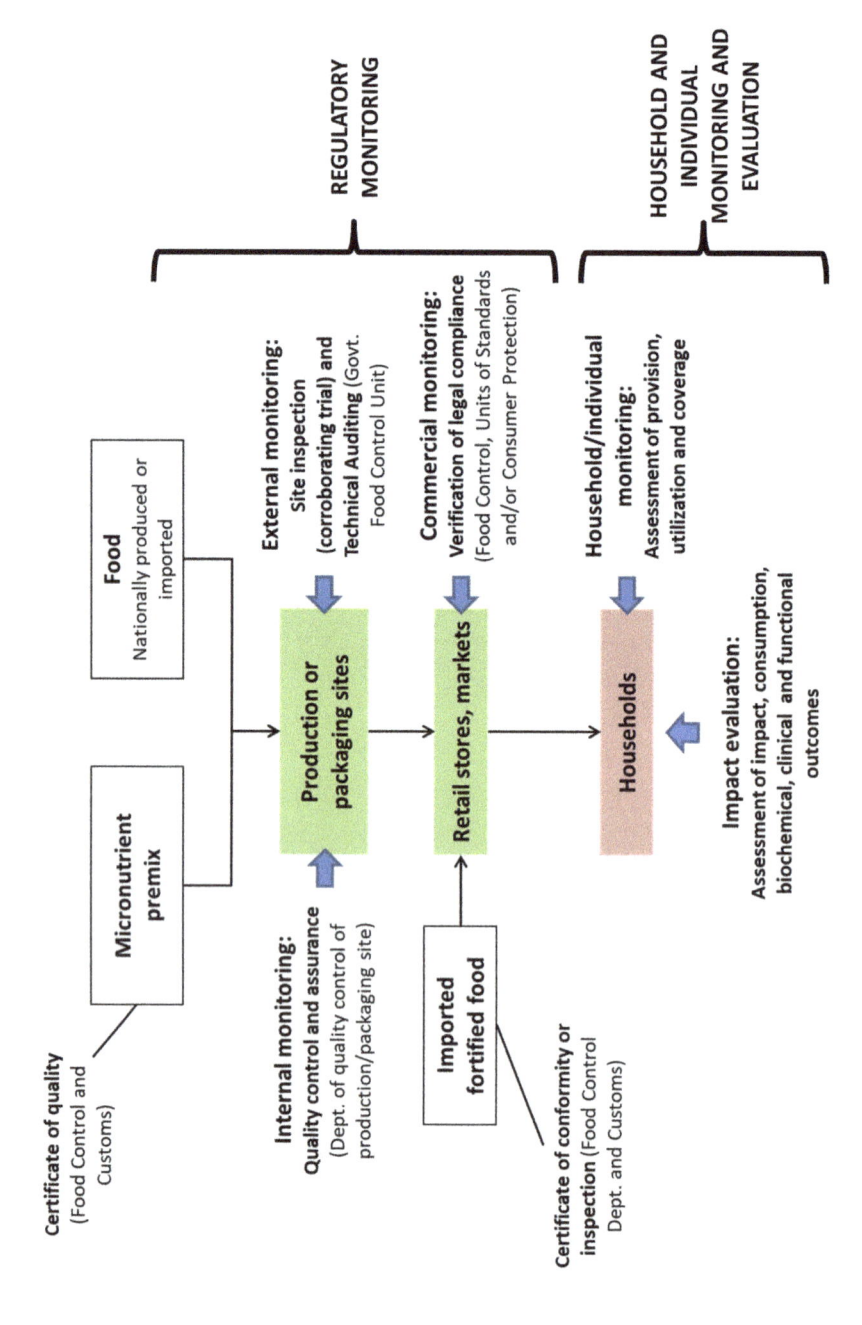

Fig. 18 Monitoring and evaluation of food fortification and its public health effects. Based on Allen et al., 2006.

food would be at risk of absorbing too much of the added nutrient, especially if their intake from other sources is already high before the fortification. Intake of the fortificant must therefore be estimated for all levels of consumption of the vehicle food.

Negative effects of universal fortification with iron have occurred in the past. In Iran, during a pilot project to study the effects of flour fortification with iron, an increase in markers of oxidative stress in non-anaemic men was found after 16 weeks of the intervention (Pouraram et al., 2012).

A thorough situation analysis and a safety assessment are therefore needed before the development of a fortification programme to determine the best approach to take. If the amount of the vehicle foods consumed varies widely, the necessary level of fortificant to reach the desirable intake in consumers with the lowest intake might put high consumers at an unacceptable risk of excessive intake. In this case, it might be preferable to choose a lower fortification dosage and select one or more additional food vehicles that are consumed by persons at risk of inadequate intake of the nutrient to be added (Allen et al., 2006).

The safety assessment must take into account all potential sources of the nutrient including supplements, and this can present a challenge when many different products are fortified, especially on a voluntary basis, and consumed simultaneously. Defining maximum levels of added nutrients is therefore particularly important for market-led fortification as some foods may be consumed in high amounts by population groups for which the UL is lower than for other groups, such as young children in the case of breakfast cereals. This issue has been presented as an objection to the universal fortification of flour with folic acid, which would benefit women of childbearing age but might be detrimental to older adults suffering from vitamin B_{12} deficiency by hindering the diagnosis of anaemia caused by cobalamin deficiency and exacerbating neurological and cognitive disorders (Selhub & Rosenberg, 2016).

3.6.3 Salt Iodization

Iodine deficiency is common in many parts of the world, especially with low levels of iodine in the soil, and adverse health effects and disorders resulting from insufficient iodine intake have long been known, ranging from miscarriage, congenital anomalies, neurocognitive impairment and increased perinatal morbidity in the foetus and newborn to impaired physical and mental development, hypothyroidism, goitre and other disturbances in older children, adolescents and adults. A widely used and practical method to assess iodine status is the measurement of urinary iodine concentration (UIC) based on the fact that over 90% of iodine ingested with food is excreted through the kidneys. At population level, a median UIC between 100 and 199 µg/l is considered optimal, even though lower values do not allow the diagnosis of iodine deficiency in individuals. Values from 20–49 µg/l indicate a moderate and below 20 µg/l a severe iodine deficiency (Eastman & Zimmermann, 2018).

In light of the high prevalence of iodine deficiency, the addition of iodine to table salt was the first fortification measure, dating back to the early 1920s when it was introduced in Switzerland and the US state of Michigan to prevent and cure goitre (Zimmermann, 2008). Other countries followed and currently (as of 2021), 147 have legislation for the universal iodization of table salt, 126 of which have mandatory legislation and 21 voluntary. Fortification of salt also includes other nutrients in some countries, mostly fluoride or, in the case of India and Ethiopia, iron (Global Fortification Data Exchange). While the average coverage of households with iodized salt has been estimated at 89% in 2021, there is high variability between countries (UNICEF, 2021b). Especially in countries with voluntary salt iodization, the level of implementation varies widely and may be insufficient. Variable coverage of households with iodized salt is even observed in high-income countries, especially in the European Region where most countries iodize table salt at least on a voluntary basis but where non-iodized salt is also available (Global Fortification Data Exchange, Žmitek & Pravst, 2016). Sales of iodized salt have even been found to decline in this region recently (European Salt Producers Association, 2017). Moreover, mandatory iodization is restricted to table salt in many countries, whereas it is voluntary for salt used in industrially processed foods (Ohlhorst et al., 2012). There is no large-scale salt iodization in the United Kingdom, even though it is the only European high-income country with mandatory flour fortification (Global Fortification Data Exchange). Problems with the availability and use of iodized salt have also been identified in Vietnam (Codling et al., 2015).

The WHO Eastern Mediterranean Region has overall seen a positive trend with regards to the iodine status of its population and the implementation of universal salt iodization. Salt iodization is mandatory in 20 of the 22 countries of the region, making it the WHO region with the highest proportion of member countries mandatorily iodizing salt (91%). The two remaining countries, Djibouti and Syria, fortify salt at least voluntarily (Fig. 19). Progress has been made particularly in Iran and Jordan (Doggui et al., 2020).

In Iran, iodine deficiency disorders manifesting as goitre showed a high prevalence in the past, as revealed by surveys in 1968 and the 1980s. 1989 saw the establishment of the Iranian National Committee for Control of Iodine Deficiency Disorders, charged with monitoring the process of salt iodization and iodine concentrations in salt and the level of household consumption of iodized salt consumption, as well as assessing the iodine status of school children (8–10 years) through measurement of UIC, training health workers and informing the public about iodine nutrition. Following the introduction of universal salt iodization in 1993, the coverage of households with adequately iodized salt increased from 50% in 1994 to 90% only 2 years later. Accordingly, goitre prevalence declined significantly, albeit with some delay, from 68% in 1989 to 5.7% in 2007, having been below 10% since 2002 (Delshad & Azizi, 2017; Doggui et al., 2020). A recent national survey conducted from 2016 to 2017 in 13,428 8- to 10-year-old school children also showed a good supply of iodine with a mean UIC of 186 µg/l and 65.4% of the sample in the optimal UIC range of 100–290 µg/l. Very low values of <20 µg/l were detected in less than 1% of the sample and between 20 and 49.9 µg/l in only 4.1%. Notably, mean iodine supply was adequate in 30 of the 31 Iranian provinces included in the study, while mean values were below 100 µg/l (80–90 µg/l) in Northern Khorasan where the highest prevalence of mild to moderate iodine deficiency was also observed (21.5%) (Rezaie et al., 2020). Even though iodine deficiency or low urinary iodine concentrations still persist in some regions of the country, the Iranian salt iodization programme can be considered a success story within the Eastern Mediterranean Region (Doggui et al., 2020).

In Jordan, more than a third of school children (37.7%) were found to be suffering from goitre in the first national survey from 1993. Median

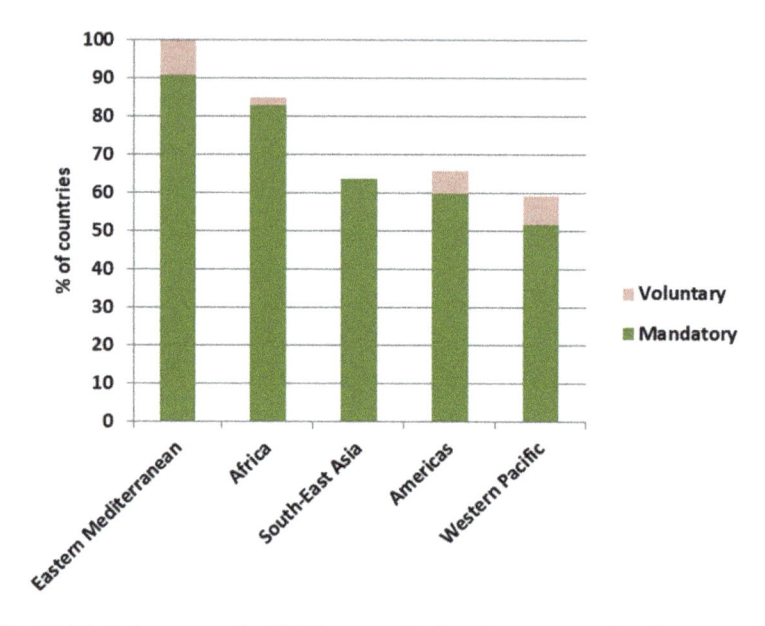

Fig. 19 Salt iodization in the WHO regions by legislation status (% of countries). Source of data: Global Fortification Data Exchange.

UIC was 40 µg/l, indicating a public health problem of iodine deficiency. Universal salt iodization was started in 1995. In 2000, median UIC in 8 to 10-year-old children had increased to 154 µg/l, even though goitre prevalence was still 32.1% (Kharabsheh et al., 2004; Doggui et al., 2020). In 2010, a survey reported a median UIC of 203 µg/l and an overall goitre prevalence of 4.9%. Household coverage with adequately iodized salt (15–40 mg/kg) was found to be sufficient at 96.4% (Ministry of Health Jordan, 2011). The iodine content of salt is internally and externally assessed monthly at the production sites and over the distribution chain.

In Saudi Arabia, iodine status of school children and adolescents based on median UIC was found to be sufficient and goitre prevalence to be low in surveys from the 1980s and 1990s, even though deficiencies were observed at the regional level (Al-Nuaim et al., 1997; Doggui et al., 2020). Mandatory universal salt iodization was launched in 2007 to improve iodine supply in the deficient parts of the country and to prevent iodine deficiency. At first, the concentration was set at 70–100 mg/kg but was reduced to 15–40 mg/kg as recommended by the WHO. A survey conducted in 2012 reported that, while adequately iodized salt was available to 69.8% of households, iodine concentrations in the majority of the analysed salt samples (70.7%) exceeded the allowed range, whereas 4.8% had concentrations <15 μg/kg. The availability of non-iodized salt at a low price was seen as a hurdle to achieving the target household coverage of ≥90% (Al-Dakheel et al., 2018). A study of school children from South-Western Saudi Arabia dating from 2013 found a median UIC of 19 μg/l and levels below 20μg/l in more than half of the participants, while none had UIC>100μg/l. Goitre was found in 24% of the children, with 5.5% having grade 2 goitre. Moreover, 22.5% of salt samples taken from the households were inadequately iodized with contents below the recommended range (Abbag et al., 2015). While, overall, iodine status is sufficient in Saudi Arabia, regional differences exist that require attention.

Iodine sufficiency was also shown in the most recent surveys in Bahrain, Kuwait and the United Arab Emirates. All 3 countries have practised mandatory salt iodization since 2007. While surveys from Kuwait and Bahrain predating the introduction of universal salt iodization already showed adequate levels of median UIC at the national level, goitre prevalence was 40% in schoolchildren from the Emirates, and the median UIC was 91 μg/l, corresponding to mild iodine deficiency, with regional differences. However, the latest survey from 2008–2009 showed a median UIC of 162 μg/l and a household coverage with iodized salt of 94% (Azizi et al., 2003; Doggui et al., 2020).

Oman introduced mandatory universal salt iodization in 1996 after iodine status was found to be insufficient in a national survey of school children from 1993–1994 (median UIC = 91 μg/l, 14.6% of samples <50 μg/l). The importation of non-iodized salt was banned in 1995. Surveys from 2004 and 2014 showed adequate iodine status (with median UIC of 223 μg/l and 194 μg/l, respectively; the former study had only included women). The prevalence of UIC <50 μg/l had fallen to 3.5% (Doggui et al., 2020).

In Afghanistan, high prevalence of goitre was repeatedly observed in the 1960s and 1990s. Salt iodization was started in 2000 and became mandatory in 2011. During the 2000s, goitre prevalence stayed high and the consumption of iodized salt was found to be low. In 2004, median UIC was <50 μg/l in children, young women and pregnant women. Only 12% of households had access to iodized salt. Two decades of civil war had left the country bereft of the means to tackle the problem appropriately. However, starting in 2003, particular efforts were taken to increase the coverage of iodized salt and eliminate iodine deficiency. The main targets were: the production, quality, distribution and marketing of iodized salt; support from the public sector and the government to improve technology, legislation and coordination and to develop a national surveillance system; and campaigns to raise consumer awareness. Salt production was successful modernized with a growth in large-scale factories. A national committee for universal salt iodization was established to support and further increase the consumption of iodized salt. The national nutrition survey from 2013 showed a significant improvement of iodine status with median UIC of 171 µg/l in school children and of 107 µg/l in women of reproductive age as well as a markedly higher household coverage of 66% (Hamid et al., 2014, Doggui et al., 2020).

In Egypt, the first reports of goitre occurrence date back to the 1930s. Iodization of salt began in 1995 and legislation for universal salt iodization was enacted in 1996, while the current law on mandatory iodization dates from 2015 (Global fortification data exchange, https://fortificationdata.org/). A survey in 2014/2015 showed the efficiency of the programme with median UIC in the adequate range (170 µg/l). However, goitre is still observed in the region of South Sinai, although this could be due to high fluorine intake rather than iodine deficiency. The household coverage of adequately iodized salt increased from 68% in 2005/2006 to 79% in 2008 and was 74.7% in 2014/2015 (Doggui et al., 2020). The most recent data from UNICEF gives 92.5% (Global fortification data exchange, https://fortificationdata.org/). A national workshop held in 2017 identified a need for continuous monitoring at the market level to reinforce the iodization programme, as well as ensuring the free access of salt producers to potassium iodate and raising awareness about iodine nutrition through education campaigns. A large number of small salt producers, many of whom are unlicensed and not applying quality control measures, pose a threat to universal salt iodization as it was found that around a quarter of salt was inadequately iodized (Ismail & Hussein, 2018).

Pakistan has a long history of iodine deficiency manifesting as goitre. A high regional variability in the prevalence of goitre has also been observed, with high occurrence particularly in the mountainous north-west. In 1994, universal salt iodization was introduced and median UIC increased to 126 µg/l in 2000 and to 158 µg/l in 2011, suggesting iodine sufficiency at the national level. However, large regional differences exist and various studies reported high proportions (>50%) of inadequately iodized salt samples (Khattak et al., 2017). The National Nutrition Survey 2018 reported the use of iodized salt by 79.6% of households across Pakistan with a slightly higher proportion in urban than in rural settings (84.4% vs. 76.7%). Regional differences were quite large, with a coverage of only 31.6% in the province of Khyber Pakhtunkhwa compared to around 90% in Islamabad Capital Territory, Punjab, Azad Jammu and Kashmir, and Gilgit Baltistan. UIC was in the sufficient range in 61.2% of 6 to 12-year-old children, while 8.4 had mild, 23% moderate and 7.3% severe deficiency (Ministry of National Health Services, Regulations and Coordinations, Government of Pakistan, 2018). Legislation is mandatory, but its full implementation faces difficulties. A major obstacle to the successful nationwide implementation of universal salt iodization is the lack of uniform legislation for all provinces of Pakistan (Khattak et al., 2017).

Mild iodine deficiency was first reported from Palestine in 1997, with large regional variation of goitre prevalence. Salt iodization was introduced in 1996. A survey from 2010 showed adequate iodine status in Palestinian school-age children with a median UIC of 193 µg/l. Adequately iodized salt was available to 86% of households compared to 37% in 1995. In 2013, this number had declined to 72% but iodine intake was still sufficient, as indicated by a median UIC of 193 µg/l in school children. A higher value was found in the Gaza Strip than in the West Bank (239 vs. 153 µg/l, respectively). In the Gaza Strip, a high percentage of the participating children had excessive UIC (35.6%) while the proportion was lower in the West Bank (12.9%) (Ministry of Health-Palestine & UNICEF, 2014). Regular monitoring of salt iodization appears advisable.

In Tunisia, iodized salt was first introduced in the north-western regions of the country where high prevalence of iodine deficiency and goitre had been observed since the first surveys in the 1970s. However, salt iodine contents were found to be low and iodine deficiency still prevalent in later studies in the 1990s. At national level, a median UIC of 158µg/l was measured in school children in 1995. In 1996, salt iodization was extended to the whole country at a level of 15–27 mg/kg. Subsequent surveys repeatedly showed adequate iodine status in school-age children. However, 2 surveys in 2012 found a high prevalence of excessive UIC particularly in the southern regions of the country and excessive iodine content in 22% of the salt samples, while only 55.8% were adequately iodized. This highlights the need for a tighter control of the iodization process to ensure adequate iodine nutrition while at the same time avoiding excessive intake (Doggui et al., 2020b).

Iodine deficiency (mean UIC <50 µg/l and goitre prevalence of 50%) was observed in Northern Iraq in 1965 and then in the 1990s in women of reproductive age and school-age children. Salt iodization was initiated in 1990 and became mandatory in 1993. However, the political instability and conflict during the 2000s caused a low availability and consumption of iodized salt. A scaling-up of iodine fortification has been pursued by a cooperation of national and international experts since 2010, but mild iodine deficiency has been observed in school-age children and pregnant women in 2011–2012 and 2013, respectively, highlighting the need for further efforts to improve iodine nutrition in Iraq (Doggui et al., 2020).

In Lebanon, iodine deficiency was identified as a public health issue by regional surveys in the 1960s. Already in 1971, a law was passed to mandate the fortification of salt with 10–200 mg/kg of iodine, but, due to the political unrest in the country, its implementation was delayed until 1995. In the first national study from 1993, mild iodine deficiency was observed in school-age children as shown by a median UIC of 60 µg/l. In 1996 and 2004, household coverage with iodized salt reached 90% and median UIC had increased to 95 µg/l by 1997, but numbers have declined more recently. In 2013–2014, median UIC had fallen to 66 µg/l and 56% of salt samples were inadequately iodized (<15 mg/kg). In 2007, a standard for food-grade salt was published and, in 2011, the legislation for salt iodization was amended with a smaller range of potassium iodate to be added (60–80 mg/kg). In 2016, a Policy Brief was issued pointing out the shortcomings of the current iodization policy and suggesting actions to improve it. For instance, a revision of the legislation was prompted as well as better monitoring, infrastructure and more training and support for the salt producing industry (Akik et al., 2016).

Morocco introduced mandatory universal salt iodization in 1995 in light of the common occurrence of iodine deficiency across the country. The level of iodine to be added was set at 80 mg/kg but this amount proved to promote excessive intakes, so that it was reduced to 15–40 mg/kg as recommended by the WHO. However, low median UIC levels were observed in the following years, especially in mountainous areas, and coverage remained unsatisfactory at 59% in 2007. More recently, it was found that the situation had not improved. The predominance of private salt manufacturers and the marketing of non-iodized salt were identified as major factors preventing the success of the USI programme (Zahidi et al., 2016; Doggui et al., 2020).

A number of surveys since the 1950s showed a high prevalence of iodine deficiency and goitre in Sudan. Iodine was first supplied through supplements in the 1970s before fortification of oil and sugar was tried. Mandatory universal salt iodization (USI) started in 1994. However, high goitre prevalence and low median UIC were still reported. By 2006, the percentage of households using iodized salt had increased to 14.4%, an improvement compared to the situation in 2000, when it had been only about 1%, but still much too low (Mahfouz et al., 2012; Doggui et al., 2020). Coverage was found to be <8% in the 2014 Multiple Indicator Cluster Survey (MICS). The fact that universal salt iodization was only implemented in ten of Sudan's eighteen provinces presents a major obstacle to the reduction of iodine deficiency. In 2015, a national committee for salt iodization was established during a national meeting held to spur the USI programme. High priority was given to the revision of the legislation and the improvement of its enforcement, as well as improvements in national salt production (Hussein, 2015). By 2018, a production plant had been created with the aim of reaching nationwide coverage of iodized salt of 90% by 2022. Standards and specifications for iodized salt were approved in 2019 and became mandatory in 2020 (Republic of Sudan, 2019; Doggui et al., 2020).

On the other hand, some countries in the region are facing the risks of excessive iodine supply. This is the case in Qatar, Somalia and Djibouti, where iodine concentration is naturally high in the groundwater and drinking water. All countries mandatorily iodize salt but the use of adequately iodized salt was found to be low in Djibouti and Somalia (1.6% and 7%, respectively). Nevertheless, high median UIC was reported in national surveys. In Qatar, on the other hand, adequately iodized salt was consumed by 87% of households and it may hence be advisable to reduce the content of iodine in salt (Doggui et al., 2020). An overview of the status of salt iodization in the countries of the region is given in Table 31.

3.6.4 Fortification of Wheat Flour, Maize Flour and Rice

In 2021, mandatory fortification of wheat flour, maize flour and/or rice was practised in 91 countries worldwide. Wheat flour is the most commonly fortified cereal with 67 countries having legislation for this product alone, one country (Papua New Guinea) only for rice, 16 countries for wheat and maize flour, 5 countries for wheat flour and rice, and just 2 countries (the USA and Costa Rica) for all 3 cereal types. In addition, 13 countries have voluntary fortification for wheat flour, and some of those with mandatory fortification of wheat flour additionally fortify maize flour or rice on a voluntary basis. Voluntary fortification is common for breakfast cereals, especially in industrialized countries where it has been found to contribute significantly to micronutrient intake in children (Hennessy et al., 2013). The most frequently added micronutrients are iron and folic acid, followed by other vitamins of the B group, while only few countries also add zinc, calcium and/or vitamin D and A.

Guidance on the fortification of wheat and maize flour with iron, folic acid, vitamin B_{12}, vitamin A and zinc is offered by a Consensus Statement from the WHO issued on the occasion of the Second Technical Workshop on Wheat Flour Fortification: Practical Recommendations for National Application that was held in the Spring of 2008 in Stone Mountain, Georgia. The focus was on these 5 micronutrients as they have particular relevance for public health in many countries. It was recommended that fortification of wheat and maize flour should be considered when these foods are industrially produced and regularly consumed by large proportions of a country's population, and that fortification should be mandated at a national level to have the most effective public health impact (WHO et al., 2009).

The choice of nutrients to add and the appropriate level should be based on a number of factors including the nutritional requirements

Table 31 Status of salt iodization in the WHO Eastern Mediterranean Region. Source of data: Doggui et al., 2020; UNICEF, 2021b.

Country	Legislation for universal salt iodization (USI)	Date of introduction of USI	Household coverage (%)	Iodine level (mg/kg) added
Afghanistan	Mandatory	2011	56.6 (2016)	≥15
Bahrain	Mandatory	1994	57.7 (2013–2014)	20–40
Djibouti	Mandatory	n.d.	79.5 (2015)	n.d.
Egypt	Mandatory	1996	92.5 (2015)	≥18
Iran	Mandatory	1990	93.5 (2000)	≥40
Iraq	Voluntary	1993	68.3 (2018)	≥20
Jordan	Mandatory	1995	88.3 (2000)	≥40
Kuwait	Mandatory	n.d.	n.d.	40–80
Lebanon	Mandatory	1995	95.3 (2004)	36–47
Libya	Mandatory	n.d.	69.1 (2007)	n.d.
Morocco	Mandatory	1995	25.0 (2014–2015)	15–40
Oman	Mandatory	1996	65.8 (2004)	20–40
Pakistan	Mandatory	1994	69.1 (2011)	≥15
Palestine	Mandatory	n.d.	88.2 (2014)	21–33 35–55 K iodate
Qatar	Mandatory	n.d.	n.d.	15–40
Saudi Arabia	Mandatory	1997	68.7 (2012)	15–40
Somalia	Mandatory	n.d.	7.5 (2009)	≥15
Sudan	Mandatory	1994	34.4 (2014)	≥15
Syria	Voluntary	1992	65.4 (2009)	18–30
Tunisia	Mandatory	1995	93.8 (2012)	15–27 25–45 K iodate
United Arab Emirates	Mandatory	n.d.	n.d.	20–40
Yemen	Mandatory	1996	48.7 (2013)	≥20

and deficiencies of the population, the usual consumption profile of industrially milled domestically produced or imported flour that could in principle be fortified, the sensory and physical effects of the fortificant nutrients on flour and flour products, additional fortification of other food vehicles, use of vitamin and mineral supplements by the target population and costs (see Table 32) (WHO et al., 2009).

In 2020, about 20% of all industrially milled grains available for human consumption worldwide were fortified. There was only a small increase compared to 2019, when this percentage amounted to about 19% while the proportion of industrially milled grains had increased by almost 2%. The numbers are higher for wheat flour, of which about 32% of the industrially milled proportion and about 26% of the total amount were fortified in 2020 compared to 30% and 24%, respectively, in 2019. However, considering that about 81% of wheat flour was industrially milled in 2020, this shows that there is still a great potential for fortification (FFI, 2021).

Among the WHO regions, the highest percentage of countries with legislation for fortification of any grain is seen in the region of the Americas, where all countries mandatorily fortify wheat flour, 6 have additional mandatory and one voluntary legislation for maize flour, and 8 countries also fortify rice (5 mandatorily, 3 voluntarily). The lowest percentage is seen for the WHO European Region, where only 8 of 53 member states fortify wheat flour mandatorily and none voluntarily. Since Brexit, no country of the European Union has any legislation for the mass fortification of grain products (see Fig. 20).

In the WHO Eastern Mediterranean Region, fortification of wheat flour dates back to 1978 when Saudi Arabia began to add iron, folic acid, thiamine, riboflavin and niacin.

In 2021, 17 of the 22 member states (77%) practiced either mandatory or voluntary fortification, and 13 do so mandatorily, while 2 members of the Gulf Cooperation Council (Qatar, and the United Arab Emirates) as well as Iraq and Sudan have voluntary legislation (see Fig. 21). In addition to mandatory wheat flour fortification, Bahrain also voluntarily enriches rice. Fortification has been discontinued in Egypt but its re-uptake is being considered (FFI, 2021). However, political instability and economic hardship currently affecting many countries in the region often compound the implementation of fortification (WHO EMRO, 2019b).

Table 32 Average levels of nutrients recommended by the WHO to consider adding to fortified wheat flour depending on extraction, fortificant chemical form and per-capita flour availability. Modified from WHO et al., 2009.

Nutrient	Extraction rate of flour	Fortificant chemical form	Level of nutrient to add (in mg/kg) by estimated average wheat flour availability (in g/day/capita)[1]			
			<75[2]	75–149	150–300	>300
Iron	Low or high	NaFeEDTA	40	40	20	15
	High	Ferrous sulfate or fumarate	60	60	30	20
	High	Electrolytic iron	NR[3]	NR[3]	60	40
Folic acid	Low or high	Folic acid	5.0	2.6	1.3	1.0
Vitamin B$_{12}$	Low or high	Cyanocobalamin	0.04	0.02	0.01	0.008
Vitamin A	Low or high	Retinyl palmitate	5.9	3.0	1.5	1.0
Zinc[4]	Low	Zinc oxide	95	55	40	30
	High	Zinc oxide	100	100	80	70

[1] These estimated levels apply if only wheat flour is used as main fortification vehicle. If other food vehicles are mass-fortified effectively, these suggested fortification levels may need to be adjusted downwards as needed.

[2] Estimated per capita consumption of <75 g/day does not enable the addition of sufficient amounts of fortificant to cover micronutrients needs for women of childbearing age. Fortification of additional food vehicles and other interventions should be considered.

[3] NR = Not Recommended because very high levels of electrolytic iron would be needed that could negatively affect sensory properties of fortified flour.

[4] Assuming 5 mg zinc intake and no additional phytate intake from other dietary sources

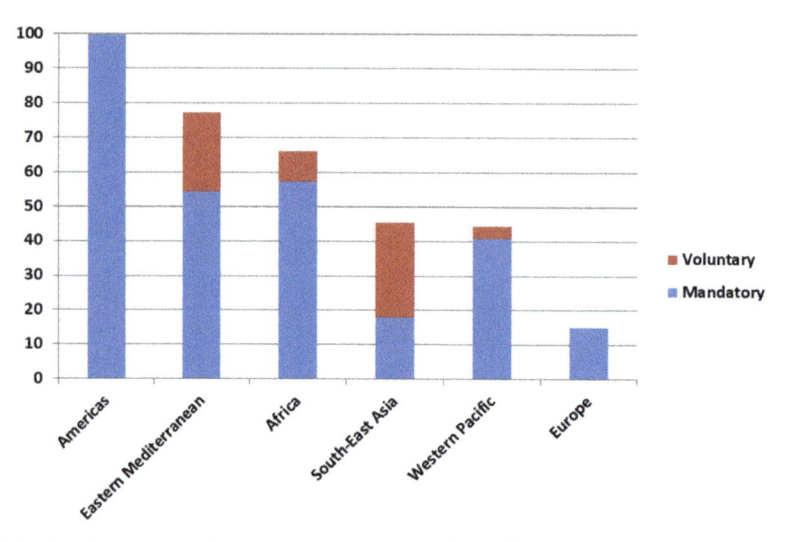

Fig. 20 Percentage of countries practising wheat flour fortification by WHO region and legislation status. Source of data: WHO EMRO, 2019b; Global Food Fortification Data Exchange.

Iron and folate are added by all countries with either mandatory or voluntary fortification legislation, followed by the B vitamins thiamine (B_1), riboflavin (B_2), and niacin that are used in 7 countries. Less common is the addition of zinc, vitamin B_{12}, vitamin A and D (see Table 33 and Fig. 22).

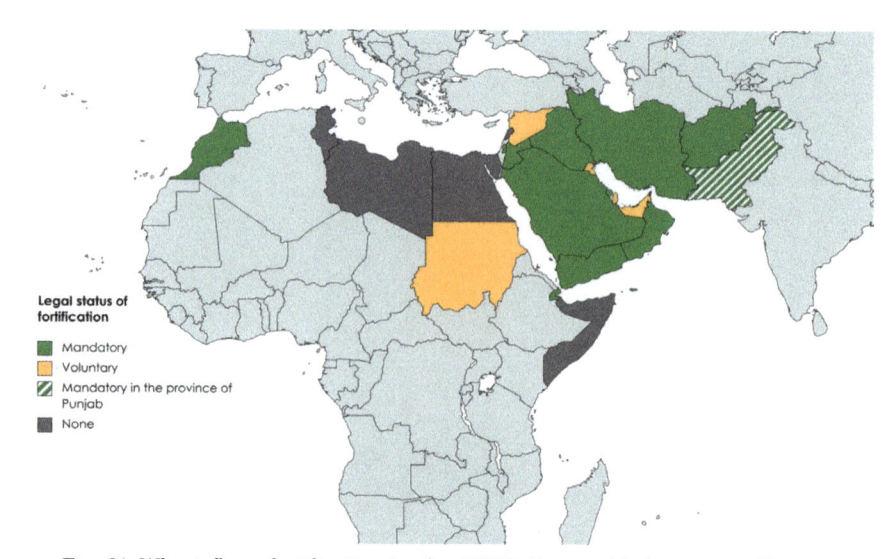

Fig. 21 Wheat flour fortification in the WHO Eastern Mediterranean Region. Source of data: WHO EMRO, 2019b; Global Food Fortification Data Exchange.

Of the Gulf Cooperation Council countries, Bahrain, Kuwait, Oman and Saudi Arabia all mandate the fortification of wheat flour with iron and folate but differ in their choice of additional nutrients. The levels of fortificants are regulated by Standard GSO194/ 2015 ICS 67.060 of the Gulf Cooperation Council Standardization Organization (GSO, 2015). Saudi Arabia is the only one of the countries (and one of 3 in the region) to also add vitamin D.

In turn, Qatar and the United Arab Emirates have voluntary wheat flour fortification. In all 6 countries, flour is almost exclusively produced by industrial mills and the rate of fortification is very high (90–100%) (WHO EMRO, 2019b). Mandatory legislation for wheat flour fortification also exists in Iran since 2007. Currently, iron and folic acid are added but the Iranian government is considering whether to include vitamin D and zinc as well. All wheat flour is industrially milled and fortified, and there is infrastructure for quality control and the evaluation and monitoring of the programme.

In Jordan, mandatory fortification of wheat flour was established in 2006. The premix contains vitamins B_1, B_2 and niacin as well as vitamin B_6, B_{12} and A, iron and zinc, and since 2010 it has also included vitamin D. The coverage of fortification is high (95%) and all flour is produced in industrial mills (WHO-EMRO, 2019b). There is also a monitoring system in place, including internal monitoring by the mills and external monitoring performed by the food fortification Technical Committee that has proven very successful. The Technical Committee is coordinated by the Nutrition Division of the Ministry of Health, but composed of members from different agencies including the Ministry of Industry and Trade, the Jordanian Food and Drugs Administration (JFDA) and provincial health inspectors (Wirth et al., 2013).

However, issues have been encountered regarding the funding of the premix that have proven challenging, especially for the subsidized bread for the refugees hosted by the country, and more trained personnel in the mills are needed. Capacity building for the evaluation of the impact of the fortification programme and improving its enforcement and monitoring, as well as improved financial support, are among the priorities for future action (WHO-EMRO, 2019b).

In Morocco, wheat flour fortification with iron and folic acid began in 2004 and became mandatory in 2006. A system for monitoring and

Table 33 Status of industrial processing and fortification of wheat flour (and rice) in the countries of the WHO EMR. Source of data: Global Fortification Data Exchange; WHO EMRO, 2019b.

Country	Proportion of cereal industrially milled (IM) and fortified (F) (%)	Legal status of fortification, year	Micronutrients added
Afghanistan	IM: 63; F: 72,7	Mandatory, 2018	Fe, folic acid, vitamin B_{12}, vitamin A
Bahrain	IM: 100; F: 95	Mandatory, 2002	Fe, folic acid
Djibouti	F: 0	Voluntary, 2012	Rice: Fe, vitamin B_1, B_2, niacin
Egypt	IM: 100; F: 95	Mandatory, 2013	Fe, Zn, folic acid
Iran	IM: 90	None	
Iraq	IM: 100; F: 100	Mandatory, 2007	Fe, folic acid, proposal for Zn and vitamin D
Jordan	IM: 100; F: 50	Mandatory, 2008	Fe, folic acid
Kuwait	IM: 100; F: 95	Mandatory, 2002	Fe, folic acid, Zn, vitamin B_1, B_2, niacin, vitamin B_6, B_{12}, vitamin A, D
Lebanon	IM: 100; F: 100	Mandatory,	Fe, folic acid, vitamin B_1, B_2, niacin
Libya	IM: 100; F: 0	None	
Morocco	IM: 100; F: 0	None	
Oman	IM: 100; F: 70	Mandatory, 2006	Fe, folic acid
	IM: 100; F: 100	Mandatory, 1996	Fe, folic acid, Zn, vitamin B_1, B_2, niacin, vitamin B_6, B_{12}, vitamin A

Country	Proportion of cereal industrially milled (IM) and fortified (F) (%)	Legal status of fortification, year	Micronutrients added
Pakistan	IM: 32; F: 14	Planned, pilot project in Punjab, 2017	Planned: Fe, folic acid, Zn, vitamin B_{12}
Palestine	IM: 100; F: 90	Mandatory, 2006	Fe, folic acid, Zn, vitamin B_1, B_2, niacin, vitamin B_6, B_{12}, vitamin A, D
Qatar	IM: 100; F: 95	Voluntary, 2015	Fe, folic acid, vitamin B_1, B_2, niacin
Saudi Arabia	IM: 100; F: 95	Mandatory, 2006	Fe, folic acid, vitamin B_1, B_2, niacin, vitamin D
Somalia	IM: 100; F: 0	None	
Sudan	IM: 80; F: 40	Voluntary, 2011, mandatory in development	Fe, folic acid, Zn, vitamin B_{12}, vitamin A
Syria	IM: 80; F: 5	Voluntary	Fe, folic acid
Tunisia	IM: 100; F: 0	None	
United Arab Emirates	IM: 100; F: 95	Voluntary, 2015	Fe, folic acid, vitamin B_1, B_2, niacin
Yemen	IM: 100; F: 95	Mandatory, 2001	Fe, folic acid

evaluation is in place, having been revised in 2015–2016. In 2019, NaFe-EDTA was substituted for the elementary iron that had been used until then to increase the bioavailability (Royaume du Maroc, 2019). All of the flour is processed in industrial mills and 70% of it is fortified (WHO-EMRO, 2019b; Global Fortification Data Exchange).

Palestine started mandatory wheat flour fortification in 2006. Together with Jordan, it adds the widest range of micronutrients in the region with iron, folic acid, zinc, as well as vitamins B_1, B_2, niacin, B_6, B_{12}, A and D. However, the compliance with the technical regulations is unsatisfactory, especially in Gaza, where only 11% of the flour is fortified and only 1.7% conforms to the standards. A somewhat better situation is seen in the West Bank, where 60% of the flour is fortified, albeit only 40% according to the standards. Major issues arise from border controls, weak monitoring, incomplete implementation of the law and insufficient funding. For instance, the costs for the premix have to be borne by the mills as subsidies are provided by the government. In Gaza, only the flour distributed by the United Nations fully complies with the fortification regulations. Subsidizing the premix is thus a priority for the future, to warrant the sustainability of the programme, along with increasing the monitoring capacity of the inspectors to improve the enforcement of the law, and capacity building for micronutrient testing (WHO-EMRO, 2019b).

Yemen and Djibouti have mandated wheat flour fortification since 2001 and 2013, respectively. In both countries, all flour is produced by industrial mills and fortification rates are high (95 to 100%).

In Afghanistan, wheat flour fortification became mandatory in 2018 after having been voluntary since 2006. About a fourth (26%) of wheat flour is industrially milled, according to the Food Fortification Initiative, with 71% of the flour being fortified; before this, most of the flour was imported (WHO EMRO, 2019b). However, with the recent political changes in the country, the further implementation of the programme is uncertain.

Iraq has begun fortifying wheat flour with iron and folic acid in 2006 with mandatory legislation and governmental financing of the premix since 2008. However, supply of the premix was discontinued in 2014. The political and economic insecurity in Iraq, electrical power shortages, lack of equipment and training of staff as well as problems with the maintenance of the predominantly private mills pose significant obstacles to the implementation of the policy. Future objectives include: the revision of the legislation on fortification; the extension of the programme to include more micronutrients; enhanced monitoring and evaluation and the maintenance of the funding (WHO EMRO, 2019b).

Syria and Sudan both have legislation for the voluntary fortification of wheat flour. In Sudan, legislation for mandatory food fortification is being prepared. A national fortification alliance providing a forum for different stakeholders, including government representatives, United Nations agencies, nongovernmental organizations and the private sector that had been established in 2005 was reactivated in 2013. Over 90% of wheat flour is processed in 6 large mills, one of which has been fortifying flour voluntarily with iron and folic acid since 2005 (WHO EMRO, 2019b). Currently, 40% of flour is fortified (Global Fortification Data Exchange). In 2017, a new 4-year food fortification project was initiated. Ensuring the sustainability of financial support for fortification is a major challenge. Future priorities include enforcing national standards for fortified flour, raising public awareness of the benefits from fortified food, obtaining industry commitment, capacity building for staff and expanding surveillance systems (WHO EMRO, 2019b).

In Syria, while 80% of flour is processed by industrial mills, only about 5% of it is currently fortified (WHO EMRO, 2019b).

Egypt had a mandatory wheat flour fortification programme in place that was discontinued in 2011 due to a lack of funding and political will, political instability leading to ministry personnel exchanges, as well as modifications of the subsidy programme for local bread. In 2019, the Ministry of Supply and Internal Trade decided to restart the programme following a comprehensive situation assessment by the Food Fortification Initiative (FFI). So far, a flour fortification committee has been established by the Government of Egypt and the FFI to guide the implementation of the programme, ensure its sustainability, develop the legal requirements for mandatory fortification and assess the situation and readiness of the mills. National monitoring guidelines were drafted with the newly established Food Safety Authority to assure compliance with the programme (WHO EMRO, 2019b).

Pakistan has currently established no mandatory fortification of wheat flour, but planning for its implementation is ongoing and a national standard for wheat flour fortification has been developed. There have been some attempts at wheat flour fortification in the past. A National Wheat Flour Fortification Programme was established in 2005 with funding support from the Global Alliance for Improved Nutrition (GAIN) but was discontinued in 2010 due to the dissolution of the Ministry of Health that had coordinated the activities. Some regional initiatives followed, and, in 2013, a national fortification alliance with GAIN support was established with the aim of bringing together relevant stakeholders from different government ministries, international and national agencies and partners for the planning and monitoring of food fortification programmes and to obtain support. Related forums have also been created at the provincial level (Zuberi et al., 2016; WHO EMRO, 2019b). In 2016, a 5-year food fortification programme (FFP) funded by the United Kingdom Department for International Development was initiated. Fortification was launched in the province of Punjab and is gradually expanded to the entire country. The programme also provides support to the milling industry. Custom duties were levied on the import of vitamin and mineral premixes, as well as sales taxes, and exemptions on custom duties were granted for the import of feeder equipment. Micronutrients that are to be added to wheat flour include iron, folic acid, zinc and vitamin B_{12}. The introduction of mandatory legislation and the allocation of government funding for the implementation and strengthening of monitoring and enforcement of legislation are the priorities for future action, together with the improvement of quality assurance and control and monitoring through training and capacity-building activities for industry and monitoring staff. Key objectives of the FFP are: to gain political commitment for ensuring governance in the development of standards, legislation and enforcement; actively involving the industry and private sector into the programme; and raise consumers' awareness of the benefits of fortified food (FFP, 2019a & b). In 2021, 992 flour mills were registered with the programme (652 in Punjab) and 14% of the flour was fortified (http://www.ffp-pakistan.org/).

No fortification programmes exist to date in Lebanon, Libya, Somalia and Tunisia.

Other staple foods that are commonly fortified are cooking oils and fats, margarine and fat spreads as well as sugar. Oils and fats generally

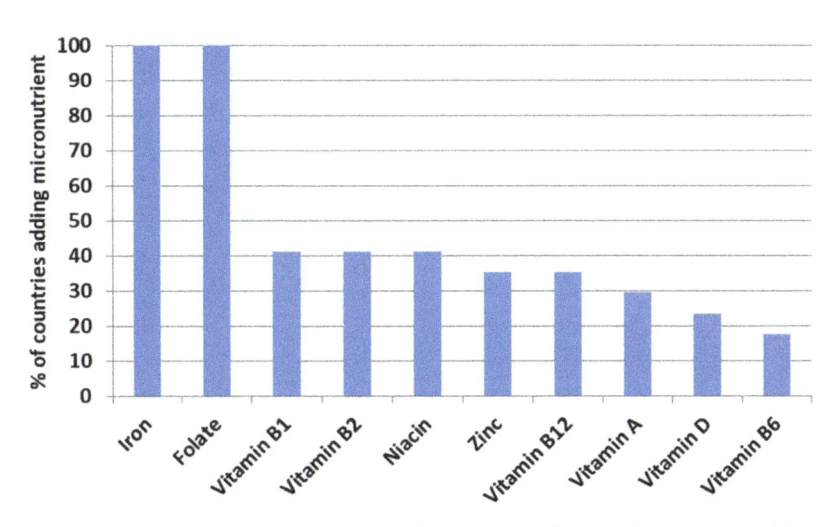

Fig. 22 Frequency of micronutrients added to wheat flour in the countries of the WHO Eastern Mediterranean Region. Source of data: Global Fortification Data Exchange.

serve as vehicles for the fat-soluble vitamins A and D as well as vitamin E in some countries. While sugar fortification is currently mostly practised in Latin America and in some countries in Sub-Saharan Africa (Mkambula et al., 2020), 44 countries as of 2021 have standards for oil fortification, 33 practising it mandatorily and 11 voluntarily. Twenty of these countries are low-income countries, but only 4 are high-income (Global Fortification Data Exchange). In most industrialized countries, margarine has been fortified with vitamin A and D, either mandatorily or voluntarily, for many decades, originally to make it equivalent to butter (IMACE, 2004). In the WHO Eastern Mediterranean Region, 5 countries (Afghanistan, Djibouti, Oman, Pakistan and Yemen) have mandatory legislation for the fortification of oil with vitamin A and vitamin D, while it is voluntary in Morocco (Global Fortification Data Exchange). Pakistan has the longest practice, dating back to 1965 and also including ghee. However, implementation and enforcement of the law have been found to be unsatisfactory so that the Food Fortification Programme, which started in 2016 with funding from the UK Department for International Development, also focuses on the improvement of oil and ghee fortification (FFP, 2019a).

3.6.5 Effectiveness of Food Fortification

The effectiveness of food fortification has been corroborated by a number of studies from countries with long-term experience of its implementation. Most evidence exists for iron and folic acid.

A comprehensive systematic review from 2013, including 201 studies from various countries all over the world and with different income levels, found significant improvements of haemoglobin and ferritin levels and reduced prevalence of anaemia after consumption of foods fortified with iron in children and women. Consumption of foods enriched with folic acid by women reduced the risks for neural tube defects (including spina bifida and anencephaly) in their children. There were also positive effects for iodine in both population groups and for vitamin A, vitamin D, calcium and zinc in children only (Das et al., 2013).

A systematic review of 18 randomized controlled trials (RCTs) in children under the age of 10 years showed that the consumption of food fortified with iron increased haemoglobin concentrations significantly (Athe et al., 2013). Another systematic review of 60 studies, most of which were conducted in children, also found a significant mean increase in haemoglobin levels and serum ferritin, and reduced risks for anaemia and iron deficiency in people consuming foods fortified with iron (Gera et al., 2012). The effect of flour fortification with iron was studied using a meta-analysis of 13 studies of government-supported, widely implemented fortification programs only. A significant positive effect on ferritin levels in women of reproductive age and in children was observed, while evidence was lower for anaemia prevalence. The authors concluded that this may be due to the fact that iron deficiency is only one of many causes of anaemia (Pachón et al., 2015).

Folic acid fortification of flour was associated with a significant decline in the incidence of neural tube defects (NTDs) in 15 of 27 studies from 9 countries included in a systematic review. The largest reductions, by 50% and more, were observed in Costa Rica, Canada, Argentina and Chile, the smallest in the USA (Castillo-Lancelotti et al., 2012).

The studies included in all these meta-analyses are limited to the extent that they differ widely in the levels, types and combinations of micronutrients as well as the food vehicles used. Many date from the time before the recommendations on food fortification by the WHO were released. However, more recent studies from Brazil and Australia reconfirm the effect of flour fortification with folic acid on NTDs. In Australia, where mandatory flour fortification with folic acid was introduced in 2007, NTD incidence was particularly reduced in the Aboriginal population in whom it had been higher, thus abolishing the former disparity (Pacheco Santos et al., 2016; D'Antoine & Bower, 2019).

Support for food fortification comes also from studies conducted in the WHO Eastern Mediterranean Region. The effects of flour fortification with iron and folic acid were observed in a pilot intervention in two Iranian provinces. Two years after the start of the programme, the mean level of ferritin in women aged 15–49 years increased significantly and the prevalence of low ferritin levels declined significantly, even though no effects were seen on haemoglobin levels or on anaemia prevalence (Sadighi et al., 2009). In the Iranian province of Golestan, flour fortification with folic acid significantly raised daily folate intake and serum folate in women aged 15–49 years, while both the prevalence of folate deficiency and the incidence of NTDs declined significantly (Abdollahi et al., 2011).

Other countries have also reported benefits from the fortification of wheat flour with iron and folic acid. In Iraq, following the implementation of food fortification together with nutritional education and supplementation, the prevalence of anaemia in women of reproductive age (15–49 years) fell from 35% to under 20% and from 26% to 21% in children under 5 years between 2008 and 2014 (WHO EMRO, 2019b). A decrease in anaemia was also observed in 15- to 49-year-old women and children under 5 years in Jordan 2000–2010 (WHO EMRO, 2019b). In Morocco, a decline in anaemia rates from 47.8% in 2006 to 29.9% in 2008 was seen in 2- to 5-year-old children (El-Hamdouchi et al., 2010) and of the prevalence of folic acid deficiency in women (Wirth et al., 2012). A decrease in the incidence of neural tube defects was reported for the period of 2008 to 2011 (Radouani et al., 2015). In Bahrain, anaemia prevalence in 6- to 18-year-old children and adolescents decreased between 2005 and 2011 after the introduction of flour fortification accompanied by nutritional education and supplementation initiatives. In pregnant women, iron-deficiency anaemia was observed less frequently, and the incidence of neural tube defects has decreased since 2000 (WHO EMRO, 2019b).

While there is solid evidence for the effectiveness of fortification with iron and folic acid to reduce the prevalence and incidence of anaemia and neural tube defects, more recently, vitamin D is gaining attention as a fortificant in light of the high prevalence of vitamin D deficiency worldwide. A recent meta-analysis supports the use of foods fortified with vitamin D to improve 25-OH levels when baseline levels are in the deficient range (<50 nmol/l) and intake of vitamin D was >10 µg/d (Dunlop et al., 2021). Food fortification with vitamin D was also evaluated by a meta-analysis of 5 studies from Iran in adults. Consumption of enriched dairy products or bread was associated with a significant increase in 25-OH levels (Nikooyeh & Neyestani, 2018).

3.6.6 Challenges and Obstacles to Food Fortification and How to Address Them

Some common challenges that can interfere with the successful implementation of food fortification as revealed by the experiences of various countries include:

- low awareness of the health impact of micronutrient deficiencies, low prioritisation and lack of political will to address the problem;
- difficulties in coordinating cooperation between agencies and government bodies from different fields and the private sector involved in the implementation and monitoring of the programme;
- limited evidence of the programme's impact and cost-effectiveness due to a lack of evaluation and research;
- lack of regulatory clarity and of technical guidance;
- insufficient or inadequate information on food consumption, nutrient status and the prevalence of micronutrient deficiencies that are required to inform public policy-making and for the evaluation of the programme's effectiveness;
- difficulties in obtaining the necessary financial and other resources for sustainable funding (e.g., for the provision of the

premix and the technical equipment as well as for maintaining monitoring);

- lack of human resources, technical equipment and know-how and low capacity to instruct and train food producers and managers as well as food inspectors;
- attaining a high coverage of fortification when production is dominated by several decentralized small-scale production sites (cereal and oil mills etc.);
- control of the appropriate fortification of imported foods, especially in the case of a high dependence on these;
- opposition from interest groups;
- failure of regulatory agencies to ensure compliance (Luthringer et al., 2015; Osendarp et al., 2018).

Costs of fortification (for the premix, the technical equipment etc.) can present a particular obstacle for small-scale food producers and processors and limit their competitiveness. High costs of the premix were named as the dominant barrier to fortification by 75% of respondents in a study assessing barriers and successes experienced by fortification systems in low- and middle-income countries from Africa and Asia (Luthringer et al., 2015). High expenses that have to be fully borne by the producers are often passed on to consumers, making the fortified products less attractive and even inaccessible to low-income groups that may benefit most from them. Manufacturers may also be tempted to deliberately under-fortify their products, particularly when external monitoring is weakly performed. This underlines the necessity of offering funding for premix along with other incentives for compliance. Adequate regulatory documents and guidelines to steer the fortification process and guide producers and controllers are also required, as well as strong and consistent penalties for violations.

A functioning cooperation between the public and private sectors together with engagement from consumers, civil society, academia, NGOs and donors is key to enable a holistic approach to food fortification. Such a cooperation is facilitated by the establishment of coordination entities like the National Fortification Alliances (NFAs) that have been created in a number of countries. NFAs act as neutral supervisors that guide the establishment, improvement and maintenance of the food fortification programme, facilitating the cooperation between the government, private sector, NGOs and civil society towards a common public health goal. By providing the leadership and managing the available budget, NFAs can help to reconcile the diverging interests of individual sectors, tackle financial constraints and increase awareness of the potential of food fortification.

Further support is provided by international actors including non-governmental technical agencies, for example the Food Fortification Initiative (FFI), the Global Alliance for Improved Nutrition (GAIN), the Iodine Global Network (IGN) and others; UN Agencies (UNICEF, FAO, WFP and WHO); academia; various donors (governmental organizations, the World Bank, the European Commission, the Bill & Melinda Gates Foundation and others) and private sector players (Hoogendoorn et al., 2016).

Regional cooperation between the countries of the WHO Eastern Mediterranean Region is recommended to allow the sharing of experiences and the propagation of new technologies and developments. A harmonized approach to food fortification taking into account individual countries' context facilitates trade, thereby increasing the access to fortified foods across the region (WHO EMRO, 2019b).

3.6.7 Biofortification — A New Approach to Micronutrient Supply

Biofortification takes a different approach to increasing the micronutrient content of foods by using agronomic and plant-breeding techniques or genetic modification (see Fig. 23). Micronutrients are thus already enriched during plant development and growth, instead of after harvest or during processing as in conventional fortification. Agronomic techniques include the application of enriched fertilizers with high solubility and bioavailability to the soil or directly on the leaves, as well as the use of beneficial microorganisms that promote plant growth and micronutrient absorption. While these techniques have been shown to increase the contents of trace elements in some crops like legume seeds, their success depends on the soil properties and the absorption by and distribution within the plant. Iron in particular has been shown to have a low bioavailability from soils. Fertilizers have to be applied repeatedly and this can have harmful effects on the environment and also reduce the absorption of other essential micronutrients while at the same time raising the cost of the procedure. Moreover, agronomic techniques only serve to increase the concentration of minerals and trace elements, but not of organic components like vitamins (Hirschi, 2009).

However, the fact that the micronutrients of many common crops show a high natural variability between varieties and growing conditions offers the potential to select varieties that are naturally richer in one or several micronutrients through conventional breeding. Genetic diversity is particularly high in local heirloom varieties that are also well adapted to their native environments and generally more resilient to climate extremes (Dwivedi et al., 2019).

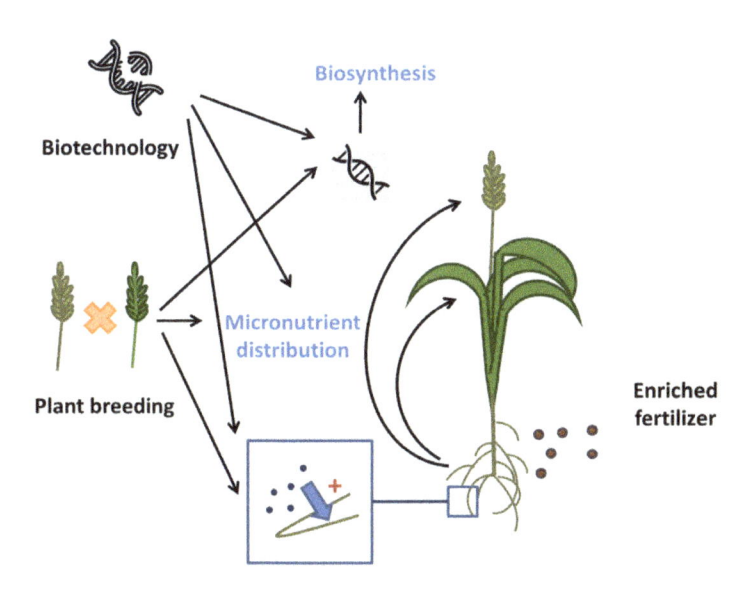

Fig. 23 Mechanisms of biofortification.

Higher micronutrient contents of crops can be achieved by increasing the absorption of trace elements from the soil, their distribution within the plant to the edible parts, as well as the reduction of antinutrients. Micronutrient storage can also be improved with regards to more bioavailable forms (White & Broadley, 2009). Crop varieties with these properties are crossbred with varieties offering other beneficial traits like high yield, drought tolerance and resistance to pests and diseases to produce new crops that are at the same time nutrient-rich and productive (Global Panel, 2015; GAIN, 2020).

Another advantage of breeding over the use of fertilizers is that the former can also increase the production of organic components like vitamins and beneficial non-nutritive compounds. A major advantage of the conventional breeding approach to biofortification is the fact that it uses intrinsic properties of the plant so that regulatory restrictions are limited. Conventionally-bred crops are generally also more accepted by consumers compared to genetically-engineered plants. Nevertheless, the success of breeding depends on the natural genetic variability of the crop in question. It also cannot introduce nutrients that are not naturally produced (Marques et al., 2021). These disadvantages can be overcome by genetic engineering that allows not only the direct potentiation or silencing of already present traits, but also the introduction of completely new ones even across species (Hirschi, 2009; Jha & Warkentin, 2020). A well-known example is Golden Rice, which was genetically modified to produce the pro-vitamin A β-carotene absent from conventional rice. Other applications include the enhanced expression of the essential amino acid methionine in beans, in which it is naturally limited (Jha & Warkentin, 2020).

However, the required technological knowledge and equipment, as well as the need for trained staff and the high costs of crop development, limit its applicability in low-income countries especially. In addition, genetically-modified crops often meet with resistance and generally have to undergo extensive regulatory approval procedures that differ between countries, thus raising the costs and time it takes for the release of bioengineered crops. For this reason, conventional breeding is often considered as the most efficient, cost-effective and sustainable approach to biofortification (Garg et al., 2018). Most of the biofortified crops released so far have been obtained through conventional breeding and this method is also applied by international and regional research initiatives on biofortification, such as HarvestPlus, a programme created by the Consultative Group on International Agricultural Research (CGIAR), or the European Union's HealthGrain (Marquez et al., 2021).

Some of the advantages and disadvantages of the different approaches to biofortification are summed up in Table 34.

Regardless of the approach taken, biofortification may be more effective than food fortification in targeting low-income subsistence farmers in remote areas, who have no access to processed and enriched foods. Global programmes like the Commercialization of Biofortified Crops (CBC) Programme of the Global Alliance for Improved Nutrition (GAIN) and HarvestPlus are dedicated to the development and propagation of biofortified crops and the creation of enabling environments for their dissemination to disadvantaged population groups.

Although the focus of these programmes lies primarily on low-income countries from sub-Saharan Africa and South-East Asia, some countries of the WHO Eastern Mediterranean Region like Pakistan, Egypt and Syria also feature among the top-priority countries for investment in the biofortification interventions listed in the HarvestPlus Biofortification Priority Index.

The index offers guidance for investments in biofortified crops by ranking the potential nutrition and health impact of the biofortification of 13 kinds of staple crops in the 128 countries included. In 2020, crops biofortified with iron, zinc and/or provitamin A were cultivated in Afghanistan, Pakistan, Syria, Egypt, Lebanon, Morocco and Tunisia. So far, most countries have not yet released biofortified crops but are testing them in the field (Fig. 24). For zinc-enriched wheat, 8 of the top 20 priority countries are from the EMR (Pakistan, Afghanistan, Syria, Egypt, Morocco, Iran, Iraq, Tunisia), and 7 for lentils fortified with iron and zinc (Syria, Morocco, Yemen, Iran, Lebanon, Pakistan, Tunisia). These two crops are the most commonly cultivated along with, to a lesser degree, pro-vitamin-A-enriched crops like maize and orange sweet potato.

While diet diversification should be the first option for improving the status of micronutrients, fortification, either of foods during processing or in the form of biofortification during crop growth, provides a valuable way to supply critical micronutrients, especially when access to healthy varied foods is limited.

Table 34 Advantages and disadvantages of biofortification techniques.

	Use of fertilizers	Classical plant breeding	Genetic engineering
Advantages	Compensation for insufficient mineral content in the soil.	Use of natural genetic variation.	No dependence upon natural variability in the gene pool.
	Simple and comparatively inexpensive.	Requires no technological expertise.	Introduction of micronutrient forms with higher bioavailability.
	Increased bioavailability of minerals through transformation into their organic forms.	Few legal constraints.	Control over distribution within the plant (targeting to edible parts).
		Higher public acceptance than genetic engineering.	Efficient and fast variety development.
Disadvantages	Only usable for certain minerals and trace elements (e.g., I, Se, to a lesser degree Zn).	Limited natural variability.	High technological and knowledge requirements.
	Dependence on soil properties (composition, pH).	It takes a long time for variety development.	High initial costs for crop development.
	No control over mineral uptake and mobility in the plant.	Risk of dependence of farmers on certain seed suppliers and loss of biodiversity.	Important regulatory constraints.
	Need for regular application of fertilizers.		Patented transgenic crops not available to poorer communities.
	Higher cost compared to conventional fertilizers.		Risk of dependence of farmers on certain seed suppliers and loss of biodiversity.
	Possible environmental harm.		Regulatory barriers.
			Low public acceptance in certain communities.

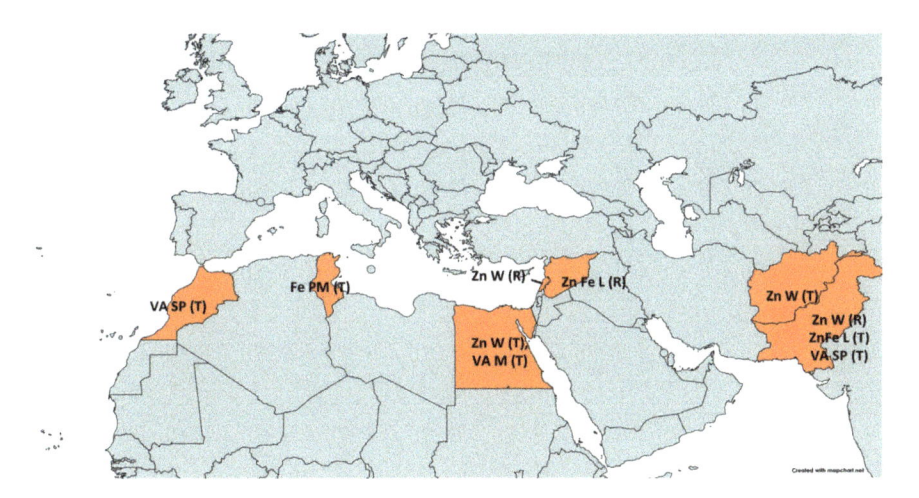

3.6 Food Fortification, Including Biofortification 241

Fig. 24 Countries of the WHO Eastern Mediterranean Region with biofortified crops released or in testing. Abbreviations: Zn W: zinc-fortified wheat, Zn Fe L: zinc- and iron-fortified lentil, Fe PM: iron-fortified pearl millet, VA M: pro-vitamin A-fortified maize, VA SP: pro-vitamin A-fortified orange sweet potato, (R): released, (T): tested. Source of data: HarvestPlus.

4. Conclusion and Outlook

The WHO Eastern Mediterranean Region is particularly affected by the multiple burdens of malnutrition. The countries of the region are currently in different phases of the nutrition transition, resulting in an increasing consumption of highly processed foods and a co-occurrence of undernourishment and micronutrient deficiencies, as well as overweight and obesity with their associated high prevalence of NCDs. The region currently has one of the highest rates of NCDs, particularly of diabetes mellitus type 2, which is expected to increase further, placing a heavy burden on healthcare systems and causing a high number of deaths and DALYs.

In addition, in a difficult natural environment that makes farming challenging, the increasing impact of climate change and the political unrest that has plagued the region for years pose a threat to food security that has further been exacerbated by the COVID-19 pandemic. As in other parts of the world, food losses and waste are significant contributors to the environmental footprint of food production in the region.

Against this background, a shift towards healthier and more sustainable diets is urgently needed for the health of the region's population and its environment. The Food Systems Summit convened by the United Nations presents a unique opportunity to set out in this direction. To support Member States, the WHO has proposed 6 game-changing actions some of which are also considered as best buys to prevent and control NCDs. To achieve the best outcome, these measures should be part of a multidimensional approach that also includes other policies and actions on health and nutrition, such as the development of national food-based dietary guidelines, public education campaigns, and investments in primary healthcare infrastructure.

The implementation of these actions in the WHO Eastern Mediterranean Region varies by action and country. The region has one of the highest rates of mandatory fortification of wheat flour and of salt iodization, which are effective measures to reduce common micronutrient deficiencies and their associated diseases such as anaemia and goitre.

The need to limit the harmful effects of a high intake of salt, sugar, saturated and especially trans-fatty acids (TFAs) is increasingly recognized in the countries of the region, many of which limit their content in foods, ban the use of major sources like partially hydrogenated fats for TFAs and forbid certain foods in settings like schools. The increasing awareness of the important role of a healthy food environment is also reflected in legislation. In addition, a number of governments are assuming their responsibility as public food procurers to ensure that diets served in public settings are healthy and sustainable.

However as summed up in Table 35 below, progress has mostly been made in a limited number of countries including the Gulf Cooperation Council Member States and the Islamic Republic of Iran, while other countries, namely those with low income levels and lacking the necessary administrative capacity, lag behind. The exchange of experiences between countries, for example in the context of workshops such as those that have previously been organized by the WHO, can help Member States overcome potential difficulties in the development and implementation of nutrition policies.

Overall, more efforts are particularly needed with regards to the implementation of the International Code on the Marketing of Breastmilk Substitutes as well as of the Recommendations on the Marketing of Unhealthy Foods and Beverages to Children.

A lack of cooperation between stakeholders has been identified as a major obstacle to the successful implementation of nutrition policies in some countries. There is often also a lack of awareness and knowledge at population level, emphasizing the importance of accompanying measures with information campaigns and education. Food labelling helps consumers to identify healthier foods, particularly in the form of easily understandable front-of-pack labels, but so far only a few countries have developed models.

For established policies, monitoring and evaluation activities have to be strengthened to ensure that implementation is properly enforced and to verify that the intended outcomes are achieved. Providing evidence for the effectiveness of a policy is also crucial to gain the support of the involved stakeholders and the public.

Cooperation between the countries of the EMR and the adoption of uniform standards and regulations for food profiling, labelling and marketing is advised to facilitate regional trade, contribute to food security and make food systems more sustainable and resilient to crises like those caused recently by the COVID-19 pandemic and the war in Ukraine.

See Online: Table 35 Actions and policies implemented or planned in the countries of the WHO Eastern Mediterranean Region.

References

Aalipour F (2019). Evaluation of salt, sodium, and potassium intake through bread consumption in Chaharmahal and Bakhtiari Province. *Int J Epidemiol Res* 6(2): 60–64, https://dx.doi.org/10.15171/ijer.2019.11

Abachizadeh K, Ostovar A, Pariani A, Raeisi A (2020). Banning advertising unhealthy products and services in Iran: A one-decade experience. *Risk Management and Healthcare Policy* 13: 965–968, https://doi.org/10.2147/rmhp.s260265

Abbag FI, Abu-Eshy SA, Mahfouz AA, Al-Fifi SA, El-Wadie H, Abdallah SM, Musa MG, Devansan CS, Patel A (2015). Iodine-deficiency disorders in the Aseer region, south-western Saudi Arabia: 20 years after the national survey and universal salt iodization. *Public Health Nutr* 18(14): 2523–2529, https://doi.org/10.1017/S1368980014003073

Abd El-Fatah NK, Abu-Elenin MM (2019). Prevalence of Stunting, Overweight and Obesity among Egyptian Primary School Children in Behera Governorate. *Food and Public Health* 9(3): 84–93, https://doi.org/10.5923/j.fph.20190903.02

Abdelkarim O, Ammar A, Soliman AMA, Hökelmann A (2017). Prevalence of overweight and obesity associated with the levels of physical fitness among primary school age children in Assiut city. *Egyptian Pediatric Association Gazette* 65(2): 43–48, https://doi.org/10.1016/j.epag.2017.02.001

Abdollahi Z, Elmadfa I, Djazayery A, Golalipour MJ, Sadighi J, Salehi F, Sadeghian Sharif S (2011). Efficacy of flour fortification with folic acid in women of childbearing age in Iran. *Ann Nutr Metab* 58: 188–196, https://doi.org/10.1159/000329726

Abduelkarem AR, Sharif SI, Bankessli FG, Kamal SA, Kulhasan NM, Hamrouni AM (2020). Obesity and its associated risk factors among school-aged children in Sharjah, UAE. *PLoS ONE* 15(6): e0234244, https://doi.org/10.1371/journal.pone.0234244

Abi Khalil, H, Hawi, M, & Hoteit, M (2022). Feeding patterns, mother-child dietary diversity and prevalence of malnutrition among under-five children in Lebanon: A cross-sectional study based on retrospective recall. *Frontiers in Nutrition* 9: 815000, https://doi.org/10.3389/fnut.2022.815000

Abolli S, Kazemi J, Hajian Motlagh Z (2021). Evaluating the quality of bread; based on the amount of salt and baking soda consumption. *J Community Health Research* 10(1): 33–40, http://dx.doi.org/10.18502/jchr.v10i1.5829

Abu Dhabi Education Council, Abu Dhabi Food Control Authority and Health Authority (2011). *School Canteen Guidelines of the Emirate of Abu Dhabi.*

AbuKhader M, Abdelraziq R, Al-Azawi M, Khamis Ali S (2020). A comparative examination of dietary sodium content in bread and its public consumption pattern in Muscat, Oman. *Nutrition & Food Science* 50(1): 116–130, https://doi.org/10.1108/NFS-02-2019-0058

Abul-Fadl A, El Atti J, Arabi A, El-Emmari L, Al-Jawaldeh A (2019). Status of breastfeeding in north african countries of the Eastern Mediterranean Region. *MCFC-Egyptian Journal of Breastfeeding (EJB)* 15: 11–40, https://doi.org/10.6084/m9.figshare.8940071.v1

Afshin A, Peñalvo JL, Del Gobbo L, Silva J, Michaelson M, O'Flaherty M et al. (2017). The prospective impact of food pricing on improving dietary consumption: A systematic review and meta-analysis. *PLoS ONE* 12(3): e0172277, https://doi.org/10.1371/journal.pone.0172277

Aguenaou H, El Ammari L, Bigdeli M, El Hajjab A, Lahmam H, Labzizi S et al. (2021). Comparison of appropriateness of Nutri-Score and other front-of-pack nutrition labels across a group of Moroccan consumers: awareness, understanding and food choices. *Arch Public Health* 79: 71, https://doi.org/10.1186/s13690-021-00595-3

Ahmed MH, Ali YA, Awadalla H, Elmadhoun WM, Noor SK, Almobarak AO (2017). Prevalence and trends of obesity among adult Sudanese individuals: Population based study. *Diabetes Metab Syndr* 11 (Suppl. 2): S963–S967, http://dx.doi.org/10.1016/j.dsx.2017.07.023

Akik C, El-Mallah C, Ghattas H, Obeid O, El-Jardali F (2016). *K2P Policy Brief: Informing Salt Iodization Policies in Lebanon to Ensure Optimal Iodine Nutrition.* Knowledge to Policy (K2P) Center, Beirut, Lebanon, April 2016.

Al-Dakheel MH, Haridi HK, Al-Bashir BM, Al-Shangiti AM, Al-Shehri SN, Hussein I (2018). Assessment of household use of iodized salt and adequacy of salt iodization: a cross-sectional National Study in Saudi Arabia. *Nutr J* 17 (1): 35, https://doi.org/10.1186/s12937-018-0343-0

Aldubayan K, Murimi M (2019). Compliance with school nutrition policy in Riyadh, Saudi Arabia: a quantitative study. *East Mediterr Health J* 25(4): 230–238, https://doi.org/10.26719/emhj.18.034

Al-Ghannami S, Al-Shammakhi S, Al Jawaldeh A, Al-Mamari F, Al Gammaria I, Al-Aamry J, Mabry R (2019). Rapid assessment of marketing of unhealthy foods to children in mass media, schools and retail stores in Oman. *East Mediterr Health J* 25(11): 820–827, https://doi.org/10.26719/emhj.19.066

Alhamad N, Almalt E, Alamir N, Subhakaran M (2015). An overview of salt intake reduction efforts in the Gulf Cooperation Council countries. *Cardiovasc*

Diagn Ther 5(3): 172–177, http://dx.doi.org/10.3978/j.issn.2223-3652.2015.04.06

Aljaadi AM, Alharbi M (2021). Overweight and obesity among Saudi children: Prevalence, lifestyle factors, and health impacts. In: Laher I (ed.), *Handbook of Healthcare in the Arab World*. 1st ed., Cham, Switzerland: Springer International Publishing, https://doi.org/10.1007/978-3-319-74365-3_187-1

Al Jawaldeh A, Al-Khamaiseh M (2018). Assessment of salt concentration in bread commonly consumed in the Eastern Mediterranean Region. *East Mediterr Health J* 24(1): 18–24, https://doi.org/10.26719/2018.24.1.18

Al Jawaldeh A, Rafii B, Nasreddine L (2018a). Salt intake reduction strategies in the Eastern Mediterranean Region. *EMHJ* 2018: 1172–1180, https://doi.org/10.26719/emhj.18.006

Al-Jawaldeh A, El Mallah C, Obeid O (2018b). Regional policies on sugar intake reduction at population levels to address obesity in the Eastern Mediterranean. *JSM Nutr Disord* 2(1): 1006, http://dx.doi.org/10.6084/m9.figshare.8247836.v1

Al-Jawaldeh A, McColl K (2020). *Protecting food security and nutrition from the impact of the COVID-19 pandemic in the Eastern Mediterranean Region: from policy to action. Adapting the regional strategy on nutrition 2020–2030*. Cairo: WHO Regional Office for the Eastern Mediterranean; 2020. Licence: CC BY-NC-SA 3.0 IGO, https://www.researchgate.net/publication/350850414_Protecting_food_security_and_nutrition_from_the_impact_of_the_COVID-19_pandemic_in_the_Eastern_Mediterranean_Region_from_policy_to_action_Adapting_the_regional_strategy_on_nutrition_2020-2030

Al-Jawaldeh A, Megally R (2020). Impact evaluation of national nutrition policies to address obesity through implementation of sin taxes in Gulf Cooperation Council countries: Bahrain, Saudi Arabia, Oman, United Arab Emirates, Kuwait and Qatar. *F1000Res* 2020, 9: 1287, http://dx.doi.org/10.12688/f1000research.27097.1

Al-Jawaldeh A, Almamary S, Mahmoud L, Nasreddine L (2020). Leveraging the Food System in the Eastern Mediterranean Region for Better Health and Nutrition: A Case Study from Oman. *Int J Environ Res Public Health* 17: 7250, https://doi.org/10.3390/ijerph17197250

Al-Jawaldeh A, Rayner M, Julia C, Elmadfa I, Hammerich A, McColl K (2020b). Improving Nutrition Information in the Eastern Mediterranean Region: Implementation of Front-of-Pack Nutrition Labelling. *Nutrients* 12: 330, https://doi.org/10.3390/nu12020330

Al-Jawaldeh A, Hammerich A, Doggui R, Engesveen K, Lang K, McColl K (2020c). Implementation of WHO recommended policies and interventions on healthy diet in the countries of the Eastern Mediterranean Region: From policy to action. *Nutrients* 12: 3700, https://doi.org/10.3390/nu12123700

Al-Jawaldeh A, Taktouk M, Doggui R, Abdollahi Z, Achakzai B, Aguenaou H (2021a). Are countries of the Eastern Mediterranean Region on track towards meeting the world health assembly target for anemia? A review of evidence. *Int J Environ Res. Public Health* 18: 2449, https://doi.org/10.3390/ijerph18052449

Al-Jawaldeh A, Taktouk M, Chatila A, Naalbandian S, Al-Thani A-AM, Alkhalaf MM et al. (2021b) Salt Reduction initiatives in the Eastern Mediterranean Region and evaluation of progress towards the 2025 Global Target: A systematic review. *Nutrients* 13: 2676, https://doi.org/10.3390/nu13082676

Al-Jawaldeh A, Taktouk M, Chatila A, Naalbandian S, Abdollahi Z, Ajlan B et al. (2021c). A systematic review of trans fat reduction initiatives in the Eastern Mediterranean Region. *Front. Nutr.* 8: 771492, https://doi.org/10.3389/fnut.2021.771492

Al-Jawaldeh A, Jabbour J (2022). Marketing of Food and Beverages to Children in the Eastern Mediterranean Region: A Situational Analysis of the Regulatory Framework. *Nutrients* (under review).

Al-kuraishy HM, Al-Gareeb AI, Atanu FO, EL-Zamkan MA, Diab HM, Ahmed AS, Al-Maiahy TJ et al. (2021). Maternal transmission of SARS-CoV-2: Safety of breastfeeding in infants born to infected mothers. *Front. Pediatr.* 9:738263, https://doi.org/10.3389/fped.2021.738263

Al-Lahham S, Jaradat N, Altamimi M, Anabtawi O, Irshid A, AlQub M (2019). Prevalence of underweight, overweight and obesity among Palestinian school-age children and the associated risk factors: a cross sectional study. *BMC Pediatrics* 19: 483, https://doi.org/10.1186/s12887-019-1842-7

Allen L, de Benoist B, Dary O, Hurrell R (eds) (2006). *Guidelines on food fortification with micronutrients*. Geneva: World Health Organization and Food and Agriculture Organization of the United Nations, http://apps.who.int/iris/bitstream/10665/43412/1/9241594012_eng.pdf

Almedawar MM, Nasreddine L, Olabi A, Hamade H, Awad E, Toufeili I et al. (2015). Sodium intake reduction efforts in Lebanon. *Cardiovasc Diagn Ther* 5(3): 178–185, http://dx.doi.org/10.3978/j.issn.2223-3652.2015.04.09

Al-Nuaim AR, Al-Mazrou Y, Kamel M, Al-Attas O, Al-Daghari N, Sulimani R (1997). Iodine Deficiency in Saudi Arabia. *Ann Saudi Med* 17(3): 293–297, https://doi.org/10.5144/0256-4947.1997.293

Al-Shehhi E, Al-Dhefairi H, Abuasi K, Al Ali N, Al Tunaiji M, Darwish E (2017). Prevalence and risk factors of obesity in children aged 2–12 years in the Abu Dhabi Islands. *World Family Medicine* 15(9): 61–74, https://doi.org/10.5742/MEWFM.2017.93103

Alsukait R, Wilde P, Bleich S, Singh G, Folta S (2019). Impact of Saudi Arabia's sugary drink tax on prices and purchases. *Curr Dev Nutr* 3 (Suppl 1): nzz034. P10-066-19, https://doi.org/10.1093%2Fcdn%2Fnzz034.P10-066-19

Al Tamimi HA (2021). The 'game changing' food systems actions: Qatar's Experience. Presentation at the Virtual Regional meeting on Creating food systems for safe, sustainable, healthy, and affordable diets in the Eastern Mediterranean Region, 16–17 August 2021.

Al-Thani M, Al-Thani A-A, Al-Chetachi W, Akram H (2017). Obesity and related factors among children and adolescents in Qatar. *Int J Basic Sci Med* 2(4): 161–165, https://doi.org/10.15171/ijbsm.2017.30

Amerzadeh M, Takian A (2020). Reducing sugar, fat, and salt for prevention and control of noncommunicable diseases (NCDs) as an adopted health policy in Iran. *Med J Islam Repub Iran* 34: 136, https://doi.org/10.47176/mjiri.34.136

Amini M, Doustmohammadian A, Ranjbar M (2021). Dietary risk reduction projects in industrial foods in Iran. *SJFST* 3(1): 1–4, http://dx.doi.org/10.47176/sjfst.3.1.1

An R (2012). Effectiveness of subsidies in promoting healthy food purchases and consumption: a review of field experiments. *Public Health Nutr* 16(7): 1215–1228, https://doi.org/10.1017/S1368980012004715

Athe R, Vardhana Rao MV, Nair KM (2013). Impact of iron-fortified foods on Hb concentration in children (<10 years): a systematic review and meta-analysis of randomized controlled trials. *Public Health Nutrition* 17(3): 579–586, https://doi.org/10.1017/S1368980013000062

Azizi F, Malik M, Bebars E, Delshad H, Bakir A (2003). Thyroid volumes in schoolchildren of the Emirates. *J Endocrinol Invest* 26: 56–60, https://doi.org/10.1007/bf03345123

Azizollaah Z, Dinarvand R, Hosseini H (2017). Nutritional traffic light labeling and taxation on unhealthy food products in Iran: Health policies to prevent non-communicable diseases. *Iran Red Crescent Med J* 19(8): e57874, http://dx.doi.org/10.5812/ircmj.57874

Babashahi M, Omidvar N, Joulaei H, Zargaraan A, Zayeri F, Veisi E et al. (2021). Scrutinize of healthy school canteen policy in Iran's primary schools: a mixed method study. *BMC Public Health* 21: 1566, https://doi.org/10.1186/s12889-021-11587-x

Backholer K, Vandevijvere S, Blake M, Tseng M (2018). Sugar-sweetened beverage taxes in 2018: a year of reflections and consolidation. *Public Health Nutr* 21(18): 3291–3295, https://doi.org/10.1017/S1368980018003324

Bandy LK, Scarborough P, Harrington RA, Rayner M, Jebb SA (2020). Reductions in sugar sales from soft drinks in the UK from 2015 to 2018. *BMC Medicine* 18: 20, https://doi.org/10.1186/s12916-019-1477-4

Belkhadir J, Brahimi M, Aguenaou H, Heikel J, El Berri H, Belakhal L, Gouaima Mazzi F, Benabed K (2021). Taxation of beverages and sweetened products in Morocco: A major achievement and a model to follow in the MENA region. *Journal of Medical and Surgical Research* VII(2): 817–820, http://dx.doi.org/10.46327/msrjg.1.000000000000176

Bin Sunaid FF, Al-Jawaldeh A, Almutairi MW, Alobaid RA, Alfuraih TM, Bensaidan FN et al. (2021). Saudi Arabia's Healthy Food Strategy: Progress & Hurdles in the 2030 Road. *Nutrients* 13: 2130, https://doi.org/10.3390/nu13072130

Bouhamida M, Benajiba N, Guennoun Y, Lachguer SA, Elhaloui NE, Zahrou F-E et al. (2020). Implementing the national strategy of salt reduction in Morocco: the baker´s perspective. *Pan African Medical Journal* 37: 337, https://doi.org/10.11604/pamj.2020.37.337.27139

Boyland E (2019). *Unhealthy food marketing: The impact on adults. A report produced for the Obesity Health Alliance*, http://obesityhealthalliance.org.uk/wp-content/uploads/2019/05/JFM-Impact-on-Adults-Boyland-May-2019-final-002.pdf

Boyland EJ, Harris JL (2017). Regulation of food marketing to children: are statutory or industry self-governed systems effective? *Public Health Nutr* 20 (5): 761–764, https://doi.org/10.1017/S136898001700046

Cairns G, Angus K, Hastings G & World Health Organization. (2009). *The extent, nature and effects of food promotion to children: a review of the evidence to December 2008*. Geneva: World Health Organization, https://apps.who.int/iris/handle/10665/44237

Campos S, Doxey J, Hammond D (2011). Nutrition labels on pre-packaged foods: A systematic review. *Public Health Nutr* 14: 1496–1506, https://doi.org/10.1017/S1368980010003290

Castillo-Lancellotti C, Tur JA, Uauy R (2012). Impact of folic acid fortification of flour on neural tube defects: a systematic review. *Public Health Nutr* 16(5): 901–911, https://doi.org/10.1017/S1368980012003576

Cecchini M, Warin L (2016). Impact of food labelling systems on food choices and eating behaviours: a systematic review and meta-analysis of randomized studies. *Obes Rev* 17(3): 201–210, https://doi.org/10.1111/obr.12364

CGIAR Research Program on Policies, and Markets (PIM) (2021). *Supporting Egypt's safety net programs for better nutrition and food security, inclusiveness, and effectiveness*. PIM Outcome Note, July 2021, Consultative Group on International Agricultural Research, https://doi.org/10.2499/p15738coll2.134530

Changing Markets Foundation (2017). *Milking it — How milk formula companies are putting profits before science*. Utrecht: Changing Markets Foundation, https://changingmarkets.org/portfolio/milking-it/

Chen X, Du J, Wu X, Cao W, Sun S (2021). Global burden attributable to high sodium intake from 1990 to 2019. *Nutr Metab Cardiovasc Dis* 31(12): 3314–3321, https://doi.org/10.1016/j.numecd.2021.08.033

Cobb LK, Anderson CAM, Elliott P, Hu FB, Liu K, Neaton JD, Whelton PK, Woodward M, Appel LJ, on behalf of the American Heart Association Council on Lifestyle and Metabolic Health (2014). Methodological issues in cohort studies that relate sodium intake to cardiovascular disease outcomes. A science advisory from the American Heart Association. *Circulation* 129: 1173–1186, https://doi.org/10.1161/CIR.0000000000000015

Cobiac LJ, Veerman L, Vos T (2013). The role of cost-effectiveness analysis in developing nutrition policy. *Annu Rev Nutr* 33: 373–393, https://doi.org/10.1146/annurev-nutr-071812-161133

Codex Committee on Food Labelling Electronic Working Group (2017). Discussion paper on consideration of issues regarding front-of-pack nutrition labelling. CX/FL 17/44/7. Agenda Item 7. Codex Alimentarius Commission, http://www.fao.org/fao-who-codexalimentarius/sh-proxy/es/?lnk=1&url=https%253A%252F%252Fworkspace.fao.org%252Fsites%252Fcodex%252FMeetings%252FCX-714-44%252FWD%252Ffl44_07e.pdf

Codex Committee on Food Labelling (2021). Proposed Draft Guidelines on Front-of-Pack Nutrition Labelling. 46th Session (virtual) 27 September-1 October and 7 October 2021. Codex Alimentarius Commission, https://ec.europa.eu/food/horizontal-topics/international-affairs/international-standards/codex-alimentarius/ccfl_en

Codling K, Quang NV, Phong L, Phuong do H, Quang ND, Bégin F, Mathisen R (2015). The Rise and Fall of Universal Salt Iodization in Vietnam: Lessons Learned for Designing Sustainable Food Fortification Programs With a Public Health Impact. *Food Nutr Bull* 36(4): 441–454, https://doi.org/10.1177/0379572115616039

Commission on Ending Childhood Obesity (2017). *Report of the Commission on Ending Childhood Obesity. Implementation plan: executive summary*. Geneva: World Health Organization (WHO/NMH/PND/ECHO/17.1). Licence: CC BY-NC-SA 3.0 IGO, https://apps.who.int/iris/handle/10665/259349

Congreso de los Estados Unidos Mexicanos (2021). Ley del Impuesto Especial sobre Producción y Servicios. Nueva Ley publicada en el Diario Oficial de la Federación el 30 de diciembre de 1980, Ultima reforma publicada DOF 12-11-2021. Cámara de Diputados del H. Congreso de la Unión, https://www.diputados.gob.mx/LeyesBiblio/pdf/LIEPS.pdf

Cowburn G, Stockley L (2005). Consumer understanding and use of nutrition labelling: A systematic review. *Public Health Nutr* 8: 21–28, https://doi.org/10.1079/phn2005666

Croker H, Packer J, Russell S, Stansfield C, Viner RM (2020). Front of pack nutritional labelling schemes: a systematic review and metaanalysis of recent evidence relating to objectively measured consumption and purchasing. *J Hum Nutr Diet* 33: 518–537, https://doi.org/10.1111/jhn.12758

Dana LM, Chapman K, Talati Z (2019). Consumers' views on the importance of specific front-of-pack nutrition information: a latent profile analysis. *Nutrients* 11(5) pii: E1158, https://doi.org/10.3390/nu11051158

D'Antoine H, Bower C (2019). Folate Status and Neural Tube Defects in Aboriginal Australians: The Success of Mandatory Fortification in Reducing a Health Disparity. *Curr Dev Nutr* 3: nzz071.

Das JK, Salam RA, Kumar R, Bhutta ZA (2013). Micronutrient fortification of food and its impact on woman and child health: a systematic review. *Systematic Reviews* 2: 67.

Delshad H, Azizi F (2017). Review of iodine nutrition in Iranian population in the past quarter of century. *Int J Endocrinol Metab* 15(4): e57758, https://doi.org/10.5812/ijem.57758

de Onis M, Onyango WA, Borghi E, Siyam Ai, Nishida C, Siekmann J (2007). Development of a WHO growth reference for school-aged children and adolescents. *Bull World Health Organ* 85(9): 660–667, https://doi.org/10.2471/BLT.07.043497

Department of Health, UK Government (2011). *Nutrient Profiling Technical Guidance.* January 2011, https://assets.publishing.service.gov.uk/government/uploads/system/uploads/attachment_data/file/216094/dh_123492.pdf

Department of Statistics/DOS and ICF (2019). *Jordan Population and Family and Health Survey 2017–18.* Amman, Jordan, and Rockville, Maryland, USA: DOS and ICF, https://dhsprogram.com/pubs/pdf/FR346/FR346.pdf

Deschasaux M, Huybrechts I, Murphy N, Julia C, Hercberg S, Srour B et al. (2018) Nutritional quality of food as represented by the FSAm-NPS nutrient profiling system underlying the Nutri-Score label and cancer risk in Europe: Results from the EPIC prospective cohort study. *PLoS Med* 15(9): e1002651, https://doi.org/10.1371/journal.pmed.1002651

Doggui R, Al-Jawaldeh H, Al-Jawaldeh A (2020). Trend of Iodine Status in the Eastern Mediterranean Region and Impact of the Universal Salt Iodization Programs: a Narrative Review. *Biol Trace Elem Res* 198(2): 390–402, https://doi.org/10.1007/s12011-020-02083-1

Drichoutis AC, Lazaridis P, Nagya R (2006). Consumers' use of nutritional labels: A review of research studies and issues. *Acad Mark Sci Rev* 2006: 1.

Ducrot P, Julia C, Méjean C, Kesse-Guyot E, Touvier M, Fezeu LK, Hercberg S, Péneau S (2016). Impact of Different Front-of-Pack Nutrition Labels on Consumer Purchasing Intentions: A Randomized Controlled Trial. *Am J Prev Med* 50(5): 627–636, https://doi.org/10.1016/j.amepre.2015.10.020

Dunlop E, Kiely M, James A, Singh T, Pham NM, Black L (2021). Vitamin D food fortification and biofortification increases serum 25-hydroxivitamin D concentrations in adults and children: An update and extended systematic review and meta-analysis of randomized controlled trials. *J Nutr* 151(9): 2622–2635, https://doi.org/10.1093/jn/nxab180

Dwivedi S, Goldman I, Ortiz R (2019). Pursuing the potential of heirloom cultivars to improve adaptation, nutritional, and culinary features of food crops. *Agronomy* 9: 441, https://doi.org/10.3390/agronomy9080441

Eastman CR, Zimmermann MB (2018). The iodine deficiency disorders. In: Feingold et al. (eds). *Thyroid Physiology and Disease*. Endotext, https://www.ncbi.nlm.nih.gov/books/NBK278943/

Ecker O, Al-Riffai P, Breisinger C, El-Batrawy R (2016). *Nutrition and Economic Development. Exploring Egypt's Exceptionalism and the Role of Food Subsidies*. Washington D.C.: International Food Policy Research Institute (IFPRI), http://dx.doi.org/10.2499/9780896292383

Edalati S, Omidvar N, Haghighian Roudsari A, Ghodsi D, Zargaraan A (2020). Development and implementation of nutrition labelling in Iran: A retrospective policy analysis. *Int J Health Plann Mgmt* 35: e28–ee44, https://doi.org/10.1002/hpm.2924

Egnell M, Talati Z, Hercberg S, Pettigrew S, Chantal J (2018). Objective understanding of front-of-package nutrition labels: An international comparative experimental study across 12 countries. *Nutrients* 10: 1542, https://dx.doi.org/10.3390%2Fnu10101542

El Ati J, Doggui R, El Ati-Hellal MA (2021). Successful pilot experiment of salt reduction in Tunisian bread: 35% gradual decrease of salt content without detection by consumers. *Int J Environ Res Public Health* 18: 1590, https://doi.org/10.3390/ijerph18041590

El Hamdouchi A, El Kari K, Rjimati L, El Haloui N, El Mzibri M, Aguenaou N, Mokhtar N (2010). Impact de l'enrichissement de la farine en fer élémentaire sur la prévalence de l'anémie chez les enfants en âge préscolaire au Maroc. *EMHJ* 16(11): 1148–1152, http://www.emro.who.int/emhj/V16/11/16_11_2010_1148_1152.pdf?ua=1

El Kardi Y, Jafri A, Anide A, Derouiche A (2017). Salt content of some fast foods in Casablanca, Morocco: Pilot study. *Nutr Clin Metab* 31(1): 82–85, https://doi.org/10.1016/j.nupar.2016.10.123

El Kishawi RR, Soo KL, Abed YA, Muda WAMW (2020). Prevalence and predictors of overweight and obesity among women in the Gaza strip-Palestine: a cross-sectional study. *BMC Public Health* 20: 864, https://doi.org/10.1186/s12889-020-08966-1

Elrayah EE, Balla SA, Abu Ahmed H (2018). Anthropometric assessment of school children in Khartoum Locality, Khartoum State, Sudan — 2014/2015. *J Biol Clin Anthropol/Anthropol. Anz.* 74/5 Suppl.: 393–401, https://doi.org/10.1127/anthranz/2018/0830

El-Said Badawi N, Barakat AA, El Sherbini SA, Fawzy HM (2013). Prevalence of overweight and obesity in primary school children in Port Said city. *Egyptian Pediatric Association Gazette* 61: 31–36, http://dx.doi.org/10.1016/j.epag.2013.04.007

Ericksen PJ (2008). Conceptualizing food systems for global environmental change research. *Global Environmental Change* 18: 234–245, https://doi.org/10.1016/j.gloenvcha.2007.09.002

Esfandiari Z, Mirlohi M, Tanha JM, Hadian M, Mossavi SI, Ansariyan A et al. (2021). Effect of face-to-face education on knowledge, attitudes, and practices toward "Traffic Light" food labeling in Isfahan society, Iran. *International Quarterly of Community Health Education* 41(3): 275–284, https://doi.org/10.1177/0272684X20916612

Esmaeili M, Abdollahi M, Abdollahi Z, Salehi F, Ajami M, Houshiarrad A (2021). Effects of trans fatty acid decreasing policy on its consumption by households in six provinces of Iran. *Iranian J Nutr Sci Food Technol* 16(2): 13–23, http://dx.doi.org/10.52547/nsft.16.2.13 (English abstract, article in Persian).

Evans CEL, Harper CE (2009). A history and review of school meal standards in the UK. *J Hum Nutr Diet* 22: 89–99, https://doi.org/10.1111/j.1365-277X.2008.00941.x

European Commission (2019). Commission Regulation (EU) 2019/649 of 24 April 2019 amending Annex III to Regulation (EC) No 1925/2006 of the European Parliament and of the Council as regards trans fat, other than trans fat naturally occurring in fat of animal origin. *Official Journal of the European Union* L110/17, http://data.europa.eu/eli/reg/2019/649/oj

European Food Information Council (EUFIC) (2018). *Global Update on Nutrition Labelling. 2018 Edition*. Brussels, https://www.eufic.org/en/healthy-living/article/global-update-on-nutrition-labelling

European Public Health Alliance (EPHA) (2016). *European Public Health Alliance. Self-regulation: a false promise for public health?* Briefing paper, https://epha.org/briefing-paper-i-self-regulation-a-false-promise-for-public-health/

European Public Health Alliance (EPHA) (2018). *Eliminating trans fats in the European Union*. Briefing paper, November 2018, https://epha.org/wp-content/uploads/2018/12/eliminating-trans-fats.pdf

European Salt Producers Association (2017). *Harmonized Salt Iodization — future policy approach to achieve the mission and vision in eliminating Iodine deficiency in Europe*. Brussels, 01.11.2017.

Eykelenboom M, van Stralen MM, Olthof MR, Schoonmade LJ, Steenhuis IHM, Renders CM, and on behalf of the PEN Consortium (2019). Political and public acceptability of a sugar-sweetened beverages tax: a mixed-method systematic review and meta-analysis. *Int J Behav Nutr Phys Act* 16: 78, https://doi.org/10.1186/s12966-019-0843-0

Fall CHD (2013). Fetal programming and the risk of non-communicable disease. *Indian J Pediatr* 80(0–1): S13–S20, https://doi.org/10.1007/s12098-012-0834-5

Fan X, Gómez MI, Coles PS (2019). Willingness to pay, quality perception, and local foods: The case of broccoli. *Agric Resource Econ Rev* 48(3): 414–432, https://doi.org/10.1017/age.2019.21

Farebrother J, Zimmermann MB, Abdallah F, Assey V, Fingerhut R, Gichohi-Wainaina WN et al. (2018). Effect of excess iodine intake from iodized salt and/or groundwater iodine on thyroid function in nonpregnant and pregnant women, infants, and children: A multicenter study in East Africa. *Thyroid* 28(9): 1–13, https://doi.org/10.1089/thy.2018.0234

FAO (2011). *Global food losses and food waste — Extent, causes and prevention. Rome: Food and Agriculture Organization of the United Nations*, http://www.fao.org/docrep/014/mb060e/mb060e00.pdf

FAO (2013a). *The State of Food and Agriculture. Food Systems for better nutrition.* Rome: Food and Agriculture Organization of the United Nations, http://www.fao.org/3/i3300e/i3300e.pdf

FAO (2013b). *Food Wastage Footprint. Impacts on natural resources. Summary report.* Rome: Food and Agriculture Organization of the United Nations, https://www.fao.org/docrep/018/i3347e/i3347e.pdf

FAO (2014). *Food and nutrition in numbers.* Rome: Food and Agriculture Organization of the United Nations, http://www.fao.org/3/a-i4175e.pdf

FAO (2015). *Regional Strategic Framework. Reducing Food Losses and Waste in the Near East & North Africa Region.* Cairo: Food and Agriculture Organization of the United Nations, https://www.fao.org/3/a-i4545e.pdf

FAO (2017a). Suite of Food Security Indicators. FAOSTAT, https://www.fao.org/faostat/en/#data/FS

FAO (2017b). *Nutrition-sensitive agriculture and food systems in practice options for intervention.* Rome: Food and Agriculture Organization of the United Nations, https://www.fao.org/3/i7848en/I7848EN.pdf

FAO (2017c). *Water for Sustainable Food and Agriculture. A report produced for the G20 Presidency of Germany.* Rome: Food and Agriculture Organization of the United Nations, https://www.fao.org/3/i7959e/i7959e.pdf

FAO (2018). *Public food procurement. Strengthening sector policies for better food security and nutrition results. Policy Guidance Note 11.* Rome: Food and Agriculture Organization of the United Nations, https://www.fao.org/3/CA2281EN/ca2281en.pdf

FAO (2022). *Information Note: The importance of Ukraine and the Russian Federation for global agricultural markets and the risks associated with the current conflict. 25 March 2022 Update.* Rome: Food and Agriculture Organization of the United Nations, https://www.fao.org/3/cb9236en/cb9236en.pdf

FAO, IFAD, UNICEF, WFP and WHO (2021). *The State of Food Security and Nutrition in the World 2021. Transforming food systems for food security, improved nutrition and affordable healthy diets for all*. Rome: FAO, https://doi.org/10.4060/cb4474en

FAO, UNDP & UNEP (2021). *A multi-billion-dollar opportunity — Repurposing agricultural support to transform food systems*. Rome: FAO, https://doi.org/10.4060/cb6562en

FAO/WHO (2015). General Principles for the Addition of Essential Nutrients to Foods. *Codex Alimentarius Commission*, CAC/GL 9–1987, https://www.fao.org/fao-who-codexalimentarius/sh-proxy/ar/?lnk=1&url=https%253A%252F%252Fworkspace.fao.org%252Fsites%252Fcodex%252FStandards%252FCXG%2B9-1987%252FCXG_009e_2015.pdf

Federici C, Detzel P, Petracca F, Dainelli L, Fattore G (2019). The impact of food reformulation on nutrient intakes and health, a systematic review of modelling studies. *BMC Nutrition* 5: 2, https://doi.org/10.1186/s40795-018-0263-6

Food Fortification Initiative (FFI) (2021). *Annual Report 2020*. Atlanta, USA: FFI, https://www.ffinetwork.org/annual-reports

Food Fortification Programme (FFP) (2019a). *Fortifying Pakistan's Future*. Policy brief, http://www.ffp-pakistan.org

Food Fortification Programme (FFP) (2019b). *Information brief for Wheat flour millers*, http://www.ffp-pakistan.org

Forouzanfar MH, Liu P, Roth GA, Ng M, Biryukov S, Marczak L et al. (2017). Global burden of hypertension and systolic blood pressure of at least 110 to 115 mm Hg, 1990–2015. *JAMA* 317(2): 165–182, https://doi.org/10.1001/jama.2016.19043

Garces-Restrepo C, Vermillion D, Muñoz G (2007). *Irrigation management transfer. Worldwide efforts and results. FAO Water report 32*. Rome: Food and Agriculture Organization of the United Nations, https://www.fao.org/docrep/010/a1520e/a1520e00.htm

Garemo M, Elamin A, Gardner A (2018). Weight status and food habits of preschool children in Abu Dhabi, United Arab Emirates: NOPLAS project. *Asia Pac J Clin Nutr* 27(6): 1302–1314, https://doi.org/10.6133/apjcn.201811_27(6).0018

Garemo M, Elamin A, Van De Venter A (2019). A review of the nutritional guidelines for children at nurseries and schools in Middle Eastern countries. *Mediterr J Nutr Metab* 12(3): 255–270, https://doi.org/10.3233/MNM-180277

Garg M, Sharma N, Sharma S, Kapoor P, Kumar A, Chunduri V, Arora P (2018). Biofortified crops generated by breeding, agronomy, and transgenic approaches are improving lives of millions of people around the world. *Front Nutr* 5: 12, https://doi.org/10.3389/fnut.2018.00012

GBD 2017 Risk Factor Collaborators (2018). Global, regional, and national comparative risk assessment of 84 behavioural, environmental and occupational, and metabolic risks or clusters of risks for 195 countries and territories, 1990–2017: a systematic analysis for the Global Burden of Disease Study 2017. *Lancet* 392(10159): 1923–1994, https://doi.org/10.1016/S0140-6736(18)32225-6

GBD 2017 Diet Collaborators (2019). Health effects of dietary risks in 195 countries, 1990–2017: a systematic analysis for the Global Burden of Disease Study 2017. *Lancet* 393: 1958–1972, https://doi.org/10.1016/S0140-6736(19)30041-8

Gera T, Sachdev HS, Boy E (2012). Effect of iron-fortified foods on hematologic and biological outcomes: systematic review of randomized controlled trials. *Am J Clin Nutr* 96: 309–324, https://doi.org/10.3945/ajcn.111.031500

Ghazavi N, Rahimi E, Esfandiari Z, Shakerian A (2020). Accuracy of the amount of trans-fatty acids in traffic light labelling of traditional sweets distributed in Isfahan, Iran. *ARYA Atheroscler* 16(2): 79–84, https://doi.org/10.22122/arya.v16i2.2005

Global Alliance for Improved Nutrition (GAIN) (2020). *The Commercialization of Biofortified Crops Programme. Expanding the reach of nutrient-enriched staples*, https://www.gainhealth.org/resources/reports-and-publications/commercialization-biofortified-crops-programme

Global Child Nutrition Foundation (GCNF) (2019). *School Meal Programs Around the World. Report Based on the Global Survey of School Meal Programs*, https://survey.gcnf.org/wp-content/uploads/2021/03/GCNF_School-Meal-Programs-Around-the-World_Report_2021_Final.pdf

Global Health Estimates (2019). *Deaths by Cause, Age, Sex, by Country and by Region, 2000–2019 (2020)*. Geneva: World Health Organization, https://www.who.int/data/gho/data/themes/mortality-and-global-health-estimates/ghe-leading-causes-of-death

Global Market Insights (2021). *Breast Milk Substitutes Market Size By Substitute Type (Milk-based Formula, Soy-based Formula, Hypoallergenic Formula), By Formula Type (Powdered, Concentrated Liquid, Ready-to-use), By Distribution Channels (Pharmacies, Retail Stores), COVID-19 Impact Analysis, Regional Outlook, Application Potential, Price Trends, Competitive Market Share & Forecast, 2021–2027.* GMI Report GMI3373.

Global Nutrition Monitoring Framework (2017). *Operational guidance for tracking progress in meeting targets for 2025.* Geneva: World Health Organization, https://apps.who.int/iris/rest/bitstreams/1093537/retrieve

Global Nutrition Report (2020). *Action on equity to end malnutrition.* Bristol, UK: Development Initiatives, https://globalnutritionreport.org/reports/2020-global-nutrition-report/

Global Panel (2015). *Biofortification: An Agricultural Investment for Nutrition. Policy Brief No. 1.* London, UK: Global Panel on Agriculture and Food Systems for Nutrition, https://www.glopan.org/download/2955/

Global Panel (2016). *Food systems and diets: Facing the challenges of the 21st century*. London, UK: Global Panel on Agriculture and Food Systems for Nutrition, https://www.glopan.org/download/2859/

Global Panel (2017). *Urban diets and nutrition: Trends, challenges and opportunities for policy action. Policy Brief No. 9*. London, UK: Global Panel on Agriculture and Food Systems for Nutrition, https://www.glopan.org/download/2899/

Global Panel (2020). *Future Food Systems: For people, our planet, and prosperity*. London, UK: Global Panel on Agriculture and Food Systems for Nutrition, https://foresight.glopan.org/

Goiana-da-Silva F, Severo M, Cruz e Silva D, Gregório MJ, Allen LN, Muc M et al. (2020) Projected impact of the Portuguese sugar-sweetened beverage tax on obesity incidence across different age groups: A modelling study. *PLoS Med* 17(3): e1003036, https://doi.org/10.1371/journal.pmed.1003036

Goodman S, Vanderlee L, Acton R, Mahamad S, Hammond D (2018). The impact of front-of-package label design on consumer understanding of nutrient amounts. *Nutrients* 10(11): 1624, https://dx.doi.org/10.3390%2Fnu10111624

Gouel C, Guimbard H (2017). *Nutrition transition and the structure of global food demand*. CEPII Working Paper. Paris: Centre d'Etudes Prospectives et d'Informations Internationales (CEPII), http://www.cepii.fr/PDF_PUB/wp/2017/wp2017-05.pdf

Grabovac I, Hochfellner L, Rieger M, Jewell J, Snell A, Weber A, Stüger HP, Schindler KE, Mikkelsen B, Dorner TE (2018). Impact of Austria's 2009 trans fatty acids regulation on all-cause, cardiovascular and coronary heart disease mortality. *Eur J Public Health* 28 (suppl. 2): 4–9, https://doi.org/10.1093/eurpub/cky147

Gregori D, Ballali S, Vögele C, Galasso F, Widhalm K, Berchialla P, Baldi I (2015). What is the value given by consumers to nutritional label information? Results from a large investigation in Europe. *J Amer Coll Nutr* 34(2): 120–125, https://doi.org/10.1080/07315724.2014.899936

Gressier M, Swinburn B, Frost G, Segal AB, Sassi F (2021). What is the impact of food reformulation on individuals' behaviour, nutrient intakes and health status? A systematic review of empirical evidence. *Obes Rev* 22: e13139, https://doi.org/10.1111/obr.13139

Griffith R, O'Connell M, Smith K (2014). *The importance of product reformulation versus consumer choice in improving diet quality*. IFS Working Papers No. W14/15, Institute for Fiscal Studies (IFS), London, http://dx.doi.org/10.1920/wp.ifs.2014.1415

Grunert KG, Wills JM (2007). A review of European research on consumer response to nutrition information on food labels. *J Public Health* 15: 385–399, https://link.springer.com/content/pdf/10.1007/s10389-007-0101-9.pdf

Guennoun Y, Bouziani A, Bajit H, El Berri H, Elammari L, Benaich S et al. (2019). Acceptance of salt reduction in bakery bread among Moroccan consumers. *Nor Afr J Food Nutr Res* 3(6): 219–228, https://doi.org/10.51745/najfnr.3.6.219-228

Guillocheau E, Legrand P, Rioux V (2019). Benefits of natural dietary trans fatty acids towards inflammation, obesity and type 2 diabetes: defining the n-7 trans fatty acid family. *OCL* 26: 46, https://doi.org/10.1051/ocl/2019047

Gulf Council Cooperation Standardization Organization (2015). GSO194/ 2015 Wheat Flour. ICS 67.060. Technical Regulation.

Hadhood SESA, Ali RAE, Mohamed MM, Mohammed ES (2017). Prevalence and correlates of overweight and obesity among school children in Sohag, Egypt. *Open Journal of Gastroenterology*, 7: 75–88, https://doi.org/10.4236/ojgas.2017.72009

Hadian Z, Feyzollahi E, Honarvar Z, Komeili-fonood R, Khosravi Darani K, Mofid V et al. (2020). Assessment of Salt (Sodium Chloride) Content in Traditional and Industrial Breads in Tehran. *Iranian Journal of Nutrition Sciences & Food Technology* 14(4): 113–122 (English abstract, article in Persian), http://nsft.sbmu.ac.ir/article-1-2457-en.html

Hamid BA (2014). Across Afghanistan children are now iodine sufficient. *IDD Newsletter* 42: 2–4, https://www.ign.org/cm_data/idd_nov14_mail.pdf

He FJ, Pombo-Rodrigues S, MacGregor GA (2014). Salt reduction in England from 2003 to 2011: its relationship to blood pressure, stroke and ischaemic heart disease mortality. *BMJ Open* 4: e004549, http://dx.doi.org/10.1136/bmjopen-2013-004549

Helen Keller International (2018). *CCNFSDU 2018: Review of the Codex Standard for Follow-Up Formula*. Washington, D.C.: Helen Keller International, https://archnutrition.org/wp-content/uploads/sites/2/2018/10/HKI-ARCH-Codex-brief.pdf

Hennessy A, Walton J, Flynn A (2013). The impact of voluntary food fortification on micronutrient intakes and status in European countries: a review. *Proc Nutr Soc* 72: 433–440, https://doi.org/10.1017/s002966511300339x

Hieke S, Wilczynski P (2011). Colour Me In — an empirical study on consumer responses to the traffic light signposting system in nutrition labelling. *Public Health Nutr* 15(5): 773–782, https://doi.org/10.1017/S1368980011002874

Hirschi KD (2009). Nutrient biofortification of food crops. *Annu Rev Nutr* 29: 401–421, https://doi.org/10.1146/annurev-nutr-080508-141143

HLPE (2017). *Nutrition and food systems. A report by the High Level Panel of Experts on Food Security and Nutrition of the Committee on World Food Security, HPLE Report 17*, Rome, https://www.fao.org/3/a-i7846e.pdf

Hoekstra AY, Chapagain AK, Mekonnen MM, Aldaya MM (2011). *The Water Footprint Assessment Manual: Setting the Global Standard*. London, Washington, D.C.: Earthscan, https://waterfootprint.org/media/downloads/TheWaterFootprintAssessmentManual_2.pdf

Hoogendoorn A, Luthringer C, Parvanta I, Garrett G (2016). *Food Fortification Global Mapping Study 2016*. European Commission, GAIN, https://www.gainhealth.org/sites/default/files/publications/documents/food-fortification-global-mapping-study-2016.pdf

Hoteit M, Zoghbi E. Al Iskandarani M, Rady A, Shankiti I, Matta J, Al-Jawaldeh A (2020). Nutritional value of the Middle Eastern diet: analysis of total sugar, salt, and iron in Lebanese traditional dishes. *F1000Research*, 9: 1254, https://doi.org/10.12688/f1000research.26278.1

Hoteit M, Ibrahim C, Saade D, Al-Jaafari M, Atwi M, Alasma, S et al. (2022a). *Correlates of sub-optimal feeding practices among under-5 children amid escalating crises in Lebanon: A national representative cross-sectional study. Children.* Basel, Switzerland, 9(6): 817, https://doi.org/10.3390/children9060817

Hoteit M, Mortada H, Al-Jawaldeh A, Ibrahim C, Mansour R (2022b). COVID-19 home isolation and food consumption patterns: Investigating the correlates of poor dietary diversity in Lebanon: a cross-sectional study. *F1000Research*, 11: 110, https://doi.org/10.12688/f1000research.75761.1

Hoteit M, Mortada H, Al-Jawaldeh A, Mansour R, Yazbeck B, AlKhalaf M et al. & Regional CORONA COOKING Survey Group (2022c). Dietary diversity in the Eastern Mediterranean Region before and during the COVID-19 pandemic: Disparities, challenges, and mitigation measures. *Frontiers in Nutrition*, 9: 813154, https://doi.org/10.3389/fnut.2022.813154

Hussein I (2015). Sudan is back on the road to universal salt iodization. *IDD Newsletter* 43(1): 16, https://www.ign.org/idd-newsletter-42015.htm

Hussein MD, Alonazi NA, Mohamed S (2018). Prevalence of obesity, overweight, underweight, and stunting among school children in Argo city, Northern Sudan. *Sudan J Paediatr* 18(2): 15–19, https://doi.org/10.24911/SJP.106-1544799078

Hyseni L, Bromley H, Kypridemos C, O'Flaherty M, Lloyd-Williams F, Guzman-Castillo M, Pearson-Stuttard J, Capewell S (2017). Systematic review of dietary trans-fat reduction interventions. *Bull World Health Organ* 95(12): 821-830G, https://dx.doi.org/10.2471%2FBLT.16.189795

ICN2 (2014a). Conference outcome document: Rome Declaration on Nutrition. Rome: Food and Agriculture Organization. Contract No.: ICN2 2014/2, http://www.fao.org/3/a-ml542e.pdf

ICN2 (2014b). Conference outcome document: Framework for Action — from commitments to action. Rome: Food and Agriculture Organization of the United Nations. Contract No.: ICN2 2014/3, https://www.fao.org/3/a-mm215e.pdf

IFPRI (2021). *Transforming food systems after COVID-19. Global Food Policy Report*. Washington, D.C.: International Food Policy Research Institute (IFPRI), https://doi.org/10.2499/9780896293991

Institute of Medicine (IOM) (US) Subcommittee on Interpretation and Uses of Dietary Reference Intakes; Institute of Medicine (US) Standing Committee on the Scientific Evaluation of Dietary Reference Intakes (2000). *DRI Dietary Reference Intakes. Applications in Dietary Assessment.* Washington, DC: National Academies Press (US), https://doi.org/10.17226/9956

Institute of Medicine of the National Academies, Committee on Food Marketing and the Diets of Children and Youth. (2006). *Food Marketing to Children and Youth: Threat or Opportunity?* Washington DC: National Academies Press (US), https://doi.org/10.17226/11514

Institut Tunisien de la Compétitivité et des Études Quantitatives (ITCEQ) (2020). *Les modifications des droits et des taxes. Année 2021.* Tunis, http://www.itceq.tn/files/finances-publiques/2021/les-modifications-des-droits-et-taxes.pdf

International Diabetes Federation (2021). *IDF Diabetes Atlas, 10th ed.* Brussels, Belgium: International Diabetes Federation, https://diabetesatlas.org/atlas/tenth-edition/

International Food Policy Research Institute (IFPRI) (2021). *2021 Global Food Policy Report: Transforming Food Systems after COVID-19.* Washington, DC: International Food Policy Research Institute, https://doi.org/10.2499/9780896293991

International Margarine Association of the Countries of Europe (IMACE) (2004). *Code of practice on vitamin A & D fortification of margarines and fat spreads.* Brussels: IMACE.

The Iodine Global Network (2021). *Global scorecard of iodine nutrition in 2020 in the general population based on school-age children (SAC).* Ottawa, Canada: IGN, https://www.ign.org/cm_data/Global-Scorecard-2020-3-June-2020.pdf

IPC. Yemen Acute Malnutrition Analysis January 2020–March 2021. Issued February 2021, https://reliefweb.int/sites/reliefweb.int/files/resources/IPC_Yemen_Acute_Malnutrition_2020Jan2021Mar.pdf

Ipsos (2020). *IFBA Audit 2019 Compliance Monitoring Report for the International Food & Beverage Alliance on UAE & KSA advertising in television, print and internet.* May 2020, https://ifballiance.org/wp-content/uploads/2020/10/GCC-IFBA-AUDIT-2019-KSA-and-UAE.pdf

Ismail MB, Hussein I (2018). Sustaining universal salt iodization in Egypt: program successes and challenges. *IDD Newsletter* 46(1): 12–13, https://www.ign.org/newsletter/idd_feb18_egypt.pdf

Jafari M, Mohammadi M, Ghazizadeh H, Nakhaee N (2016). Feasibility and outcome of reducing salt in bread: A community trial in Southern Iran. *Global Journal of Health Science* 8(12): 163–169, https://doi.org/10.5539/gjhs.v8n12p163

Jensen JD, Smed S, Aarup L, Nielsen E (2015). Effects of the Danish saturated fat tax on the demand for meat and dairy products. *Public Health Nutr* 19(17): 3085–3094, https://doi.org/10.1017/s1368980015002360

Jha AB, Warkentin TD (2020). Biofortification of pulse crops: Status and future perspectives. *Plants* 9: 73, https://doi.org/10.3390/plants9010073

Joint FAO/WHO Food Standards Programme Codex Alimentarius Commission. Forty-second Session, Geneva, Switzerland, 7–12 July 2019. *Report of the Fortieth Session of the Codex Committee on Nutrition and Foods for Special Dietary Uses*, Berlin, Germany, 26–30 November 2018.

Joint statement by the UN Special Rapporteurs on the Right to Food, Right to Health, the Working Group on Discrimination against Women in law and in practice, and the Committee on the Rights of the Child in support of increased efforts to promote, support and protect breast-feeding. 11/17/2016, https://www.ohchr.org/en/NewsEvents/Pages/DisplayNews.aspx?NewsID=20871&LangID=E

Jones A, Neal B, Reeve B, Ni Mhurchu C, Thow AM (2019). Front-of-pack nutrition labelling to promote healthier diets: current practice and opportunities to strengthen regulation worldwide. *BMJ Global Health* 4: e001882, https://doi.org/10.1136/bmjgh-2019-001882

Jradi H, Al Mughthem A, Bawazir AA (2020). Does the current scope of nutrition labelling provided in the Saudi markets cope with the increasing trend of chronic disease? *Research Square*, https://doi.org/10.21203/rs.2.23201/v1

Julia C, Hercberg S (2017). Development of a new front-of-pack nutrition label in France: the five-colour Nutri-Score. *Public Health Panorama* 3(4): 712–725, https://apps.who.int/iris/bitstream/handle/10665/325207/php-3-4-712-725-eng.pdf?sequence=1&isAllowed=y

Julia C, Blanchet O, Méjean C, Péneau S, Ducrot P, Allès B et al. (2016). Impact of the front-of-pack 5-colour nutrition label (5-CNL) on the nutritional quality of purchases: an experimental study. *Int J Behav Nutr Phys Act* 13: 101, https://doi.org/10.1186/s12966-016-0416-4

Kaigang L, Haynie D, Palla H, Lipsky L, Iannotti RJ, Simons-Morton B (2016). Assessment of adolescent weight status: Similarities and differences between CDC, IOTF, and WHO references. *Prev Med* 87: 151–154, https://doi.org/10.1016/j.ypmed.2016.02.035

Kakisu E, Tomchinsky E, Lipps MV, Fuentes J (2018). Analysis of the reduction of trans-fatty-acid levels in the foods of Argentina. *Int J Food Sci Nutr* 69(8): 928–937, https://doi.org/10.1080/09637486.2018.1428537

Kanter R, Vanderlee L, Vandevijvere S (2018). Front-of-package nutrition labelling policy: global progress and future directions. *Public Health Nutr* 21: 1399–1408, https://doi.org/10.1017/S1368980018000010

Kaushik I, Grewal RB (2017). Trans fatty acids: Replacement technologies in food. *Advances in Research* 9(5): 1–14, https://doi.org/10.9734/AIR/2017/33297

Kelly B, Vandevijvere S, Freeman B, Jenkin G (2015). New media but same old tricks: Food marketing to children in the digital age. *Curr Obes Rep* 4(1): 37–45, https://doi.org/10.1007/s13679-014-0128-5

Kelly S, Swensson LFJ (2017). *Leveraging institutional food procurement for linking small farmers to markets: Findings from WFP's Purchase for Progress initiative and Brazil's food procurement programmes. FAO Agricultural Development Economics Technical Study 1*. Rome: Food and Agriculture Organization, http://www.fao.org/3/i7636e/i7636e.pdf

Kharabsheh S, Belbesi A, Qarqash W, Azizi F (2004). Goiter prevalence and urinary iodine excretion in schoolchildren of Jordan. *Int J Vitam Nutr Res* 74(4): 301–304, https://doi.org/10.1024/0300-9831.74.4.301

Khattak RM, Khan Khattak MN, Ittermann T, Völzke H (2017). Factors affecting sustainable iodine deficiency elimination in Pakistan: A global perspective. *J Epidemiol* 27: 249–257, http://dx.doi.org/10.1016/j.je.2016.04.003

Kim BF, Santo RE, Scatterday AP, Fry JP, Synka CM, Cebron SR et al. (2020). Country-specific dietary shifts to mitigate climate and water crises. *Global Environmental Change* 62: 101926, https://doi.org/10.1016/j.gloenvcha.2019.05.010

Kingdom of Bahrain Ministry of Health, Information and eGovernment Authority, WHO (2018). *Bahrain National Health Survey 2018*, https://www.data.gov.bh/en/ResourceCenter/DownloadFile?id=3470

KIT Royal Tropical Institute (2019). *Afghanistan Health Survey 2018*. RMNCAH Directorate / MoPH, 2019, https://www.kit.nl/wp-content/uploads/2019/07/AHS-2018-report-FINAL-15-4-2019.pdf

Lebanon Nutrition Sector (2022). *National Nutrition SMART Survey Report 2021*, https://www.unicef.org/mena/media/15741/file/National%20Nutrition%20SMART%20Survey%20Report%20.pdf

Leppo K, Ollila E, Peña S, Wismar M, Cook S (eds) (2013). *Health in All Policies. Seizing opportunities, implementing policies*. Helsinki: Ministry of Social Affairs and Health Finland, https://www.euro.who.int/__data/assets/pdf_file/0007/188809/Health-in-All-Policies-final.pdf

Lobstein T, Landon J, Lincoln P (2007). *Misconceptions and misinformation: The problems with Guideline Daily Amounts (GDAs). A review of GDAs and their use for signalling nutritional information on food and drink labels*. London: National Heart Forum, https://www.heartforum.org.uk/downloads/NHFGDAreport.pdf

Loloei S, Pouraram H, Majdzadeh R, Takian A, Goshtaei M, Djazayery A (2019). Policy analysis of salt reduction in bread in Iran. *AIMS Public Health*, 6(4): 534–545, https://doi.org/10.3934/publichealth.2019.4.534

Lopez Villar J (2015). *Tackling Hidden Hunger: Putting Diet Diversification at the Centre*. Penang, Malaysia: Third World Network, https://www.twn.my/title2/books/pdf/TacklingHiddenHunger.pdf

Luthringer CL, Rowe LA, Vossenaar M, Garrett GS (2015). Regulatory Monitoring of Fortified Foods: Identifying Barriers and Good Practices. *Glob Health Sci Pract* 3(3): 446–461, https://dx.doi.org/10.9745%2FGHSP-D-15-00171

Machín L, Aschemann-Witzel J, Curutchet MR, Giménez A, Ares G (2018). Does front-of-pack nutrition information improve consumer ability to make healthful choices? Performance of warnings and the traffic light system in a simulated shopping experiment. *Appetite* 121: 55–62, https://doi.org/10.1016/j.appet.2017.10.037

Mahfouz MS, Gaffar AM, Bani IA (2012). Iodized salt consumption in Sudan: present status and future directions. *J Health Popul Nutr* 30: 431–438.

Marques E, Darby HM, Kraft J (2021). Benefits and limitations of non-transgenic micronutrient biofortification approaches. *Agronomy* 11: 464, https://doi.org/10.3390/agronomy11030464

Mason H, Shoaibi A, Ghandour R, O'Flaherty M, Capewell S, Khatib R et al. (2014). A cost effectiveness analysis of salt reduction policies to reduce coronary heart disease in four Eastern Mediterranean countries. *PLoS ONE* 9(1): e84445, https://doi.org/10.1371/journal.pone.0084445

Mateo-Sagasta J, Zadeh SM, Turral H (2017). *Water pollution from agriculture: a global review. Executive summary*. Rome: Food and Agriculture Organization of the United Nations; Colombo, Sri Lanka: International Water Management Institute (IWMI). CGIAR Research Program on Water, Land and Ecosystems (WLE), http://www.fao.org/3/a-i7754e.pdf

McCrudden C (2004). Using public procurement to achieve social outcomes. *Natural Resources Forum* 28: 257–267.

McLean RM (2014). Measuring population sodium intake: a review of methods. *Nutrients* 6: 4651-4662, https://dx.doi.org/10.3390%2Fnu6114651

Meltzer HM, Aro A, Andersen NL, Koch B, Alexander J (2003). Risk analysis applied to food fortification. *Public Health Nutr* 6(3): 281–290, https://doi.org/10.1079/phn2002444

Micha R, Mozaffarian D (2008). Trans Fatty Acids: Effects on cardiometabolic health and implications for policy. *Prostaglandins Leukot Essent Fatty Acids* 79(3–5): 147–152, https://dx.doi.org/10.1016%2Fj.plefa.2008.09.008

Miller DD, Welch RM (2013). Food system strategies for preventing micronutrient malnutrition. *Food Policy* 42: 115–128, https://doi.org/10.1016/j.foodpol.2013.06.008

Milman N, Byg K-E, Ovesen L, Kirchhoff M, Jürgensen KS-L (2003). Iron status in Danish women 1984–1994: a cohort comparison of changes in iron stores and the prevalence of iron deficiency and iron overload. *Eur J Haematol* 71: 51–61, https://doi.org/10.1034/j.1600-0609.2003.00090.x

Ministère de la Protection des consommateurs, Gouvernement du Grand-Duché de Luxembourg (2021). 7 pays européens se sont engagés à faciliter le déploiement du Nutri-Score. Communiqué de Presse, 12 février 2021, https://gouvernement.lu/dam-assets/documents/actualites/2021/02-fevrier/CO-Nutri-Score.pdf

Ministère de la Santé, République Tunésienne (2018). *Stratégie Nationale Multisectorielle de Prévention et Contrôle des Maladies Non Transmissibles (MNT) 2018–2025*, https://extranet.who.int/ncdccs/Data/TUN_B11_Strat%C3%A9gie%20Nationale%20MNT%2018-25_Finale%20(derni%C3%A8re%20version%20juin%202018).pdf

Ministère de la Santé, DPRF/DPE/SEIS, Royaume du Maroc (2018). *Enquête Nationale sur la Population et la Santé Familiale (ENPSF) 2017–2018*. Rabat, Maroc, https://www.sante.gov.ma/Documents/2020/03/Rapport%20ENPSF%202018%202i%C3%A8me%20%C3%A9dition.pdf

Ministry of Education and Higher Education, Emirate of Qatar (2016). *List of food items in school canteens*. Doha, Qatar, https://extranet.who.int/nutrition/gina/en/node/63352

Ministry of Food, Agriculture and Fisheries in Denmark, Danish Technical University, National Food Institute (2014). *Danish data on trans fatty acids in foods*. Glostrup, Søborg, https://www.foedevarestyrelsen.dk/Publikationer/Alle%20publikationer/2014004.pdf

Ministry of Health, Kingdom of Bahrain (2019). *National Action Plan for control and prevention of Non communicable diseases (2019–2030)*, https://extranet.who.int/nutrition/gina/sites/default/filesstore/BHR_2019_National%20Action%20Plan%20for%20control%20and%20prevention%20of%20Non%20communicable%20diseases%20%282019-2030%29%20%20.pdf

Ministry of Health, Kingdom of Bahrain, Gulf Health Council, United Nations Development Programme, World Health Organization, Secretariat of the UN Inter-Agency Task Force on NCDs (2020). *The case for investment in prevention and control of non-communicable diseases in Bahrain*. October 2020, https://bahrain.un.org/en/download/64179/122828

Ministry of Health Jordan, Global Alliance for Improved Nutrition (GAIN), United States Centers for Disease Control and Prevention (CDC), United Nations Children's Fund (UNICEF)-Jordan (2011). *National Micronutrient Survey*, Jordan 2010, https://www.gainhealth.org/sites/default/files/publications/documents/national-micronutrient-survey-jordan-2010.pdf

Ministry of Health, Kingdom of Saudi Arabia, Institute of Health Metrics and Evaluation, University of Washington (2013). *Saudi Health Interview Survey*. Riyadh, Saudi Arabia, http://www.healthdata.org/sites/default/files/files/Projects/KSA/Saudi-Health-Interview-Survey-Results.pdf

Ministry of Health, Sultanate of Oman (2016). *National plan for the prevention and control of chronic non-communicable diseases 2016–2025*, https://extranet.who.int/nutrition/gina/en/node/39383

Ministry of Health, Sultanate of Oman, UNICEF (2017). *Oman National Nutrition Survey 2017*. Ministry of Health: Muscat, Oman, https://groundworkhealth.org/wp-content/uploads/2020/04/ONNS_Report_2017.pdf

Ministry of Health FGS, FMS, Somaliland, UNICEF, Brandpro, GroundWork (2020). *Somalia Micronutrient Survey 2019*. Mogadishu, Somalia, https://www.unicef.org/somalia/media/1681/file/Somalia-Micronutient-Survey-2019.pdf

Ministry of Health-Palestine & UNICEF (2014). *Palestinian Micronutrient Survey (PMS) 2013. Final Report*. Ministry of Health: West Bank, Palestine.

Ministry of Health and Prevention, United Arab Emirates (2017). *National Action Plan in Nutrition*, https://extranet.who.int/nutrition/gina/sites/default/filesstore/ARE%202017%20National%20Strategy%20Plan%20in%20Nutrition.pdf

Ministry of Health and Prevention, United Arab Emirates (2017). *National Plan to Combat Childhood Obesity*, United Arab Emirates, https://extranet.who.int/nutrition/gina/sites/default/filesstore/ARE_2017_National%20Plan%20to%20Combat%20Childhood%20Obesity%20United%20Arab%20Emirates.pdf

Ministry of National Health Services, Regulations and Coordinations, Government of Pakistan (2018). *National Nutrition Survey 2018. Key findings report*, https://www.unicef.org/pakistan/media/1951/file/Final%20Key%20Findings%20Report%202019.pdf

Ministry of Public Health of Afghanistan & UNICEF (2013). National Nutrition Survey Afghanistan 2013. *Survey Report; Ministry of Public Health*: Kabul, Afghanistan, https://www.humanitarianresponse.info/sites/www.humanitarianresponse.info/files/assessments/Report%20NNS%20Afghanistan%202013%20%28July%2026-14%29.pdf

Ministry of Public Health, Emirate of Qatar (2017). *Qatar National Nutrition and Physical Activity Action Plan 2017–2022*, https://extranet.who.int/nutrition/gina/sites/default/filesstore/QAT_2017_Action%20Plan%202017-2022-FINAL.pdf

Miracolo A, Sophiea M, Mills M, Kanavos P (2021). Sin taxes and their effect on consumption, revenue generation and health improvement: a systematic literature review in Latin America. *Health Policy and Planning*, 36: 790–810, https://doi.org/10.1093/heapol/czaa168

Mkambula P, Mbuya MNN, Rowe LA, Sablah M, Friesen VM, Chadha M (2020). The unfinished agenda for food fortification in low-and middle-income countries: Quantifying progress, gaps and potential opportunities. *Nutrients* 12: 354, https://doi.org/10.3390/nu12020354

Moazzem Hossain SM, Leidman E, Kingori J, Al Harun A, Bilukha OO (2016). Nutritional situation among Syrian refugees hosted in Iraq, Jordan, and Lebanon: cross-sectional surveys. *Confl Health* 10: 26, https://doi.org/10.1186/s13031-016-0093-6

Mohammadi-Nasrabadi F, Zargaraan A, Salmani Y, Abedi A, Shoaie E, Esfarjani F (2021). Analysis of fat, fatty acid profile, and salt content of Iranian restaurant foods during the COVID-19 pandemic: Strengths, weaknesses, opportunities, and threats analysis. *Food Sci Nutr* 9(11): 6120–6130, https://doi.org/10.1002/fsn3.2563

Monteiro CA, Cannon G, Lawrence M, Costa Louzada ML, Pereira Machado P (2019). *Ultra-processed foods, diet quality, and health using the NOVA classification system*. Rome: FAO, https://www.fao.org/3/ca5644en/ca5644en.pdf

Moslemi M, Kheirandish M, Mazaheri R, Hosseini H, Jannat B, Mofid V et al. (2020). National food policies in the Islamic Republic of Iran aimed at prevention of noncommunicable diseases. *East Mediterr Health J* 26(12): 1556–1564, https://doi.org/10.26719/emhj.20.024

Muller L, Ruffieux B (2020). What makes a front-of-pack nutritional labelling system effective: The impact of key design components on food purchases. *Nutrients* 12: 2870, https://doi.org/10.3390/nu12092870

Mhurchu CN, Gorton D (2007). Nutrition labels and claims in New Zealand and Australia: a review of use and understanding. *Aust N Z J Public Health* 31(2): 105–112, https://doi.org/10.1111/j.1753-6405.2007.00026.x

Nutrition Technical Rapid Response Team (2017). *Report on the Knowledge, Attitudes and Practices (KAP) survey Infant and Young Child Feeding*, Syria, 2017, https://www.humanitarianresponse.info/en/operations/whole-of-syria/document/report-knowledge-attitudes-and-practices-kap-survey-infant-and

Nasreddine L, Ayoub JJ, Al-Jawaldeh A (2018). Review of the nutrition situation in the Eastern Mediterranean Region. *EMHJ* 24(1): 77–91, http://applications.emro.who.int/EMHJ/v24/01/EMHJ_2018_24_01_77_91.pdf

Nasreddine L, Taktouk M, Dabbous M, Melki J (2019) The extent, nature, and nutritional quality of foods advertised to children in Lebanon: the first study to use the WHO nutrient profile model for the Eastern Mediterranean Region. *Food Nutr Res* 63: 1604, http://dx.doi.org/10.29219/fnr.v63.1604

Neto B, Rodríguez Quintero R, Wolf O, Sjögren P, Lee P, Eatherley D (2016). *Revision of the EU Green Public Procurement Criteria for Food and Catering Services*. EUR 28050 EN, https://doi.org/10.2791/099130

Nikooyeh B, Neyestani TR (2018). Efficacy of food fortification with vitamin D in Iranian Adults: A systematic review and meta-analysis. *Nutrition and Food Sciences Research* 5(4): 1–6, http://dx.doi.org/10.29252/nfsr.5.4.1

Nilson A, Piza J (1998). Food fortification: A tool for fighting hidden hunger. *Food Nutr Bull* 19: 49–60, https://doi.org/10.1177%2F156482659801900109

Obeid O (2016). Lebanon rallies to fight IDD. *IDD Newsletter* 2/2016, https://www.ign.org/newsletter/idd_may16_lebanon_1.pdf

OECD (2016). *Stocktaking report on MENA public procurement systems*. MENA-OECD Network on Public Procurement, https://www.oecd.org/gov/ethics/Stocktaking_MENA_Public_Procurement_Systems.pdf

OECD (2020). *Improving the E-procurement Environment in Tunisia: Supporting vulnerable groups in gaining better access to TUNEPS*. Paris, https://www.oecd.org/mena/governance/improving-e-procurement-environment-tunisia-en.pdf

OECD (2021). *Agricultural Policy Monitoring and Evaluation 2021: Addressing the Challenges facing Food Systems*. Paris: OECD Publishing, https://doi.org/10.1787/2d810e01-en

Office of Communication UK (2004). *Childhood obesity — Food advertising in context: children's food choices, parents' understanding and influence, and the role of food promotion*, https://www.ofcom.org.uk/__data/assets/pdf_file/0020/19343/report2.pdf

Ohlhorst SD, Slavin M, Bhide JM, Bugusu B (2012). Use of iodized salt in processed foods in select countries around the world and the role of food processors. *Compr Rev Food Sci Food Safety* 11: 233–284, https://doi.org/10.1111/j.1541-4337.2011.00182.x

Omidvar N, Babashahi M, Abdollahi Z, Al-Jawaldeh A (2021). Enabling Food Environment in Kindergartens and Schools in Iran for Promoting Healthy Diet: Is It on the Right Track? *Int J Environ Res Public Health* 18: 4114, https://doi.org/10.3390/ijerph18084114

Osendarp SJM, Martinez H, Garrett GS, Neufeld LM, De-Regil LM, Vossenaar M, Darnton-Hill I (2018). Large-Scale Food Fortification and Biofortification in Low- and Middle-Income Countries: A Review of Programs, Trends, Challenges, and Evidence Gaps. *Food Nutr Bull* 39 (2): 315–331, https://doi.org/10.1177/0379572118774229

Oteng A-B, Kersten S (2020). Mechanisms of action of trans fatty acids. *Adv Nutr* 11: 697–708, https://doi.org/ https://doi.org/10.1093/advances/nmz125

Pacheco Santos LM, Reyes Lecca RC, Cortez-Escalante JJ, Niskier Sanchez M, Rodrigues HG (2016). Prevention of neural tube defects by the fortification of flour with folic acid: a population-based retrospective study in Brazil. *Bull World Health Organ* 94: 22–29, https://doi.org/ http://dx.doi.org/10.2471/BLT.14.15136

Pachón H, Spohrer R, Mei Z, Serdula MK (2015). Evidence of the effectiveness of flour fortification programs on iron status and anemia: a systematic review. *Nutr Rev* 73 (11): 780–795, https://doi.org/10.1093/nutrit/nuv037

Pernitez-Agan S, Wickramage K, Yen C, Dawson-Hahn E, Mitchell T, Zenner D (2019) Nutritional profile of Syrian refugee children before resettlement. *Confl Health* 13: 22, https://doi.org/10.1186/s13031-019-0208-y

Peymani P, Joulaie H, Zamiri N, Ahmadi SM, Dinarvand R, Hosseini H et al. (2012). Iran's experience on reduction of trans-fatty acid content in edible oils. *Middle-East Journal of Scientific Research* 11(9): 1207–1211, https://doi.org/10.5829/idosi.mejsr.2012.11.09.64197

Pfeuffer M, Jahreis G (2018). Trans fatty acids. Origin, metabolism, health risks. *Ernahrungs Umschau* 65(12): 196–203, https://doi.org/10.4455/eu.2018.047

Piwoz EG, Huffman SL (2015). The impact of marketing of breast-milk substitutes on WHO-recommended breastfeeding practices. *Food Nutr Bull* 36 (4): 373–386, https://doi.org/10.1177/0379572115602174

Poore J, Nemecek T (2018). Reducing food's environmental impacts through producers and consumers. *Science* 360: 987–992, https://doi.org/10.1126/science.aaq0216

Pope DH, Karlsson JO, Baker P, McCoy D (2021). Examining the environmental impacts of the dairy and baby food industries: Are first-food systems a crucial missing part of the healthy and sustainable food systems agenda now underway? *Int J Environ Res Public Health* 18: 12678, https://doi.org/10.3390/ijerph182312678

Popkin B (2006). Global nutrition dynamics: the world is shifting rapidly toward a diet linked with noncommunicable diseases. *Am J Clin Nutr* 84: 289–298, https://doi.org/10.1093/ajcn/84.1.289

Popkin B (2015). Nutrition transition and the global diabetes epidemic. *Curr Diab Rep* 15(9): 64, https://doi.org/10.1007/s11892-015-0631-4

Popkin BM, Ng SW (2021). Sugar sweetened beverage taxes: Lessons to date and the future of taxation. *PLoS Med* 18(1): e1003412, https://doi.org/10.1371/journal.pmed.1003412

Pouraram H, Elmadfa I, Dorosty AR, Abtahi M, Neyestani TR, Sadeghian S (2012). Long-term consequences of iron-fortified flour consumption in nonanemic men. *Ann Nutr Metab* 60 (2): 115–121, https://doi.org/10.1159/000336184

Pouraram H, Djazayery A, Mohammad K, Parsaeian M, Abdollahi Z, Dorosty Motlagh A et al. (2018). Second National Integrated Micronutrient Survey in Iran: Study design and preliminary findings. *Arch Iran Med* 21 (4): 137–144, http://www.aimjournal.ir/PDF/aim-21-137.pdf

Powles J, Fahimi S, Micha R, Khatibzadeh S, Shi P, Ezzati M, Engell RE, Lim SS, Danaei G, Mozaffarian D; Global Burden of Diseases Nutrition and Chronic Diseases Expert Group (NutriCoDE) (2013). Global, regional and national sodium intakes in 1990 and 2010: a systematic analysis of 24 h urinary sodium excretion and dietary surveys worldwide. *BMJ Open* 3 (12): e003733, https://doi.org/10.1136/bmjopen-2013-003733

Public Health England (2018). *Salt targets 2017: Progress report. A report on the food industry's progress towards meeting the 2017 salt targets.* London, https://assets.publishing.service.gov.uk/government/uploads/system/uploads/attachment_data/file/765571/Salt_targets_2017_progress_report.pdf

Radouani MA, Chahid N, Benmiloud L, El Ammari L, Kharbach A, Rjimati L et al. (2015). Prevalence of neural tube defects: Moroccan study 2008–2011. *Open Journal of Pediatrics*, 5: 248–255, http://dx.doi.org/10.4236/ojped.2015.53038

Radzicki MJ (2007). *Introduction to system dynamics. A systems approach to understanding complex policy issues.* Washington, DC: US Department of Energy, https://web.nmsu.edu/~lang/files/mike.pdf

Ratnayake WMN, L'Abbe MR, Mozaffarian D (2009). Nationwide product reformulations to reduce trans fatty acids in Canada: when trans fat goes out, what goes in? *Eur J Clin Nutr* 63: 808–811, https://doi.org/10.1038/ejcn.2008.39

Regulation (EU) No 1169/2011 of the European Parliament and of the Council of 25 October 2011 on the provision of food information to consumers, amending Regulations (EC) No 1924/2006 and (EC) No 1925/2006 of the European Parliament and of the Council, and repealing Commission Directive 87/250/EEC, Council Directive 90/496/EEC, Commission Directive 1999/10/EC, Directive 2000/13/EC of the European Parliament and of the Council, Commission Directives 2002/67/EC and 2008/5/EC and Commission Regulation (EC) No 608/2004. *Official Journal of the European Union* L 304/18, http://data.europa.eu/eli/reg/2011/1169/oj

Republic of Sudan (2019). *Memorandum of Agreement on Universal Salt Iodization in Sudan 2019–2022,* https://www.unicef.org/sudan/media/2231/file/USI_MOA%202019-2022.pdf

République Tunisienne Ministère de la Santé, Institut National de la Santé (2019). *La Santé des Tunisiens. Résultats de l'Enquête. Tunisian Health Examination Survey-2016.* Institut National de la Santé: Tunis, Tunisia, http://www.santetunisie.rns.tn/images/rapport-final-enquete2020.pdf

Restrepo BJ, Rieger M (2016a). Trans fat and cardiovascular disease mortality: Evidence from bans in restaurants in New York. *J Health Econ* 45: 176–196.

Restrepo BJ, Rieger M (2016b). Denmark's policy on artificial trans fat and cardiovascular disease. *Am J Prev Med* 50 (1): 69–76, https://doi.org/10.1016/j.jhealeco.2015.09.005

Rezaie M, Dolati S, Hariri Far A, Abdollahi Z, Sadeghian S (2020). Assessment of iodine status in Iranian students aged 8–10 years: Monitoring the National Program for the Prevention and Control of Iodine Deficiency Disorders in 2016. *Iran J Public Health* 49(2): 377–385, https://www.ncbi.nlm.nih.gov/pmc/articles/PMC7231715/pdf/IJPH-49-377.pdf

Rollins NC, Bhandari N, Hajeebhoy N, Horton S, Lutter CK, Martines JC, Piwoz EG, Richter LM, Victora CG, on behalf of The Lancet Breastfeeding Series Group (2016). Why invest, and what it will take to improve breastfeeding practices? *Lancet* 387: 491–504, https://doi.org/10.1016/S0140-6736(15)01044-2

Royaume du Maroc (2019). Arrêté conjoint du ministre de l'agriculture, de la pêche maritime, du développement rural et des eaux et forêts et du ministre de la santé n°441-19 du 9 kaada 1440 (12 juillet 2019) fixant les caractéristiques des farines de blé tendre enrichies d'un composé fer-vitamines. Bulletin Officiel. Cent-huitième année, N° 6810, 5 moharrem 1441 (5 septembre 2019). Edition de Traduction Officielle. ISSN 0851-1217, p. 1854. Rabat,

2019, http://www.onssa.gov.ma/images/reglementation/reglementation-sectorielle/vegetaux-et-produits-dorigine-vegetaux/Produits-dorigine-vegetale/Produits_alimentaires/ARR.441-19.FR.pdf

Sadighi J, Mohammad K, Sheikholeslam R, Amirkhani MA, Torabi P, Salehi F, Abdolahi Z (2009). Anaemia control: Lessons from the flour fortification programme. *Publ Health* 123: 794–799, https://doi.org/10.1016/j.puhe.2009.09.024

Sánchez-Romero LM, Penko J, Coxson PG, Fernández A, Mason A, Moran AE, Ávila-Burgos L, Odden M, Barquera S, Bibbins-Domingo K (2016). Projected impact of Mexico's sugar-sweetened beverage tax policy on diabetes and cardiovascular disease: A modeling study. *PLoS Med* 13 (11): e1002158, https://doi.org/10.1371/journal.pmed.1002158

Saudi Arabia General Authority for Statistics. *Household Health Survey 2017*, https://www.stats.gov.sa/sites/default/files/household_health_survey_2017_1.pdf

Schorling E, Niebuhr D, Kroke A (2017). Cost-effectiveness of salt reduction to prevent hypertension and CVD: a systematic review. *Public Health Nutr* 20 (11): 1993–2003, https://doi.org/10.1017/s1368980017000593

Selhub J, Rosenberg IH (2016). Excessive folic acid intake and relation to adverse health outcome. *Biochimie* 126: 71–78, https://doi.org/10.1016/j.biochi.2016.04.010

Skeaff CM (2009). Feasibility of recommending certain replacement or alternative fats. *Eur J Clin Nutr* 63: S34–S49, https://doi.org/10.1038/sj.ejcn.1602974

Sudan-WHO (2012). *Global school-based student health survey (GSHS)*. WHO, https://www.who.int/publications/m/item/2012-gshs-fact-sheet-sudan

Stender S, Astrup A, Dyerberg J (2008). Ruminant and industrially produced trans fatty acids: health aspects. *Food Nutr Res* 52: 10.3402, https://doi.org/10.3402/fnr.v52i0.1651

Stender S, Astrup A, Dyerberg J (2012). A trans European Union difference in the decline in trans fatty acids in popular foods: a market basket investigation. *BMJ Open* 2(5): e000859, https://doi.org/10.1136/bmjopen-2012-000859

Taha AA, Marawan HM (2015). Socio-behavioral determinants of overweight and obesity in Egyptian primary school children. *J Child Adolesc Behav* 3: 236, https://doi.org/10.4172/2375-4494.1000236

Taher A, Al Saffar L, Al Jamri A (2019). Prevalence of overweight and obesity amongst Bahraini adolescents aged 12–15 years attending primary care health centers. *J Bahrain Med Soc* 31(1): 37–43, https://doi.org/10.26715/jbms.2019.1_26022019b

Teng AM, Jones AC, Mizdrak A, Signal L, Genç M, Wilson N (2019). Impact of sugar-sweetened beverage taxes on purchases and dietary intake: Systematic review and meta-analysis. *Obes Rev* 20: 1187–1204, https://doi.org/10.1111/obr.12868

Tuomilehto J, Jousilahti P, Rastenyte D, Moltchanov V, Tanskanen A, Pietinen P, Nissinen A (2001). Urinary sodium excretion and cardiovascular mortality in Finland: a prospective study. *Lancet* 357: 848–851, https://doi.org/10.1016/s0140-6736(00)04199-4

Uauy R, Aro A, Clarke R, Ghafoorunissa R, L'Abbé M, Mozaffarian D, Skeaff M, Stender S, Tavella M (2009). WHO Scientific Update on trans fatty acids: summary and conclusions. *Eur J Clin Nutr* 63: S68–S75, https://doi.org/10.1038/ejcn.2009.15

United Arab Emirates Ministry of Health and Prevention (2018). *UAE National Health Survey Report 2017–2018.* Dubai, https://cdn.who.int/media/docs/default-source/ncds/ncd-surveillance/data-reporting/united-arab-emirates/uae-national-health-survey-report-2017-2018.pdf?sfvrsn=86b8b1d9_1&download=true

UNEP (Westhoek H, Ingram J., Van Berkum S., Özay L., Hajer M) (2016). *Food Systems and Natural Resources. A Report of the Working Group on Food Systems of the International Resource Panel.* United Nations Environment Programme, https://www.resourcepanel.org/file/133/download?token=6dSyNtuV

UNEP (2021). *Food Waste Index Report 2021.* Nairobi: United Nations Environment Programme, https://wedocs.unep.org/bitstream/handle/20.500.11822/35280/FoodWaste.pdf

United Nations General Assembly (2016). United Nations Decade of Action on Nutrition (2016–2025). Resolution 70/259 adopted by the General Assembly on 1st April 2016. 70th session. New York: United Nations, https://digitallibrary.un.org/record/827411

UNICEF (2017). *Report on the knowledge, attitudes and practices (KAP) survey infant and young child feeding (IYCF).* Syria, https://www.humanitarianresponse.info/sites/www.humanitarianresponse.info/files/documents/files/iycf_kap_survey_report_syria_vf_1.pdf

UNICEF (2021a). *Syria Crisis — Humanitarian Situation Report (January–March 2021),* https://reliefweb.int/sites/reliefweb.int/files/resources/UNICEF%20Syria%20Humanitarian%20Situation%20Report%20-%20Jan%20-%20March%202021.pdf

UNICEF, Division of Data, Analysis, Planning and Monitoring (2021b). *UNICEF Global Databases on Iodized salt.* New York, United Nations Children's Fund, https://data.unicef.org/topic/nutrition/iodine/

UNICEF, WHO (2018). *Implementation guidance: protecting, promoting and supporting breastfeeding in facilities providing maternity and newborn services — the revised Baby-friendly Hospital Initiative.* Geneva: World Health Organization. Licence: CC BY-NC-SA 3.0 IGO, https://apps.who.int/iris/bitstream/handle/10665/272943/9789241513807-eng.pdf?sequence=19&isAllowed=y

UNICEF, WHO (2019). *Low birthweight (LBW) estimates, 2019 Edition*, https://www.unicef.org/media/53711/file/UNICEF-WHO%20Low%20birthweight%20estimates%202019%20.pdf

United Nations Committee on the Rights of the Child (CRC) (1989). *Convention on the Rights of the Child*, https://www.ohchr.org/sites/default/files/crc.pdf

United Nations Committee on the Rights of the Child (CRC) (2013a). General comment No. 15 (2013) on the right of the child to the enjoyment of the highest attainable standard of health (art. 24), CRC/C/GC/15, https://www.refworld.org/docid/51ef9e134.html

United Nations Committee on the Rights of the Child (CRC) (2013b). General comment No. 16 (2013) on State obligations regarding the impact of the business sector on children's rights, CRC/C/GC/16, https://www.refworld.org/docid/51ef9cd24.html

United Nations Children's Fund (UNICEF), World Health Organization, International Bank for Reconstruction and Development/The World Bank (2021). *Levels and trends in child malnutrition: key findings of the 2021 edition of the joint child malnutrition estimates.* Geneva: World Health Organization. Licence: CC BY-NC-SA 3.0 IGO, https://apps.who.int/iris/rest/bitstreams/1344826/retrieve

UNICEF/WHO/World Bank (2021). Joint Child Malnutrition Estimates Database, April 2021, https://data.unicef.org/resources/dataset/malnutrition-data/

UNHCR/UNICEF/WFP/Save the Children (2017). *Interagency Nutrition Surveys amongst Syrian Refugees in Jordan. Final Report*, https://data2.unhcr.org/en/documents/download/53758

United Nations Standing Committee on Nutrition (UNSCN) (2014). *The nutrition sensitivity of agriculture and food policies. A synthesis of eight country case studies.* Geneva: UNSCN, https://www.unscn.org/files/Publications/Country_Case_Studies/UNSCN_Synthesis_Report_March_16_final.pdf

Vallgårda S, Holm L, Jensen JD (2015). The Danish tax on saturated fat: why it did not survive. *Eur J Clin Nutr* 69: 223–226, https://doi.org/10.1038/ejcn.2014.224

Van Berkum S, Dengerink J, Ruben R (2018). *The food systems approach: sustainable solutions for a sufficient supply of healthy food.* Wageningen: Wageningen Economic Research, Memorandum 2018–2064, http://library.wur.nl/WebQuery/wurpubs/fulltext/451505

Van Tulleken C, Wright C, Brown A, McCoy D, Costello A (2020). Marketing of breastmilk substitutes during the COVID-19 pandemic. *Lancet* 396: e58, https://doi.org/10.1016/S0140-6736(20)32119-X

Vartiainen E (2018). The North Karelia Project: Cardiovascular disease prevention in Finland. *Global Cardiology Science and Practice* 2018(2): 13, https://doi.org/10.21542/gcsp.2018.13

Vaz JS, Maia MFS, Neves PAR, Santos TM, Vidaletti LP, Victora C (2021). Monitoring breastfeeding indicators in high-income countries: Levels, trends and challenges. *Matern Child Nutr* 2021; 17: e13137, https://doi.org/10.1111/mcn.13137

Vyth E, Steenhuis IHM, Roodenburg AJC, Brug J, Seidell JC (2010). Front-of-pack nutrition label stimulates healthier product development: a quantitative analysis. *Int J Behav Nutr Phys Act* 7: 65, https://doi.org/10.1186/1479-5868-7-65

Walters DD, Phan LTH, Mathisen R (2019). The cost of not breastfeeding: global results from a new tool. *Health Policy Plan* 34(6): 407–417, https://doi.org/10.1093/heapol/czz050

Wang Q, Afshin A, Yawar Yakoob M, Singh GM, Rehm CD, Khatibzadeh S et al. (2016). Impact of nonoptimal intakes of saturated, polyunsaturated, and trans fat on global burdens of coronary heart disease. *J Am Heart Assoc* 5: e002891, https://doi.org/10.1161/JAHA.115.002891

Weiderpass E, Botteri E, Longenecker JC, Alkandari A, Al-Wotayan R, Al Duwairi Q, Tuomilehto J (2019). The prevalence of overweight and obesity in an adult Kuwaiti population in 2014. *Front Endocrinol* 10: 449, https://doi.org/10.3389/fendo.2019.00449

White PJ, Broadley MR (2009). Biofortification of crops with seven mineral elements often lacking in human diets — iron, zinc, copper, calcium, magnesium, selenium and iodine. *New Phytologist* 182: 49–84, https://doi.org/10.1111/j.1469-8137.2008.02738.x

Wirth JP, Laillou A, Rohner F, Northrop-Clewes CA, Macdonald B, Moench-Pfanner R (2012). Lessons learned from national food fortification projects: Experiences from Morocco, Uzbekistan, and Vietnam. *Food Nutr Bull* 33 (4, supplement): S281-S291, https://doi.org/10.1177%2F15648265120334S304

Wirth JP, Nichols E, Mas'd H, Barham R, Johnson QW, Serdula M (2013). External Mill Monitoring of Wheat Flour Fortification Programs: An Approach for Program Managers Using Experiences from Jordan. *Nutrients* 5: 4741–4759, https://doi.org/10.3390/nu5114741

World Cancer Research Fund International (2018). Building momentum: lessons on implementing a robust sugar sweetened beverage tax, www.wcrf.org/buildingmomentum

World Cancer Research Fund International, American Institute for Cancer Research (2018). *Diet, nutrition, physical activity and cancer: a global perspective. Continuous Update Project Expert Report*, https://www.wcrf.org/dietandcancer/contents

WFP (2020). *State of School Feeding Worldwide 2020*. Rome: World Food Programme. ISBN 978-92-95050-04-4, https://www.wfp.org/publications/state-school-feeding-worldwide-2020

WHO (1981). *International Code of Marketing of Breast-milk Substitutes*. Geneva: World Health Organization, https://apps.who.int/iris/bitstream/handle/10665/40382/9241541601.pdf?sequence=1&isAllowed=y

WHO (1994). *Infant and young child nutrition. Forty-seventh World Health Assembly. 47.5*. Geneva: World Health Organization, https://apps.who.int/iris/bitstream/handle/10665/177049/WHA47_1994-REC-1_eng.pdf?sequence=1&isAllowed=y

WHO (2006). *WHO child growth standards: length/height-for-age, weight-for-age, weight-for-length, weight-for-height and body mass index-for-age: methods and development*. World Health Organization: Geneva, https://apps.who.int/iris/bitstream/handle/10665/43413/924154693X_eng.pdf?sequence=1&isAllowed=y

WHO (2008a). *Indicators for assessing infant and young child feeding practices: conclusions of a consensus meeting held 6–8 November 2007 in Washington D.C., USA*. Geneva: World Health Organization, http://whqlibdoc.who.int/publications/2008/9789241596664_eng.pdf

WHO (2008b). *2008–2013 Action plan for the global strategy for the prevention and control of noncommunicable diseases*. Geneva: World Health Organization, https://www.paho.org/en/file/30828/download?token=bLVke8Da

WHO (2010). *Set of recommendations on the marketing of foods and non-alcoholic beverages to children*. Geneva: World Health Organization, http://whqlibdoc.who.int/publications/2010/9789241500210_eng.pdf

WHO (2011). *Haemoglobin concentrations for the diagnosis of anaemia and assessment of severity. Vitamin and Mineral Nutrition Information System*. Geneva: World Health Organization (WHO/NMH/NHD/MNM/11.1), http://www.who.int/vmnis/indicators/haemoglobin.pdf

WHO (2012a). *A framework for implementing the set of recommendations on the marketing of foods and non-alcoholic beverages to children*. Geneva: World Health Organization, https://apps.who.int/iris/bitstream/handle/10665/80148/9789241503242_eng.pdf?sequence=1&isAllowed=y

WHO (2012b). *Guideline: sodium intake for adults and children*. Geneva: World Health Organization, https://apps.who.int/iris/rest/bitstreams/110243/retrieve

WHO (2013). *Global Action Plan for the prevention and control of noncommunicable diseases 2013–2020*. Geneva: World Health Organization, https://apps.who.int/iris/rest/bitstreams/442296/retrieve

WHO (2014). *Comprehensive implementation plan on maternal, infant and young child nutrition*. Geneva: World Health Organization, https://apps.who.int/iris/handle/10665/113048

WHO (2016a). International statistical classification of diseases and related health problems (ICD-10). 10th ed, https://icd.who.int/browse10/2016/en

WHO (2016b). *SHAKE the salt habit — technical package for salt reduction.* Geneva: World Health Organization, http://apps.who.int/iris/bitstream/10665/250135/1/9789241511346-eng.pdf

WHO (2017a). *'Best buys' and other recommended interventions for the prevention and control of noncommunicable diseases. Updated (2017) appendix 3 of the Global Action Plan for the Prevention and Control of Noncommunicable Diseases 2013–2020.* Geneva: World Health Organization, https://www.who.int/ncds/management/WHO_Appendix_BestBuys_LS.pdf

WHO (2017b). *Guidance on ending the inappropriate promotion of foods for infants and young children: implementation manual.* Geneva: World Health Organization. Licence: CC BY-NC-SA 3.0 IGO, https://apps.who.int/iris/bitstream/handle/10665/260137/9789241513470-eng.pdf

WHO (2018a). *Marketing of breast-milk substitutes: national implementation of the international code, status report 2018.* Geneva: World Health Organization. Licence: CC BY-NC-SA 3.0 IGO, https://apps.who.int/iris/rest/bitstreams/1137996/retrieve

WHO (2018b). *Global nutrition policy review 2016–2017: country progress in creating enabling policy environments for promoting healthy diets and nutrition.* Geneva: World Health Organization, https://apps.who.int/iris/rest/bitstreams/1161738/retrieve

WHO (2019a). *Leading causes of death and disability 2000–2019: A visual summary,* https://www.who.int/data/stories/leading-causes-of-death-and-disability-2000-2019-a-visual-summary

WHO (2019b). *Guiding principles and framework manual for front-of-pack labelling for promoting healthy diet.* Geneva: World Health Organization, https://www.who.int/publications/m/item/guidingprinciples-labelling-promoting-healthydiet

WHO (2020). *Marketing of breast-milk substitutes: national implementation of the international code, status report 2020.* Geneva: World Health Organization. Licence: CC BY-NC-SA 3.0 IGO, https://apps.who.int/iris/rest/bitstreams/1278635/retrieve

WHO (2021a). *REPLACE trans fat. An action package to eliminate industrially-produced trans-fatty acids.* Geneva: World Health Organization. Licence: CC BY-NC-SA 3.0 IGO, https://apps.who.int/iris/bitstream/handle/10665/331301/WHO-NMH-NHD-18.4-eng.pdf

WHO (2021b). *Countdown to 2023: WHO report on global trans fat elimination 2021.* Geneva: World Health Organization. Licence: CC BY-NC-SA 3.0 IGO, https://apps.who.int/iris/rest/bitstreams/1389769/retrieve

WHO (2021c). *Action framework for developing and implementing public food procurement and service policies for a healthy diet.* Geneva: World Health Organization. Licence: CC BY-NC-SA 3.0 IGO, https://apps.who.int/iris/rest/bitstreams/1332396/retrieve

World Health Organization. Global Database on the Implementation of Nutrition Action (GINA). Policy — The Palestinian National Regulation for Marketing of Breast-milk Substitutes (2012), https://extranet.who.int/nutrition/gina/sites/default/filesstore/PSE%202012%20The%20Palestinian%20National%20Regulation%20for%20Marketing%20of%20Breast-milk%20Substitutes%20.pdf

WHO Regional Office for the Eastern Mediterranean (2015). *Report on the Technical consultation on salt and fat reduction strategies in the Eastern Mediterranean Region. Tunis, Tunisia, 30–31 March.* Cairo: World Health Organization, Regional Office for the Eastern Mediterranean, https://apps.who.int/iris/bitstream/handle/10665/253419/IC_Meet_Rep_2015_EN_16339.pdf?sequence=1&isAllowed=y

WHO Regional Office for the Eastern Mediterranean (2017a). *Nutrient profile model for the marketing of food and non-alcoholic beverages to children in the WHO Eastern Mediterranean Region.* Cairo: World Health Organization, Regional Office for the Eastern Mediterranean, https://apps.who.int/iris/bitstream/handle/10665/255260/EMROPUB_2017_en_19632.pdf?sequence=1&isAllowed=y

WHO Regional Office for the Eastern Mediterranean Region (2017b). Standardizing food composition tables, reflecting sugar, trans fat, saturated fat and salt contents. Report of a regional meeting on 20th to 22nd September 2016 in Rabat, Morocco. *EMHJ* 23 (1): 51–52, https://apps.who.int/iris/bitstream/handle/10665/251837/IC_Meet_Rep_2016_EN_19232.pdf?sequence=1&isAllowed=y

WHO, Regional Office for the Eastern Mediterranean (2018). *Implementing the WHO recommendations on the marketing of food and non-alcoholic beverages to children in the Eastern Mediterranean Region.* Cairo: World Health Organization. Regional Office for the Eastern Mediterranean, https://apps.who.int/iris/bitstream/handle/10665/328213/EMROPUB_2018_2248_en.pdf?sequence=1&isAllowed=y

WHO, Regional Office for the Eastern Mediterranean (2019a). *Strategy on nutrition for the Eastern Mediterranean Region 2020–2030.* Cairo: World Health Organization, Regional Office for the Eastern Mediterranean, https://applications.emro.who.int/docs/9789290222996-eng.pdf

WHO, Regional Office for the Eastern Mediterranean (2019b). *Wheat flour fortification in the Eastern Mediterranean Region / World Health Organization.* Cairo: World Health Organization, Regional Office for the Eastern Mediterranean, https://apps.who.int/iris/bitstream/handle/10665/311730/EMROPUB_2019_EN_22339.pdf?sequence=1&isAllowed=y

WHO Regional Office for Europe (2013). *Marketing of foods high in fat, salt and sugar to children: update 2012–2013.* Copenhagen: World Health Organization, https://www.euro.who.int/__data/assets/pdf_file/0019/191125/e96859.pdf

WHO Regional Office for Europe (2014). *European Food and Nutrition Action Plan 2015–2020*. Copenhagen: World Health Organization, https://www.euro.who.int/__data/assets/pdf_file/0008/253727/64wd14e_FoodNutAP_140426.pdf

WHO Regional Office for Europe (2016). *Tackling food marketing to children in a digital world: trans-disciplinary perspectives*. Copenhagen: World Health Organization, https://www.euro.who.int/__data/assets/pdf_file/0017/322226/Tackling-food-marketing-children-digital-world-trans-disciplinary-perspectives-en.pdf

WHO Regional Office for Europe (2018). *Evaluating implementation of the WHO set of recommendations on the marketing of foods and non-alcoholic beverages to children. Progress, challenges and guidance for next steps in the WHO European Region*. Copenhagen: World Health Organization, https://www.euro.who.int/__data/assets/pdf_file/0003/384015/food-marketing-kids-eng.pdf

WHO/FAO (2003). *Diet, nutrition and the prevention of chronic diseases. Report of a joint WHO/FAO expert consultation. WHO Technical Report Series No. 916*. Geneva: World Health Organization, http://whqlibdoc.who.int/trs/WHO_TRS_916.pdf

WHO, FAO, UNICEF, GAIN, MI, FFI (2009). *Recommendations on wheat and maize flour fortification. Meeting Report: Interim Consensus Statement*. Geneva: World Health Organization, (http://www.who.int/nutrition/publications/micronutrients/wheat_maize_fort.pdf

WHO, UNICEF (2017a). *NetCode toolkit. Monitoring the marketing of breast-milk substitutes: protocol for ongoing assessments*. Geneva: World Health Organization. Licence: CC BY-NC-SA 3.0 IGO, https://apps.who.int/iris/rest/bitstreams/1092573/retrieve

WHO, UNICEF (2017b). *NetCode toolkit. Monitoring the marketing of breast-milk substitutes: protocol for periodic monitoring systems*. Geneva: World Health Organization. Licence: CC BY-NC-SA 3.0 IGO, https://apps.who.int/iris/bitstream/handle/10665/259695/9789241513494-eng.pdf?sequence=1&isAllowed=y

Wong MMY, Arcand J, Leung AA, Thout SR, Campbell NRC, Webster J (2017). The science of salt: A regularly updated systematic review of salt and health outcomes (December 2015–March 2016). *J Clin Hypertens* 19, 322–332, https://doi.org/10.1111/jch.12970

Wyness LA, Butriss JL, Stanner SA (2011). Reducing the population's sodium intake: the UK Food Standards Agency's salt reduction programme. *Public Health Nutr* 15 (2): 254–261, https://doi.org/10.1017/S1368980011000966

Yazzie D, Tallis K, Curley C, Sanderson PR, Eddie R, Behrens TK, et al. (2020). The Navajo Nation Healthy Diné Nation Act: A Two Percent Tax on Foods of Minimal-to-No Nutritious Value, 2015–2019. *Prev Chronic Dis* 17: 200038, https://doi.org/10.5888/pcd17.200038

Zahidi A, Zahidi M, Taoufik J (2016). Assessment of iodine concentration in dietary salt at household level in Morocco. *BMC Public Health* 16: 418, https://doi.org/10.1186/s12889-016-3108-8

Zargaraan A, Dinarvand R, Hosseini H (2017). Nutritional traffic light labelling and taxation on unhealthy food products in Iran: health policies to prevent non-communicable diseases. *Iran Red Crescent Med J* 19: e57874, https://doi.org/10.5812/ircmj.57874

Zdruli P (2014). Land Resources of the Mediterranean: Status, Pressures, Trends and Impacts on Future Regional Development. *Land Degrad Develop* 25 (4): 373–384, https://doi.org/10.1002/ldr.2150

Zendeboodi F, Sohrabvandi S, Khanniri E, Nikmaram P, Fanood R, Khosravi K et al. (2021). Salt content of processed foods in the Islamic Republic of Iran, and compliance with salt standards. *East Mediterr Health J* 27(7): 687–692, https://doi.org/10.26719/2021.27.7.687

Zimmermann MB (2008). Research on Iodine Deficiency and Goiter in the 19th and Early 20th Centuries. *J Nutr* 138: 2060–2063, https://doi.org/10.1093/jn/138.11.2060

Žmitek K, Pravst I (2016). Iodization of salt in Slovenia: Increased availability of non-iodized salt in the food supply. *Nutrients* 8: 434, https://doi.org/10.3390/nu8070434

Zuberi S, Mehmood R, Gazdar H (2016). *Review of agri-food value chain interventions aimed at enhancing consumption of nutritious food by the poor: Pakistan.* LANSA Working Paper 7, Brighton: Leveraging Agriculture for Nutrition in South Asia (LANSA), https://opendocs.ids.ac.uk/opendocs/bitstream/handle/20.500.12413/12167/LANSA%20Working%20Paper%20Value%20Chains%20Pak.pdf?sequence=1&isAllowed=y

Websites

United Nations Sustainable Development Goals, https://www.un.org/sustainabledevelopment

United Nations Food Systems Summit 2021, https://www.un.org/en/food-systems-summit/

UN Comtrade Database, https://comtrade.un.org/data/

The Local: German retailers embrace ugly food, https://www.thelocal.de/20131013/52371/

EcoWatch: French Supermarket Limits Food Waste by Selling Ugly Produce, https://www.ecowatch.com/french-supermarket-limits-food-waste-by-selling-ugly-produce-1881928868.html#toggle-gdpr

Lebanese Food Bank, https://lebanesefoodbank.org/

WHO Noncommunicable Disease Surveillance, Monitoring and Reporting: Global school-based student health survey, https://www.who.int/teams/noncommunicable-diseases/surveillance/systems-tools/global-school-based-student-health-survey

WCRF. Taxes on sugar–sweetened beverages and energy drinks — Mexico. NOURISHING database, https://policydatabase.wcrf.org/level_one?page=nourishing-level-one#step2=2#step3=315 https://www.fooddrinktax.eu/article/denmark-abolishes-excise-duty-on-soft-drinks/

Reuters: Italy delays contested new sugar and plastic taxes until 2023, https://www.reuters.com/world/europe/italy-delays-contested-new-sugar-plastic-taxes-until-2023-2021-10-21/

Health Star Rating System, http://www.healthstarrating.gov.au

Food Drink Europe: Reference intakes, http://www.referenceintakes.eu

Facts Up Front, http://www.factsupfront.org

Ministry of Economy and Commerce, Emirate of Qatar (2017). Ministry of Economy and Commerce in cooperation with the Ministry of Public Health launches initiative to regulate data relating to food and beverage menus of restaurants and cafes, https://www.nutritics.com/downloads/resources/Food%20and%20Bev%20data.pdf

Qatar Tribune (1 March 2017). New guidelines for foods & beverages at health facilities, https://www.qatar-tribune.com/news-details/id/51203

Global Fortification Data Exchange, https://fortificationdata.org/

Food Fortification Programme, http://www.ffp-pakistan.org/

Harvest Plus Biofortification Priority Index, https://www.harvestplus.org/knowledge-market/in-the-news/harvestplus-updates-biofortification-priority-index-more-crops-and

WHO. Global Health Observatory Data Repository. Prevalence of thinness among children and adolescents, BMI < -2 standard deviations below the median (crude estimate): Estimates by Country, https://apps.who.int/gho/data/view.main.NCDBMIMINUS205-19Cv

WHO. Global Health Observatory Data Repository. Prevalence of overweight among children and adolescents, BMI > +1 standard deviations above the median (crude estimate): Estimates by Country, https://apps.who.int/gho/data/view.main.BMIPLUS1C05-19v

WHO. Global Health Observatory Data Repository. Prevalence of obesity among children and adolescents, BMI > +2 standard deviations above the median (crude estimate): Estimates by Country, https://apps.who.int/gho/data/view.main.BMIPLUS2C05-19v

Index

Abu Dhabi 45, 47, 129, 131, 138–139, 198, 204
adolescents 7–8, 12, 31, 36–38, 42, 47–50, 54, 59–62, 73–74, 76, 95, 106, 148–149, 171, 208, 212, 214, 233
advergames 97
Afghanistan xxi, xxii, 16, 32, 34, 37–38, 40, 43–44, 48–49, 54–55, 58, 62–67, 71, 118, 146, 164, 168, 215, 221, 226, 228, 231, 239
Africa 9, 14, 17–19, 117, 168, 171, 185, 193, 231, 235, 239
Aleppo 66, 68
Algeria 179
anaemia 22, 53–56, 86, 211, 232–234, 244
animal food products 8, 17, 186, 205
anthropogenic greenhouse gas emissions 24, 25, 111. *See also* carbon dioxide
Argentina 168, 175, 232
Argo 38, 51
Asia 9, 14–15, 17–18, 110, 148, 174, 235, 239
Asia-Pacific Region 9, 110
Australasia 110
Australia 129, 132, 233
Austria 168

Baby-friendly Hospital Initiative (BFHI) 113
back-of-pack (BOP) information 125–126
Bahrain xxi, xxii, 16, 32, 35, 38, 40–41, 43–44, 48–49, 55, 58, 72, 76, 88, 91–92, 107, 118, 148, 151–156, 196, 168, 170–171, 215, 199, 201, 44, 214, 221, 225–226, 233
Bangladesh 168
Beirut 33, 45, 69, 150
Belgium 128

Bill & Melinda Gates Foundation 236
biofortification 205, 236–241
blue water footprint 18
body mass index (BMI) 36–37, 39–40, 43, 47, 49–50
Brazil 233
breastfeeding 23, 63, 64, 65, 66, 67, 68, 82, 95, 64, 109, 110, 111, 112, 113, 115, 116, 122. *See also* lactating women
early initiation of 65–66
exclusive 63–65, 109–110
breastmilk substitutes xxi, 27, 78, 82, 95, 105, 110–114, 118–120
breastmilk substitutes (BMS) 110–112, 118–119
Brexit 222

Canada 168, 175, 197, 232
cancer xxii, 77, 135, 145
carbon dioxide 15, 16, 183, 186, 191. *See also* anthropogenic greenhouse gas emissions
carbon footprint 15–17, 25
cardio-vascular disease (CVD) 144
cash-based transfers (CBT) 195
Chad 168
children under 5 years 33, 36, 47, 61, 65
Chile 90, 131, 232
climate change xix, xx, 4, 20–21, 81, 84, 175, 243
Codex Alimentarius Committee on Food Labelling 127–128
combined moderate acute malnutrition (cMAM) 36
Commercialization of Biofortified Crops (CBC) 239
complementary feeding 66, 68
coronary heart disease 77, 165–166
coronary heart disease (CHD) 166, 171

Costa Rica 220, 232
COVID-19 pandemic xix, 7–8, 11, 34, 47, 72, 76, 111, 195, 243, 245

Democratic Republic of Congo 197
Denmark 88, 93, 166–168, 175
diabetes xxii, xxiii, 91, 166, 243
diet diversity 67, 183, 194, 198, 205
diet pattern 81, 93
disability-adjusted life-years (DALYs) 7, 146–147, 171, 243
Djibouti xxi, 8, 16, 32–35, 38, 40, 44, 46, 48–49, 55, 57–58, 64, 118, 148, 154, 179, 213, 219, 221, 226, 228, 231

Eastern Mediterranean and North African Region 77, 146, 148
Eastern Mediterranean Region (EMR) xxi, xxii, xxiii, 8, 13, 15–16, 21, 27–29, 31–33, 36, 39, 43, 45, 51, 55, 57–58, 63–65, 71, 77–78, 81–82, 88, 92, 101–102, 105, 117–120, 138–139, 142, 148–149, 151, 153–154, 156, 161, 163–164, 168–171, 174, 177, 179, 182, 192–193, 195–196, 201, 213, 221–222, 224, 226, 231, 233, 236, 239, 241, 243–245
ECHO (Commission on Ending Childhood Obesity) (WHO) 96
Ecuador 131
Egypt xxi, xxiii, 8, 16, 20, 32, 34, 36, 38, 40, 43–44, 46–50, 55–56, 58, 64, 76–77, 85–86, 91, 105–106, 118, 149, 153–156, 170–171, 179, 192–193, 195, 216, 221–222, 226, 229, 239
endothelial dysfunction 166
energy intake (EI) 171, 173
e-procurement 184–185
  KONEPS 185
  TUNEPS 184–185
estimated average requirement (EAR) 208
Ethiopia 168, 212
European Commission 116, 168, 236
European Union (EU) 25, 100, 125, 130, 168, 222, 238

fast food 73, 75, 88, 96, 160
fertilizer 4–5, 9, 16–17, 21–22, 24, 236–238, 240
Finland 131, 144, 189
  Finnish Heart symbol 131
fiscal policies xxi, 27, 78, 82–84, 87, 94
folate 36, 53, 59–62, 224–225, 233
folic acid 53, 57, 62, 208, 211, 220, 222, 225–230, 232–234
food advertising 100, 105, 106, 107, 108, 109, 120, 153. *See also* food marketing; marketing impact; marketing level of exposure; marketing power

Food and Agriculture Organization of the United Nations (FAO) xix, xxii, 1, 7–9, 11, 13–15, 17–22, 24, 83–84, 87, 112, 166, 184, 189, 205–206, 208, 236
food environment 2, 244
food fortification 205, 207–210, 225, 229–230, 232–236, 239
  dosage 207–208, 211
  effectiveness 206–209, 220, 223, 232, 234, 238–239
  flour 207, 211–212, 220, 222–226, 228–233, 223
  fortificants 207–208, 211, 222–223, 225, 234
  household coverage 214–216, 218, 221
  mandatory 57, 206–207, 212–213, 215–222, 224–225, 227–231, 233, 58
  monitoring 207–209, 213, 216–218, 225, 228–230, 234–235, 245
  safety 207, 209, 211
  voluntary 57–58, 211–212, 220–222, 224–225, 228–229, 231
Food Fortification Initiative (FFI) 222, 229, 236
food fortification programme (FFP) 230–231
food labelling xxi, 2, 26, 27, 78, 82, 101, 112, 113, 115, 125, 126, 127, 128, 129, 130, 131, 132, 133, 134, 135, 137, 138, 139, 140, 141, 142, 143, 145, 151, 152, 153, 161, 162, 166, 169, 170, 172, 173,

182, 207, 244, 245. *See also* health symbols (for nutrition labelling); warning symbols (for nutrition labelling)
food loss 4, 13–15, 19–20, 24, 180, 243
food marketing xxi, 1, 26, 27, 78, 82, 95, 96, 97, 98, 99, 100, 101, 102, 105, 106, 107, 108, 109, 110, 111, 112, 113, 114, 117, 118, 119, 120, 132, 138, 139, 143, 182, 153, 173, 216, 219, 196, 214, 217, 244, 104. *See also* food advertising; marketing impact
; marketing level of exposure
; marketing power
food price xix, xxii, 2, 4–5, 8–10, 18–19, 25, 83–86, 89–90, 94, 132, 143, 175, 183–184, 215
food reformulation xxi, 26–27, 78, 82, 89–90, 127, 132–133, 135, 143–146, 151–154, 159, 167, 169–170, 174–177, 180
food security xxii, 1–2, 4, 8–9, 11, 19, 21, 24–25, 36, 81, 83, 86, 183, 198, 243, 245
food subsidies 4, 10–11, 83–86, 94, 228–229
food supply chain 2, 4, 13, 20, 24
food systems xx, xxi, xxiii, 1–5, 8–9, 11–13, 18, 20, 23–27, 77, 81–83, 87, 179–182, 193, 200, 245
food taxes 26, 83, 86, 88, 89, 90, 91, 92, 93, 94, 151, 230, 93. *See also* sin taxes
food waste xxi, 1, 11, 13–20, 24, 27, 185–187, 191, 195
Food Waste Index 15–16
France 73, 128, 140, 157
front-of-pack labels (FOPL) 26, 101, 126–132, 134–142, 153, 166, 169, 244
fruit and vegetable intake 7, 10, 23, 67–68, 71–77, 85–86, 119, 143, 181, 187, 205

Gaza Strip 37, 43, 54, 59–60, 73–74, 217, 228
Germany 93, 128
Global acute malnutrition (GAM) 35–36
Global Alliance for Improved Nutrition (GAIN) 230, 236, 238–239

Global Health Observatory (GHO) 33, 36–40, 43–44, 47–49, 54–55
globalization 8, 10
Global School-Based Student Health Survey (GSHS) 37, 51, 76
Greece 35, 47
Green Apple symbol 141
greenhouse gas (GHG) emissions 15, 17–18
green water footprint 18
Guideline Daily Amount (GDA) 129–130, 134, 140
Gulf Cooperation Council (GCC) 8, 35, 43, 45, 47–48, 71, 88, 91, 105, 125, 138, 155, 168, 170–171, 222, 225, 244

Hama 66, 68
HarvestPlus 238–239, 241
Healthier Choice Logo 129, 131
Health in all policies (HiAP) 189
Health Star Rating 129, 131–132, 134, 139–140
health symbols (for nutrition labelling) 131, 132, 138, 140. *See also* food labelling; Nordic Keyhole symbol; Finnish Heart symbol; Weqaya health logo
healthy diet xxi, 9, 11–12, 23, 25–27, 71, 78, 82, 84–85, 88, 94, 96, 112, 134–135, 180, 182, 187–190, 199
height-for-age z-score (HAZ) 34
Helen Keller International 112–113
HFSS foods (High in Fat, Salt and Sugar) 95–96, 100
hydrogenated fats 77, 164, 244
hypertension 77, 143–147, 152, 164

Idlib 66, 68
India 168, 212
Indonesia 18
insulin resistance 166
Integrated Food Security Phase Classification (IPC) 36, 42, 64
International Code of Marketing of Breast-milk Substitutes 111, 113

International Food Policy Research Institute (IFPRI) 8, 11–12
International Fund for Agricultural Development (IFAD) xix, 7–8
International Obesity Taskforce (IOTF) 49–50
iodine 53, 57, 58, 208, 211, 212, 213, 214, 215, 216, 217, 218, 219, 220, 232. *See also* salt iodization
Iodine Global Network (IGN) 57, 236
iodization. *See also* iodine
Iran xxi, 16, 20, 32, 34–35, 37–38, 40, 44, 46, 48–49, 55–56, 58, 61, 63–64, 85, 91–92, 105–106, 118, 126, 131, 138–142, 148–149, 153–156, 162–163, 168, 170–176, 196, 198, 201, 211, 213, 221, 225–226, 233–234, 239, 244
Iranian Institute of Standards and Industrial Research (ISIRI) 155, 160
Iranian National Standards Organization 162–163, 172
Iraq xxi, 16, 20, 32, 34–36, 38, 40, 44, 46–49, 55, 57–58, 64, 76, 85, 118, 149, 154, 156, 179, 195–196, 218, 221–222, 226, 228, 233, 239
iron 36, 53, 56–57, 175, 205, 208, 211–212, 220, 222–223, 225, 228–230, 232–234, 239, 241
irrigation 21, 24
Israel 88, 131
Italy 93

Jordan xxi, 8, 16, 32, 34–35, 38, 40, 43–44, 46–49, 55–56, 58, 64–65, 67, 76, 105, 118, 138, 142, 149, 153–155, 192, 156, 170–171, 213, 199, 201, 33, 214, 221, 225–226, 228, 233

Kazakhstan 88
Kellogg's 107, 174
Khartoum 38, 46, 51, 64
Kuwait xxi, 16, 32–34, 38, 40–41, 44, 46, 48–49, 54–55, 58, 64, 76, 85, 88, 91–92, 118, 148–149, 153–156, 160, 168, 170–172, 179, 192, 199, 202, 215, 221, 225–226

lactating women 31, 42, 59, 60, 73, 74. *See also* breastfeeding
Latin America 17, 148, 231
Lebanon xxi, 8, 16, 20, 32–35, 38, 40–41, 44–45, 47–49, 55–58, 65, 69, 72, 76, 108, 118, 138, 148, 150, 154–155, 157, 161, 171, 179, 193, 196–198, 202, 218, 221, 226, 230, 239
Libya xxi, 8, 16, 32, 34, 38, 40, 44–46, 48–49, 55, 57–58, 118, 164, 179, 195, 221, 226, 230
local food production 23, 25, 86, 89, 101, 108, 113, 119, 173, 175, 177, 180, 182–183, 186–187, 189, 193, 195, 229, 237
low birth weight 31–32
Luxembourg 128

malnutrition xix, xxii, 8, 10, 12, 19, 27, 31, 34–36, 40, 42, 45–46, 51, 64, 77, 81–82, 110, 164, 180, 194, 243
marketing impact 95, 96, 97, 98, 99, 100, 105. *See also* food advertising; food marketing;
marketing level of exposure;
marketing power
marketing level of exposure 95, 97, 98, 99. *See also* food advertising; food marketing; marketing impact;
marketing power
marketing power 97, 99. *See also* food advertising; food marketing; marketing impact;
marketing level of exposure
Mars 107, 174
Mauritania 179
MENA (Mediterranean and North Africa) region 17, 179, 185, 195–196
Mexico 88, 90–91, 131
Middle East 59, 171, 185, 193
minimum dietary diversity (MDD) 66
minimum meal frequency (MMF) 66
monitoring 15, 20, 57, 97, 98, 99, 100, 107, 113, 114, 115, 116, 126, 136, 137, 152, 153, 154, 155, 162, 164, 171, 172, 176, 189, 199, 200. *See also* food fortification: monitoring

Moroccan National Survey on Population and Family Health (ENPSF), 46, 66
Morocco xxi, 8, 16, 32, 34, 38, 40, 44, 48–49, 55, 58, 64, 66, 68, 88, 91–92, 105, 118, 138–139, 148, 150, 153–154, 157, 160–161, 169–171, 192, 219, 202, 93, 221, 225–226, 231, 233, 239

Near East & North Africa Region 9, 19
Nestlé 107, 174
NetCode 112–118
NetCode Ongoing Monitoring System Protocol 114
NetCode Periodic Protocol 114
NetCode Toolkit 114
Netherlands, the 18, 128
neural tube defects (NTDs) 232–233
New York 46, 168
New Zealand 129, 132
niacin 208, 222, 224–228
Niger 197
Nigeria 168
non-communicable diseases (NCD) 41, 82, 84–85, 95–96, 101, 107, 127, 143–144, 151, 164, 168, 172–173, 176, 187, 191, 197, 202, 243
Nordic Keyhole symbol 129, 131
North Africa 17–19, 171, 185, 193
North African, Western and Central Asian Region 13, 16–18
North American and European Region 13
North American Region 17, 110
North Karelia Project 144
nutrient profile models 100, 182, 196
Nutri-Score system 128–131, 133–135, 139
nutritional transition xxii, 5, 35, 43, 71, 243
nutrition information 125, 127, 161, 173

obesity xix, xxii, 7, 10, 31, 41, 43–51, 63, 71, 76–77, 81–82, 86, 89–90, 95–96, 112–113, 126, 143–144, 176, 187, 191, 196, 243
Oceania 17, 148

Oman xxi, xxii, 16, 20, 32, 34, 38, 40–42, 44, 46, 48–49, 55–56, 58, 61–62, 64–65, 67, 73, 76, 88, 91–92, 107, 109, 117–118, 148, 150, 153–155, 157, 161, 168, 170, 179, 196, 199, 202, 215, 221, 225–226, 231
Organisation for Economic Co-operation and Development (OECD) 9, 25, 83–84, 179, 186
overweight xix, xxii, 7, 10, 31, 35, 39, 41, 43–51, 63, 71, 76–77, 86, 191, 243
oxidative stress 166, 211

Pakistan xxi, xxiii, 8, 16, 32, 34, 37–38, 40, 44, 48–50, 54–55, 57–59, 64, 66–67, 77, 105, 118, 142, 150, 216, 154, 164, 169–170, 46, 217, 221, 227, 229, 231, 239
Palestine, Occupied Territories of xxi, 16, 32–34, 37, 39, 42–43, 46, 50, 54–55, 58–60, 64–65, 68, 73–74, 76, 91, 115, 117–118, 148, 150–151, 154, 157, 203, 217, 55, 217, 221, 227–228
Papua New Guinea 220
partially hydrogenated vegetable oil (PHO) 166, 169, 204
Peru 131
Philippines, the 168
plant-based nutrition 5
Poland 88
Portugal 90, 136
pregnant women 31, 42–43, 53–57, 59–61, 73–74, 120, 55, 215, 218, 233
public food procurement 19, 182–183, 186–190, 193, 198, 200–201
Punjab 142, 164, 169–170, 217, 227, 230

Qatar xxi, xxii, 16, 32, 35, 38, 40, 44, 48–49, 55, 57–58, 64, 76, 85, 88, 91–92, 107, 118, 140, 153–155, 158, 196–197, 162, 168, 170, 219–221, 199–201, 203, 46, 225, 227

refugees 12, 35–36, 41, 47, 55–56, 65, 197–198, 225
REPLACE action framework (WHO) 166–167

Riyadh 106, 141, 197
Russia 8–9
  invasion of Ukraine 8–9

salt xxii, 23, 26, 57, 71, 75, 76, 77, 81, 85, 88, 95, 97, 98, 105, 106, 107, 125, 128, 130, 131, 132, 138, 140, 141, 143, 144, 145, 147, 148, 149, 151, 152, 153, 154, 155, 156, 157, 158, 159, 160, 161, 162, 163, 164, 174, 175, 176, 177, 181, 182, 197, 198, 200, 201, 202, 203, 204, 207, 212, 213, 214, 215, 216, 217, 218, 219, 220, 221, 244, 151. *See also* sodium
  in bread 152, 154–164, 175–176
salt iodization 57–58, 212–221, 244
saturated fat (SF) 88
saturated fatty acids (SFA) 106, 144, 165, 175, 202, 204
Saudi Arabia, Kingdom of xxi, xxii, 8, 16, 20, 32, 34–35, 37–38, 40–41, 44, 46, 48–49, 55, 58, 62, 74, 76, 88, 91–92, 106–107, 118, 138–139, 141, 150, 153–154, 158, 162, 168, 170–174, 179, 196–197, 199, 204, 214–215, 221–222, 225, 227
Saudi Food and Drug Administration (SFDA) 140, 162, 172–173, 204
school-age children 7, 36–39, 47–48, 50, 58, 61, 148, 195, 217–218
school meal programmes 192–194, 196
severe acute malnutrition (SAM) 35–36
SHAKE Technical Package for salt reduction (WHO) 152–153
Singapore 129, 131
sin taxes 88, 89, 90, 91, 93. *See also* food taxes
sodium 76, 77, 125, 129, 134, 138, 141, 142, 143, 144, 145, 147, 148, 149, 151, 152, 154, 161, 163, 165, 182, 187. *See also* salt
solid food introduction 67–69
Somalia xxi, xxii, 8, 16, 32, 34, 37–38, 40, 43–45, 48–49, 54–55, 58, 60, 219, 221, 227, 33, 230, 46, 33–34
South Africa 168
South Korea 184–185
Spain 128

Sri Lanka 168
steatohepatitis 166
stroke 77, 146–147
stunting 33–36, 57, 86
Sub-Saharan Africa 9, 14, 17, 148, 231
Sudan xxi, xxii, 8, 16, 32, 34, 37–39, 43, 45, 50–51, 55, 58, 63–64, 67–68, 119, 148, 151, 219, 221, 64, 46, 218, 227, 229
sugar xxii, 10, 23, 26, 67, 71, 73, 76–77, 81, 84–86, 88–93, 95–98, 102, 105–109, 125, 128–132, 134, 138, 140–141, 143–145, 165, 174, 182, 187, 219, 198, 200–204, 104, 227, 230–231, 104
sugar-sweetened beverages (SSBs) 88, 90–93
Sustainable Development Goals (SDG) xix, xx, 15, 27, 179
sustainable diet xx, xxi, 27, 78, 82, 188–189, 243
Sweden 93, 131
Switzerland 57, 128, 212
Syria xxi, 16, 32, 34–36, 38, 41, 44, 46–49, 55–58, 64–66, 68, 119, 151, 179, 195, 197–198, 213, 221, 227, 229, 239

thinness 36
tolerable upper level of intake (UL) 209, 211
traffic-light system 129–131, 133–134, 138–141, 200, 203
trans-fatty acids (TFAs) 77, 141–142, 144, 164–177, 187, 198–199, 201–202, 244, 204
Tunisia xxi, 8, 16, 20, 32–34, 38, 41–42, 44, 46, 48–49, 55, 58, 64, 74, 86, 91, 119, 138–140, 148, 151, 153–155, 159, 162, 170–171, 179, 184–185, 192–195, 204, 217, 221, 227, 230, 239
Turkey 35, 47, 96

UK Food Standards Agency (FSA) 96, 131, 135
UK Office of Communications 131–132
Ukraine xxii, 8–9
  war in xix, xxii, 8, 245
undernutrition 10, 36
underweight 31, 33–43, 51

UNESCO 37
UNICEF xix, 7–8, 31–38, 40–42, 45–47, 60–62, 65, 67–68, 113, 73–74, 212, 216–217, 221, 113–114, 236, 64, 46, 33–34
United Arab Emirates xxi, xxii, 16, 20, 32–33, 35, 38, 41, 43–45, 48–49, 54–55, 58, 63, 75–77, 85, 88, 91, 93, 107–108, 119, 138, 151, 153–155, 195, 159, 168, 170–171, 173, 215, 221, 196, 204, 44, 33, 214, 225, 227
United Nations Development Programme (UNDP) 83–84, 87
United Nations Environmental Programme (UNEP) 1–2, 4–5, 10–11, 13, 15–16, 21, 24, 83–84, 87
United Nations Food Systems Summit xx, xxiii, 26, 78, 81, 243
United Nations (UN) xix, xx, xxiii, 1, 8, 14, 26, 34, 45, 78, 81, 110, 185, 189, 198, 228–229, 236, 243
United States of America , 57, 88, 91, 93, 100, 212, 33, 220, 232
universal salt iodization (USI) 219, 221
urbanization xxii, 4, 10, 26
urinary iodine concentration (UIC) 57, 212–219
urinary sodium excretion 76, 148
Uruguay 131
U.S. Centers for Disease Control and Prevention (CDC) 37, 39, 49–50

Vietnam 212
vitamin A 36, 53, 57, 59–61, 68, 209, 220, 224, 226–227, 231–232, 238, 241
vitamin B12 59–62, 211, 220, 224, 226–227, 230
vitamin D 53, 57, 59–62, 208, 220, 225–227, 231–232, 234

warning symbols (for nutrition labelling) 130, 131, 132, 134, 139. *See also* food labelling
wasting 33–36, 86
water use efficiency 21
weight-for-age z-score (WAZ) 34
weight-for-height z-score (WHZ) 34–36, 45, 47
Weqaya health logo 129, 131, 138–139
West Bank 37, 59–60, 73–74, 217, 228
Western and Central Asia 17–18
women of reproductive age 40–41, 54, 59, 61–62, 71, 216, 218, 232–233
World Bank 33–34, 36, 45–46, 88, 236
World Food Programme (WFP) xix, 7–8, 35, 47, 192–195, 197–198, 236
World Health Assembly 56, 63, 111–112, 114
World Health Organization (WHO) xix, xxi, xxii, xxiii, 7–8, 10–11, 13, 15–16, 23, 25, 27–29, 31–34, 36–41, 43–51, 54–58, 63–66, 68, 71, 77–78, 81–82, 85, 88, 91–92, 96–102, 105–108, 110, 112–115, 117–118, 120, 125–128, 135–140, 142, 144, 182, 147–149, 151–153, 156, 164–171, 174, 213, 187, 214, 188–190, 192–193, 195–198, 201, 33, 212–214, 219–226, 228–233, 236, 239, 241, 44, 55, 104

Yemen xxi, xxii, 8, 16, 32–34, 36–38, 41–42, 44–46, 48–49, 54–55, 58, 64, 119, 154, 164, 179, 195, 221, 227–228, 231, 239

zinc 36, 53, 57, 59–61, 205, 220, 223–225, 228, 230, 232, 239, 241

About the Team

Alessandra Tosi was the managing editor for this book.

Lucy Barnes performed the copy-editing, proofreading and indexing.

Jeevanjot Kaur Nagpal designed the cover. The cover was produced in InDesign using the Fontin font.

Luca Baffa typeset the book in InDesign and produced the paperback and hardback editions. The text font is Tex Gyre Pagella; the heading font is Californian FB.

Luca produced the EPUB, AZW3, PDF, HTML, and XML editions — the conversion is performed with open source software such as pandoc (https://pandoc.org/) created by John MacFarlane and other tools freely available on our GitHub page (https://github.com/OpenBookPublishers).

This book need not end here...

Share

All our books — including the one you have just read — are free to access online so that students, researchers and members of the public who can't afford a printed edition will have access to the same ideas. This title will be accessed online by hundreds of readers each month across the globe: why not share the link so that someone you know is one of them?

This book and additional content is available at:

https://doi.org/10.11647/OBP.0322

Donate

Open Book Publishers is an award-winning, scholar-led, not-for-profit press making knowledge freely available one book at a time. We don't charge authors to publish with us: instead, our work is supported by our library members and by donations from people who believe that research shouldn't be locked behind paywalls.

Why not join them in freeing knowledge by supporting us: https://www.openbookpublishers.com/support-us

Follow @OpenBookPublish

Read more at the Open Book Publishers **BLOG**

You may also be interested in:

Forests and Food
Addressing Hunger and Nutrition Across Sustainable Landscapes

Bhaskar Vira, Christoph Wildburger and
Stephanie Mansourian (eds)

https://doi.org/10.11647/10.11647/OBP.0085

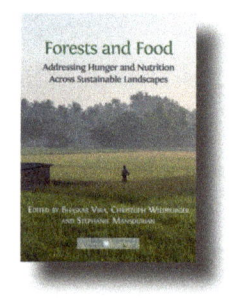

Global Warming in Local Discourses
How Communities around the World Make Sense of Climate Change

Michael Brüggemann and Simone Rödder (eds)

https://doi.org/10.11647/10.11647/OBP.0212

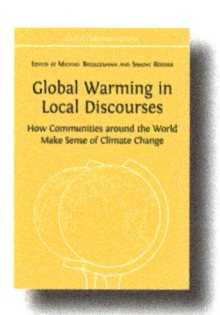

Non-communicable Disease Prevention
Best Buys, Wasted Buys and Contestable Buys

Wanrudee Isaranuwatchai, Rachel A. Archer, Yot Teerawattananon and Anthony J. Culyer (eds)

https://doi.org/10.11647/10.11647/OBP.0195

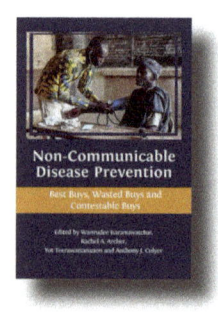